Prosthodontics

Editors

LISA A. LANG
LILY T. GARCÍA

DENTAL CLINICS OF NORTH AMERICA

www.dental.theclinics.com

April 2019 • Volume 63 • Number 2

ELSEVIER

1600 John F. Kennedy Boulevard • Suite 1800 • Philadelphia, Pennsylvania, 19103-2899

http://www.dental.theclinics.com

DENTAL CLINICS OF NORTH AMERICA Volume 63, Number 2
April 2019 ISSN 0011-8532, ISBN: 978-0-323-68244-2

Editor: John Vassallo; j.vassallo@elsevier.com
Developmental Editor: Laura Fisher

Dental Clinics of North America (ISSN 0011-8532) is published quarterly by Elsevier Inc., 360 Park Avenue South, New York, NY 10010-1710. Months of issue are January, April, July, and October. Business and Editorial Offices: 1600 John F. Kennedy Boulevard, Suite 1800, Philadelphia, PA 19103-2899. Periodicals postage paid at New York, NY and additional mailing offices. Subscription prices are $304.00 per year (domestic individuals), $603.00 per year (domestic institutions), $100.00 per year (domestic students/residents), $366.00 per year (Canadian individuals), $782.00 per year (Canadian institutions), $424.00 per year (international individuals), $782.00 per year (international institutions), and $200.00 per year (international and Canadian students/residents). International air speed delivery is included in all *Clinics* subscription prices. All prices are subject to change without notice. **POSTMASTER:** Send address changes to *Dental Clinics of North America*, Elsevier Health Sciences Division, Subscription Customer Service, 3251 Riverport Lane, Maryland Heights, MO 63043. **Customer Service (orders, claims, online, change of address): Elsevier Health Sciences Division, Subscription Customer Service, 3251 Riverport Lane, Maryland Heights, MO 63043. Tel: 1-800-654-2452 (U.S. and Canada). Fax: 314-447-8029. E-mail: journalscustomerservice-usa@elsevier.com (for print support); journalsonlinesupport-usa@elsevier.com (for online support).**

Reprints. For copies of 100 or more, of articles in this publication, please contact the Commercial Reprints Department, Elsevier Inc., 360 Park Avenue South, New York, NY 10010-1710. Tel.: 212-633-3874; Fax: 212-633-3820; E-mail: reprints@elsevier.com.

The Dental Clinics of North America is covered in *MEDLINE/PubMed (Index Medicus), Current Contents/Clinical Medicine, ISI/BIOMED* and *Clinahl*.

Contributors

EDITORS

LISA A. LANG, DDS, MS, MBA
Chair, Division of Restorative and Prosthetic Dentistry, The Ohio State University College of Dentistry, Columbus, Ohio

LILY T. GARCÍA, DDS, MS, FACP
Associate Dean for Education, University of Iowa College of Dentistry and Dental Clinics, Iowa City, Iowa

AUTHORS

REVA MALHOTRA BAREWAL, DDS, MS
Clinical Assistant Professor, Department of Pulmonology and Critical Care, Oregon Health and Science University, Portland, Oregon

MARKUS B. BLATZ, DMD, PhD
Professor of Restorative Dentistry and Chairman, Department of Preventive and Restorative Sciences, Assistant Dean for Digital Innovation and Professional Development, University of Pennsylvania School of Dental Medicine, Philadelphia, Pennsylvania

MATTHEW S. BRYINGTON, DMD, MS
Assistant Director for Graduate Prosthodontics, Department of Restorative Dentistry, West Virginia University, School of Dentistry, Morgantown, West Virginia

STEPHEN D. CAMPBELL, DDS, MMSc, FACP
Professor, Department of Restorative Dentistry, University of Illinois at Chicago College of Dentistry, Chicago, Illinois

JULIAN CONEJO, DDS, MSc
Visiting Scholar, Department of Preventive and Restorative Sciences, University of Pennsylvania School of Dental Medicine, Philadelphia, Pennsylvania

RYAN COOK, DDS, MS
Chair, Associate Professor, Department of Restorative Sciences, School of Dentistry, University of North Carolina at Chapel Hill, Chapel Hill, North Carolina

LYNDON F. COOPER, DDS, PhD
Associate Dean for Research, Department Head of Oral Biology, University of Illinois at Chicago, College of Dentistry, Chicago, Illinois

INGEBORG J. DE KOK, DDS, MS
Associate Professor, Department of Restorative Sciences, University of North Carolina, Chapel Hill, North Carolina

IBRAHIM S. DUQUM, DDS, MS
Associate Professor, Director, Division of Prosthodontics, Department of Restorative Sciences, University of North Carolina, Chapel Hill, North Carolina

DAVID L. GUICHET, DDS
Private Practice, Providence Prosthodontics Dental Group, Orange, California

LAUREN H. KATZ, DDS
Fellow, Department of Restorative Sciences, University of North Carolina, Chapel Hill, North Carolina

JIYEON J. KIM, DMD, MS
Clinical Assistant Professor, Department of Restorative Dentistry, University of Illinois at Chicago, Chicago, Illinois

KENT L. KNOERNSCHILD, DMD, MS, FACP
Professor, Program Director, Advanced Education Program in Prosthodontics, Department of Restorative Dentistry, University of Illinois at Chicago College of Dentistry, Chicago, Illinois

DAMIAN J. LEE, DDS, MS
Program Director and Assistant Professor, Advanced Prosthodontics Program, Division of Restorative and Prosthetic Dentistry, The Ohio State University College of Dentistry, Columbus, Ohio

DIANA LEYVA DEL RIO, DDS, MS
Graduate Research Assistant, Oral Biology, The Ohio State University College of Dentistry, Columbus, Ohio

KEVIN LIM, DMD, MS
Assistant Professor, Department of Restorative Sciences, School of Dentistry, University of North Carolina at Chapel Hill, Chapel Hill, North Carolina

WEI-SHAO LIN, DDS
Associate Professor, Department of Prosthodontics, Indiana University School of Dentistry, Indianapolis, Indiana

DEAN MORTON, BDS, MS
Indiana Dental Association Professor, Chair, Department of Prosthodontics, Indiana University School of Dentistry, Indianapolis, Indiana

KAMOLPHOB PHASUK, DDS, MS
Clinical Assistant Professor, Department of Prosthodontics, Indiana University School of Dentistry, Indianapolis, Indiana

WALDEMAR D. POLIDO, DDS, MS, PhD
Clinical Professor, Department of Oral Surgery and Hospital Dentistry, Indiana University School of Dentistry, Indianapolis, Indiana

PAOLA C. SAPONARO, DDS, MS
Division of Restorative and Prosthetic Dentistry, The Ohio State University College of Dentistry, Columbus, Ohio

ROBERT R. SEGHI, DDS, MS
Professor, Division of Restorative and Prosthetic Dentistry, The Ohio State University College of Dentistry, Columbus, Ohio

GHADEER THALJI, DDS, PhD
Associate Professor, Department of Restorative Sciences, University of Illinois at Chicago, Chicago, Illinois

Contents

Preface: Changing Face of Prosthodontics xi

Lisa A. Lang and Lily T. García

Update on Perio-Prosthodontics 157

Ryan Cook and Kevin Lim

Knowledge of the periodontal-restorative interface is critical in the fabrication of restorations that are functional and esthetic. Understanding biological principles allows the clinician to predict how the periodontium will respond to restorative therapy. Factors that influence the response to therapy in the periodontal-restorative interface are periodontal biotype, gingival architecture, alveolar crest position, gingival margin position, and gingival zenith.

The Current State of Chairside Digital Dentistry and Materials 175

Markus B. Blatz and Julian Conejo

This article describes and illustrates the current state of chairside computer-aided design computer-aided manufacturing technologies and materials. It provides a historical background and discusses the different components of the chairside digital workflow: intraoral scanners, design software, milling machines, and sinter furnaces. The material range available for chairside digital dentistry is broad and includes polymethyl methacrylates, composite resins, and a large variety of ceramics. Clinical applications and success rates of the different material groups are summarized and discussed based on the current scientific evidence.

Prosthodontic Management of Implant Therapy: Esthetic Complications 199

Lyndon F. Cooper, Ingeborg J. De Kok, Ghadeer Thalji, and Matthew S. Bryington

The essential promise of implant dentistry is the ability to imperceptibly replace missing teeth. To achieve this, careful planning, execution, and maintenance is required by the dentist and patient to maintain a long-term esthetic and functional result. Unfortunately, as a result of biological, prosthetic, and iatrogenic factors, unesthetic results can occur. This article explores the potential causes for the unesthetic dental implant and the possible solutions that may improve the clinical situation. Whereas relatively simple errors may be corrected through prosthetic means, greater complications may require surgical intervention to achieve the desired result.

Management of Implant/Prosthodontic Complications 217

Ingeborg J. De Kok, Ibrahim S. Duqum, Lauren H. Katz, and Lyndon F. Cooper

Dental implants continue to grow in popularity because they are a predictable treatment to replace missing teeth. They have a high success rate; however, they are still associated with some clinical complications. This article discusses a diverse range of complications related to the restorative and mechanical aspects of dental implants and the management of such complications, as well as potential factors contributing to them.

Biomaterials: Ceramic and Adhesive Technologies **233**

Robert R. Seghi and Diana Leyva del Rio

This review highlights ceramic material options and their use. The newer high-strength ceramics in monolithic form have gained popularity despite the lack of long-term clinical data to support this paradigm shift. Although there are some encouraging clinical data available, there is a need to develop laboratory simulation models that can help predict long-term clinical performance for ceramic and adhesive cements.

Management of Edentulous Patients **249**

Damian J. Lee and Paola C. Saponaro

Edentulism, defined as the complete loss of all dentition, is a worldwide phenomenon. Edentulism occurs because of biologic disease processes, such as dental caries, periodontal diseases, trauma, and oral cancer. Edentulism is accompanied by several comorbidities that can significantly influence an individual. Although the rate of edentulism is declining, the number of edentulous patients continues to rise because of the increase in population. The management of edentulous patient has been addressed since the early days of dentistry. This article describes complete dentures and their maintenance, and advanced technology in complete dentures, and in implant-retained and implant-supported prosthesis.

Revisiting the Removable Partial Denture **263**

Jiyeon J. Kim

The partial edentulous population is increasing because of an increasing aging population, increased life expectancy, and individuals retaining more teeth at an older age. Therefore, the need for fixed and removable partial denture (RPD) therapy will remain high and will continue into the future. RPDs provide minimally invasive, cost-effective, timely care, and are preferred to fixed dental prostheses using teeth or implant therapy in many clinical scenarios. This article discusses RPD classification systems to review basic concepts and special framework design considerations, and explores advancements in the field such as implant-assisted RPD, CAD/CAM RPD, and new polymer framework materials.

Making the Best Clinical Decisions for Patients: The Pros-CAT Protocol™ **279**

Kent L. Knoernschild and Stephen D. Campbell

The Pros-CAT protocol critical appraisal method uses accepted strategies to identify and summarize best evidence to support patient care through evidence-based analysis that includes assessing the patient; developing a concise clinical question; conducting a literature search to identify pertinent research; critically appraising the identified literature for validity, reliability, and applicability to the patient situation; synthesizing the literature into a meaningful conclusion using an organized method; and applying that synthesis to the patient's need. The Pros-CAT protocol is applicable for practicing clinicians, dental students, postgraduate students, and residents. The Pros-CAT index compares evidence strength for patient applicability.

Obstructive Sleep Apnea: The Role of Gender in Prevalence, Symptoms, and Treatment Success **297**

Reva Malhotra Barewal

The purpose of this article is to provide an overview of known similarities and differences between genders relative to presenting symptoms, demographics, and severity of obstructive sleep apnea. There is a relationship of risk of disease occurrence relative to stages of reproductive life of a woman, indicating that chronologic age might not be as important as timing of pregnancy and menopausal transition. The current understanding of gender differences in treatment success and compliance with oral appliance therapy is limited and requires further investigation.

Consideration for Contemporary Implant Surgery **309**

Dean Morton, Kamolphob Phasuk, Waldemar D. Polido, and Wei-Shao Lin

The advancement of technology often provides clinicians and patients better clinical alternatives to achieve optimal treatment outcomes. Computer-guided options allow clinicians to realize the virtual prosthodontically driven surgical plan, facilitating more predictable implant placement. Although the use of technology does not mean the clinicians can forgo the fundamental treatment principles when treating a patient, proper assessment and diagnostic approach from prosthodontic, surgical, and radiographic perspectives are still essential for a successful clinical outcome. The purpose of this article is to review the fundamental concepts for the use of computer-guided surgery to facilitate prosthodontic treatment.

Digital Workflows in the Management of the Esthetically Discriminating Patient **331**

David L. Guichet

Traditional methods of designing and creating restorations are being increasingly replaced by digital processes. Software and hardware platforms for esthetic restoration design allow for local computer-aided design/computer-aided manufacturing (CAD/CAM) production. These systems are becoming ubiquitous and their strengths can be applied to the management of the esthetically discerning patient. This article takes a critical look at the effectiveness of digital workflows, including digital treatment planning using multiple datasets, linked digital workflows, digital restorative design, milled prototypes, and minimally veneered zirconia restorations. A complete digital workflow can be used in the treatment of the esthetically discriminating prosthodontic rehabilitation patient.

DENTAL CLINICS OF NORTH AMERICA

FORTHCOMING ISSUES

July 2019
Unanswered Questions in Implant Dentistry
Mohanad Al-Sabbagh, *Editor*

October 2019
Caries Management
Sandra Guzmán-Armstrong, Margherita Fontana, Marcelle Nascimento, and Andrea Zandona, *Editors*

January 2020
Oral Diseases for the General Dentist
Orrett E. Ogle and Arvind Babu Rajendra Santosh, *Editors*

RECENT ISSUES

January 2019
Evidence-Based Dentistry
Robert J. Weyant, *Editor*

October 2018
Orofacial Pain
Steven D. Bender, *Editor*

July 2018
Emerging ImagingTechnologies in Dentomaxillofacial Radiology
Rujuta A. Katkar and Hassem Geha, *Editors*

Preface
Changing Face of Prosthodontics

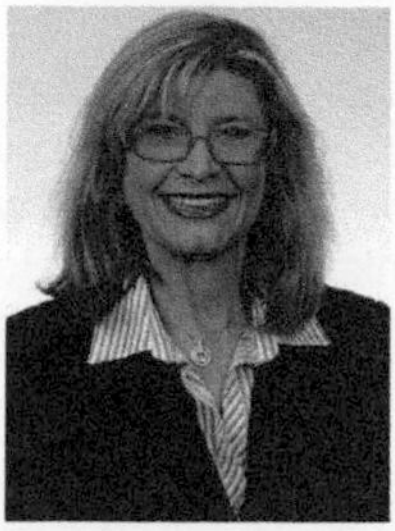

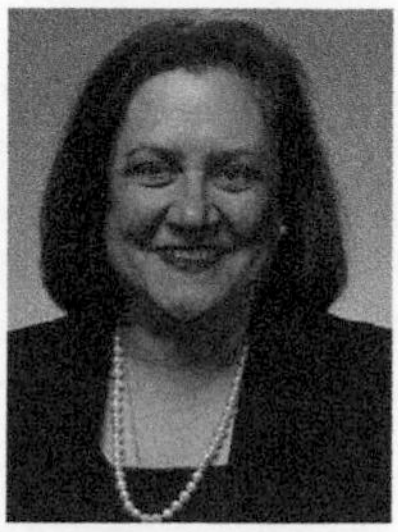

Lisa A. Lang, DDS, MS, MBA   Lily T. García, DDS, MS
Editors

Over the last three decades, advances in technology changed the world around us. Technological advances influence our personal lives and that of our patients, occurring at a faster pace due to changes in communication technology that drive how society accesses information and influences societal demands. The exponential advances in dentistry, in particular, in Prosthodontics, reflect increasing demands for optimal esthetic results, high-quality precision, shorter treatment time, treatment decisions based on predictable outcomes, and evidence-based treatment approaches driving research and technology. While rehabilitating patients to a restored state of function and comfort remains a mainstay, patients expect to have improved quality of life and highly esthetic restorations with the latest biomaterials and technologies.

In order for general dentists and prosthodontists to fulfill the needs of their patients, each must commit professionally to understanding foundational knowledge of classic prosthodontic principles and practice and translating those fundamental principles in an era of advancing digital technologies and biomaterials. This integration must occur in all areas of the discipline. The technology explosion has resulted in improved materials, practices, and technologies that allow us to evaluate, diagnose, and treat patients in an environment that did not exist 40 years ago.

As masters of diagnosis and treatment planning, we now have the tools to do this in a digital world. We have the ability to image the patient from pretreatment to completion of treatment, evaluating, diagnosing, planning, and executing treatment virtually. We may now not only plan the surgical placement of implants but also execute the surgical placement by means of surgical guides made using digital technologies. Implants, which were once limited to the edentulous mandible, are now used in every imaginable type of rehabilitation. With this unlimited use in more complex situations comes an increase in complications. The purpose of this issue is to provide fundamental knowledge in current topics of interest affecting the dynamic discipline and specialty of prosthodontics. As guest editors, we would like to thank our friends and colleagues

Dent Clin N Am 63 (2019) xi–xii
https://doi.org/10.1016/j.cden.2019.01.001
0011-8532/19/© 2019 Published by Elsevier Inc.

from around North America who so graciously agreed to contribute their time and efforts to bring the reader the best possible science and clinical rationale in prosthodontics. This issue of *Dental Clinics of North America* represents the highest levels of expertise that spans the new and old disciplines of prosthodontics: fixed, removable, and implant prosthodontics, the periodontal-prosthodontics connection, ceramic and adhesive technologies, sleep apnea, various aspects of the digital workflow, and the Pro-CAT evidence-based dentistry.

We would like to express our deepest gratitude to our colleagues who have demonstrated a level of professional commitment to excellence which is reflected in this publication. It is a privilege to experience a unique and rare occasion to collaborate with this group of prominent individuals. Finally, we would like to thank Laura Fisher, John Vassallo, and the Elsevier staff for all their help during the process and *Dental Clinics of North America* for affording us this wonderful opportunity.

Lisa A. Lang, DDS, MS, MBA
Chair, Division of Restorative and Prosthetic Dentistry
The Ohio State University College of Dentistry
305 West 12th Avenue
Postle Hall Room 3020
Columbus, OH 43210, USA

Lily T. García, DDS, MS
Associate Dean for Education
University of Iowa College of Dentistry and Dental Clinics
801 Newton Road, DSB N310
Iowa City, IA 52242-1010, USA

E-mail addresses:
Lang.513@osu.edu (L.A. Lang)
lily-garcia@uiowa.edu (L.T. García)

Update on Perio-Prosthodontics

Ryan Cook, DDS, MS*, Kevin Lim, DMD, MS

KEYWORDS

- Periodontal biotype • Restorative margin position • Alveolar crest
- Gingival architecture • Gingival margin • Gingival zenith

KEY POINTS

- Knowledge of biological principles allows the clinician to predict periodontal response to restorative therapy.
- Factors that influence the periodontal-restorative interface in both implant and tooth-borne restorations include periodontal biotype, gingival architecture, alveolar crest position, gingival margin position, and gingival zenith.
- Identification of alveolar crest position is critical in determining the location of the restorative margin.
- Resolution of periodontal inflammation before restorative therapy is paramount in predicting the periodontal response.

INTRODUCTION

Understanding the periodontal-restorative interface allows for fabrication of restorations that are both functional and esthetic. Diagnosis and treatment planning, which integrates biological and mechanical principles, allows the clinician to predict the periodontal response to therapy in both implant and tooth-borne fixed prosthodontics. Factors that influence the periodontal-restorative interface are periodontal biotype, gingival architecture, alveolar crest position, gingival margin position, and gingival zenith.

Periodontal Biotype and Gingival Architecture

Periodontal biotype has been evaluated and discussed throughout the dental literature from its relation to anatomy to its effect on therapy. Periodontal biotype plays a critical role in gingival esthetics and treatment outcomes in the periodontal-restorative interface.

Disclosure Statement: The authors have nothing to disclose.
Department of Restorative Sciences, School of Dentistry, University of North Carolina at Chapel Hill, 335 Brauer Hall CB 7450, Chapel Hill, NC 27599, USA
* Corresponding author.
E-mail address: ryancookddsms@unc.edu

Dent Clin N Am 63 (2019) 157–174
https://doi.org/10.1016/j.cden.2018.11.001

Hirschfield[1] first observed a thin alveolar contour and made the clinical observation that a thin bony contour was accompanied by a thin gingival form. Ochsenbein and Ross[2] classified the gingival anatomy as flat or pronounced scalloped, relating a flat gingiva to a square tooth form and pronounced scalloped gingiva to a tapering tooth form. Weisgold[3] demonstrated an increased susceptibility to recession in individuals with a thin, scalloped gingival architecture. This theory was further supported by studies demonstrating that central incisors with a narrow crown had a greater prevalence of recession than incisors with a wide, square form.[4,5]

De Rouck and colleagues[6] illustrated the presence of 2 distinct gingival biotypes. The first, which occurred in one-third of the study population and was most prominent among women, was classified as having a thin gingival biotype, slender tooth form, narrow zone of keratinized tissue, and a high gingival scallop. The second, which occurred in two-thirds of the study population and mainly among men, was classified as having a thick gingival biotype, quadratic tooth form, broad zone of keratinized tissue, and a flat gingival margin.

Cook and colleagues[7] demonstrated that clinically there are 2 distinct periodontal biotypes. A thin periodontal biotype is associated with a thin labial plate and an apical alveolar crest when compared with a thick/average periodontal biotype. An accurate tool to diagnosis periodontal biotype is the ability (thin periodontal biotype) or inability (thick/average periodontal biotype) to visualize the periodontal probe through the gingival sulcus.

Diagnosis of periodontal biotype influences the treatment planning of many esthetic procedures. Periodontal biotype evaluation can be a valuable tool in establishing patient expectations in many complex esthetic procedures by allowing the clinician to predict therapeutic outcomes.

Alveolar Crest Position

Becker and colleagues[8] used human skulls to measure the vertical distance between the interproximal bony crest and the buccal crest of bone at the midfacial point on the same tooth and developed the following classification system: flat with a mean distance 2.1 mm (standard deviation of 0.51 mm); scalloped with a mean distance 2.5 mm (standard deviation of 0.56 mm); and pronounced scalloped with a mean distance 4.1 mm (standard deviation of 0.60 mm).

Kois[9] suggested a classification system related to periodontal biotype involving the relationship between the cementoenamel junction (CEJ) and the crest of the bone:

1. Normal crest: midfacial alveolar crest is 3 mm and proximal alveolar crest is 3 to 4.5 mm apical to the CEJ—85% of population.
2. High crest: midfacial alveolar crest is less than 3 mm and proximal alveolar crest is 3 mm apical to the CEJ—2% of population.
3. Low crest: midfacial alveolar crest is greater than 3 mm and proximal alveolar crest is greater than 4.5 mm apical to the CEJ—13% of population.

Position of the Gingival Margin

Gingival margin position is critical when determining ideal gingival esthetics. There are 2 categories of ideal gingival esthetics: strong and soft. In the strong configuration, the gingival margins of the maxillary center incisors, lateral incisor, and canines coincide on a horizontal plane (**Fig. 1**). In the soft configuration, the gingival margins of the maxillary center incisors and canines coincide, whereas the gingival margin of the lateral incisors is slightly below this horizontal line (**Fig. 2**). Other factors such as

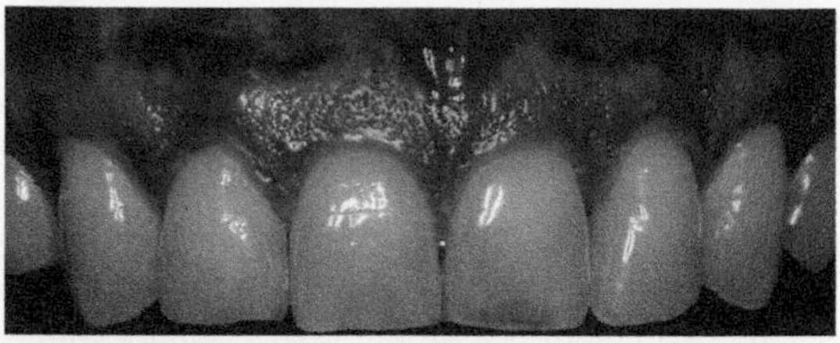

Fig. 1. Strong gingival margin position.

maxillary/mandibular lip position, tooth form (tapered, square), and gender may play a role in gingival margin position.[10]

Gingival Zenith

Gingival zenith location is an important aspect of gingival esthetics because it establishes the visional illusion of the tooth's long axis. The gingival zenith is located distal to the long axis of the maxillary central incisors and canines. Maxillary lateral incisors display a symmetric gingival height of contour and a gingival zenith at the mesial-distal midline.[11] Lateral incisors can display the most gingival zenith variation (0.4 mm).[12]

Implant Restorations and the Periodontal-Restorative Interface

The diagnosis and treatment planning of maxilla anterior implant restorations is a complex process involving the merger of form, function, and esthetics. Successful treatment outcomes require clinicians to pay close attention to the periodontal-restorative interface during diagnosis and treatment planning to ensure restorations mimic natural dentition. This detailed thought process is evident when evaluating anterior implant restorations, where the difference between treatment success and failure may be tenths of millimeters. Understanding how the periodontium responds to therapy is critical to achieving a successful esthetic outcome.

Diagnosis and treatment planning of anterior implant restorations involves evaluation of the 4 Ps:

- Periodontal biotype
- Position of the gingival margin and gingival zenith
- Placement of implant
- Position of the alveolar crest

Periodontal biotype

Diagnosis of periodontal biotype allows clinicians to predict clinical outcomes by relating the soft tissue morphology to the underlying bony anatomy. Patients with a

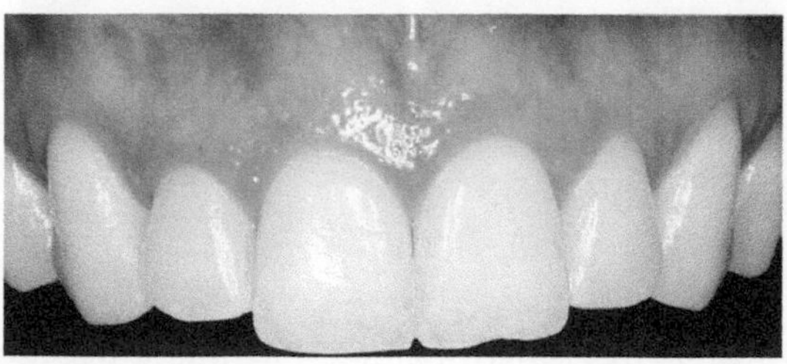

Fig. 2. Soft gingival margin position.

thin periodontal biotype differ from patients with a thick/average periodontal biotype in that they present with a thinner labial plate (**Fig. 3**) and an alveolar crest position that is located more apical in relation to the CEJ (**Fig. 4**).[7] Periodontal biotype can be diagnosed by the ability to visualize the periodontal probe (**Fig. 5**) through the gingival sulcus in thin biotype and the inability to visualize the probe (**Fig. 6**) in a thick biotype.[6] Periodontal biotype has been shown to affect soft tissue esthetic outcomes around anterior implants. Patients with a thin periodontal biotype have more interproximal and midfacial recession postimplant placement than a patient with a thick periodontal biotype.[13,14] Diagnosis of periodontal biotype is essential in treatment planning of anterior implant restorations. Patients with a thin periodontal biotype can be challenging due to their clinical presentation. Patients who present with a thin periodontal biotype may require additional therapy such as hard and soft tissue augmentation.

Position of the gingival margin and gingival zenith

Evaluation of the preexisting gingival margin position is critical in the diagnosis and treatment planning of anterior implant restorations. Ideal gingival esthetics is associated with the gingival margins of the maxillary central incisors and canines being on the same horizontal plane as if an imaginary line connected them. The lateral incisors are either along the same horizontal line or 0.5 to 1.0 mm inferior (**Fig. 7**).[15,16] If a vertical line bisected the midline of the maxillary anterior teeth, the location of the gingival zenith position would be found 1.0 mm distally for central incisors, 0.4 mm distally for the lateral incisors, and 0 mm for canines (**Fig. 8**). The gingival zenith level in an apical-coronal direction of lateral incisors relative to the gingival tangential zenith line joining adjacent central incisor and canine is approximately 1 mm.[12]

When evaluating the gingival margin position in anterior implant restorations, it is pertinent to compare the adjacent and contralateral teeth. With this in mind, the

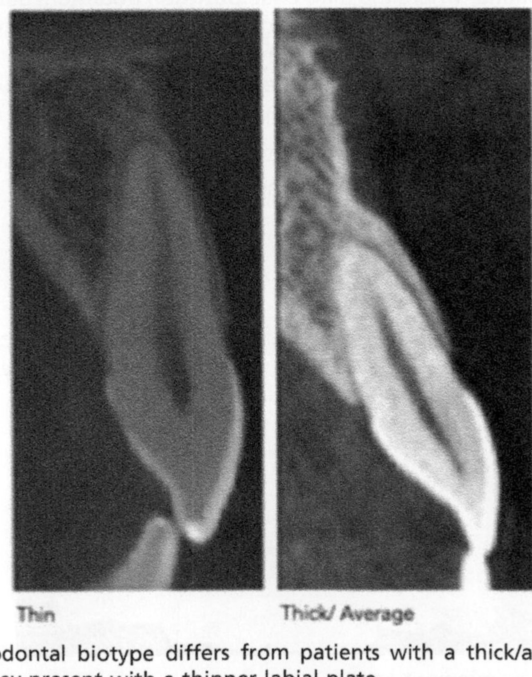

Fig. 3. Thin periodontal biotype differs from patients with a thick/average periodontal biotype in that they present with a thinner labial plate.

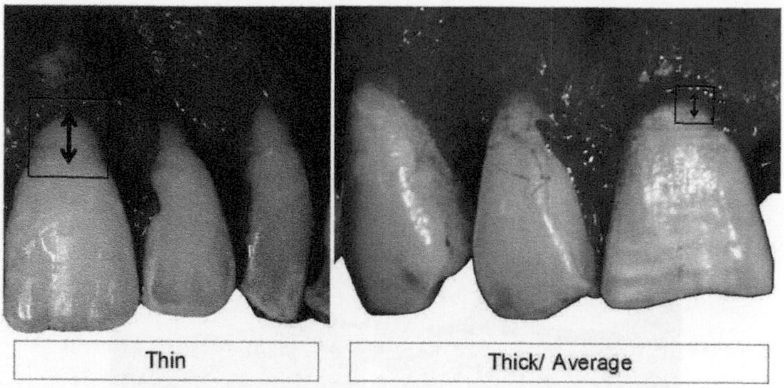

Fig. 4. Thin periodontal biotype differs from patients with a thick/average periodontal biotype in that they present with an alveolar crest position that is located more apical in relation to the CEJ.

proposed implant gingival margin can be classified as being superior, equal or inferior to the adjacent or contralateral tooth (**Fig. 9**). Diagnosis of the existing gingival margin position assists the clinician in sequencing the treatment plan.

Placement of the implant

Planning the position of an anterior implant is critical to the esthetic and functional prognosis. Diagnosis and treatment planning begins with a conventional or digital full-contour wax-up. A diagnostic wax-up allows the clinician to diagnose the amount of restorative space and interimplant space, and establish the proposed gingival margin position.

Adequate horizontal and vertical space between teeth and implants is essential to achieve an esthetic outcome. The horizontal space needed between a tooth and an implant is 1.5 to 2 mm (**Fig. 10**) and between 2 adjacent implants is 3 mm (**Fig. 11**).[17–19] The vertical distance from the alveolar crest to the restorative contact position between a tooth and an implant will be 4.5 mm (**Fig. 12**) and between 2 adjacent implants is 3.4 mm (**Fig. 13**).[20,21]

Identifying the gingival margin position in the diagnostic waxing allows the clinician to locate the proper labial-palatal and apical position of the implant platform. The apical distance from the planned gingival margin is 3 mm (**Fig. 14**).[22,23] The labial-palatal distance from the planned gingival margin/buccal plate is 2 mm (**Fig. 15**).[22,23]

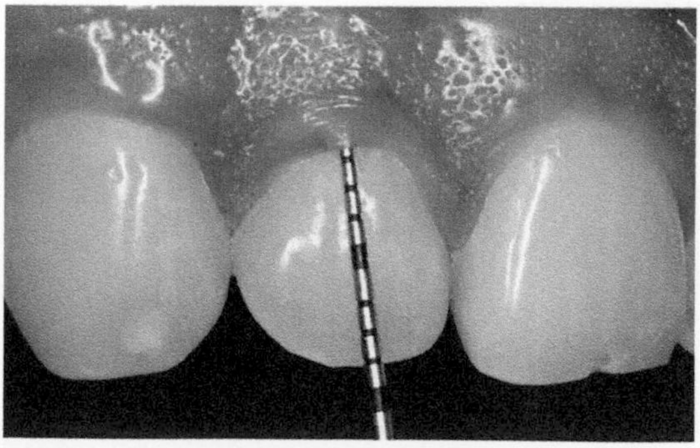

Fig. 5. Probe visible through the gingival sulcus in thin periodontal biotype.

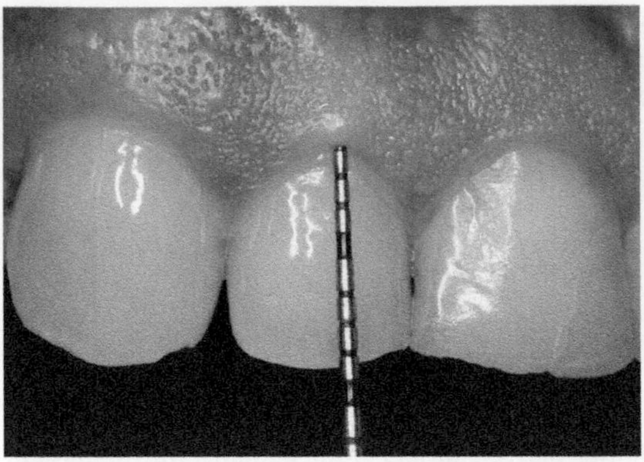

Fig. 6. Probe not visible through the gingival sulcus in thick/average periodontal biotype.

Position of the alveolar crest

Identifying the position of the alveolar crest is paramount in establishing a treatment plan. A normal alveolar crest position is approximately 3 mm apical to the CEJ and follows the anatomic scallop of the CEJ with variations in alveolar crest position.[24,25] A typical clinical presentation of a high-crest position is seen in a patient with excessive gingival display diagnosed with altered passive eruption. Altered passive eruption is diagnosed by the inability to clinically locate the CEJ through the gingival sulcus. The inability to locate the CEJ is due to the incisal position of the alveolar crest in reference to the CEJ.[26] The underlying hard tissue supports the overlaying soft tissue, resulting in long-term stability of proximal and buccal soft tissue (**Fig. 16**).

Four Ps' Influence on Treatment Planning and Treatment Sequence

The 4 Ps can assist in treatment planning and sequencing anterior implant restorations. From the diagnostic wax-up, the 3-dimensional position of the implant is determined. Once the implant position is determined, the diagnosis of periodontal biotype as thin or thick/average guides the clinician in sequencing treatment after assessing the gingival margin and alveolar crest position.

A comprehensive diagnosis and treatment plan of the periorestorative interface is essential in maxilla anterior implant restorations. Using periodontal biotype, position of the gingival margin/gingival zenith, implant placement, and position of the alveolar crest allows the clinician to sequence treatment, set realistic expectations, and enhance therapeutic outcomes.

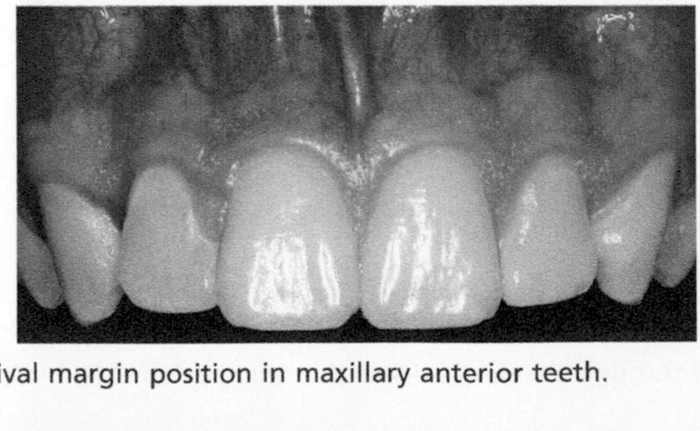

Fig. 7. Ideal gingival margin position in maxillary anterior teeth.

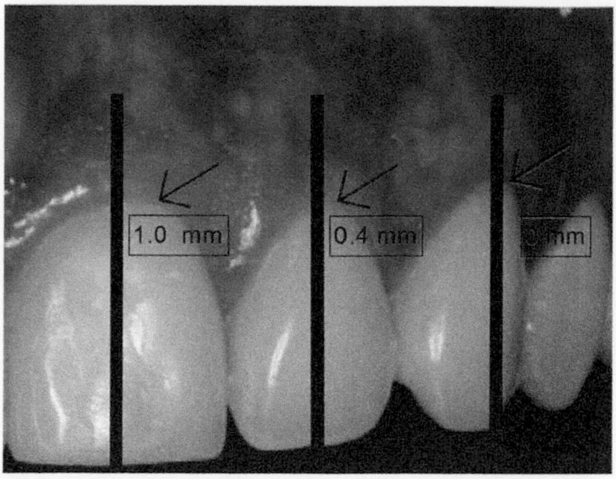

Fig. 8. Gingival zenith position from the vertical bisected midline of the central incisors, lateral incisors, and canines.

Tooth-Borne Restorations and the Periodontal-Restorative Interface

A clinician's knowledge of anatomy, form, and function of the maxillary anterior dentition is paramount in achieving optimal treatment outcomes. The simple act of placing a probe into the gingival sulcus to determine its visibility may provide an excellent clue as to the clinical periodontal biotype and the true nature of the underlying labial plate thickness.

In fixed prosthodontics, knowledge of the periodontal-restorative interface aids the clinician in preparing anterior teeth for all ceramic restorations. If the clinician diagnoses a patient with a thick/average biotype due to the inability to visualize a periodontal probe when placed into the gingival sulcus, it should inform them that the patient may be more susceptible to biologic width invasion because their alveolar crest position may be closer to the CEJ. On the other hand, if the clinician diagnoses a patient with a thin biotype due to the ability to visualize a periodontal probe when placed into the gingival sulcus, it should inform them that the patient may be more susceptible to gingival recession because the alveolar crest position may be further apical from the CEJ.

Alveolar Crest Position and Biologic Width

Classification of alveolar crest position (normal, high, and low crest)[26] may aid clinical decisions in restorative margin location and retraction technique. Treatment outcomes

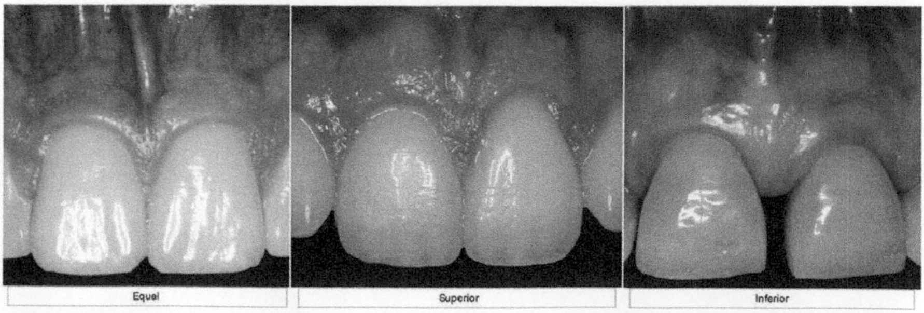

Fig. 9. Classification of gingival margin position of #9 in comparison to #8 (Equal, Superior, or Inferior).

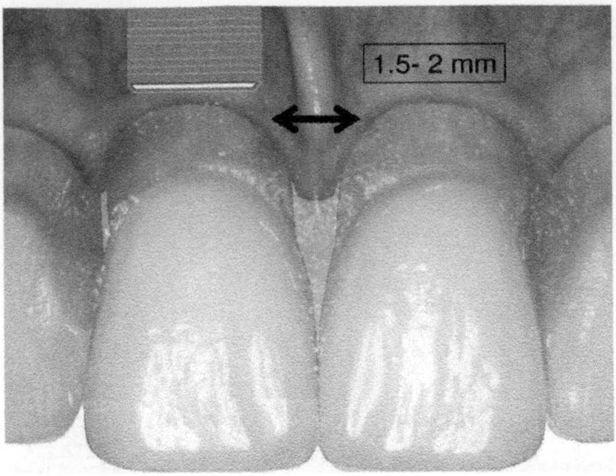

Fig. 10. Horizontal space between a tooth and an implant.

in each of the 3 crest positions suggest that clinical outcomes may be related to the gingival/alveolar crest form. Preparing intracrevicular finish lines in a patient with a high alveolar crest position may increase the susceptibility of biologic width impingement because the bony crest is positioned close to the CEJ. Conversely, when intracrevicular finish lines are prepared in a patient with a low alveolar crest position, an increased propensity for gingival recession exists resulting in exposed restorative margins.

Tarnow[27] demonstrated the relationship between the alveolar crest position and the contract point found between adjacent teeth. When the distance between the alveolar crest and the contact point is 5 mm or less, dental papilla fill is predictable. If the distance between the alveolar crest and the contact point is 6 mm, the papilla will be present 56% of the time and at a 7 mm the papilla will be present 27% of the time.[27]

Understanding the dentogingival complex is of utmost importance in mastering the periodontal-restorative interface in fixed restorations. The dentogingival complex is composed of 2 components, the connective tissue and the epithelial attachment.[28] The dimensional relationship between the periodontal tissues and crestal bone was described by Garguilo and collegues.[29] The relationship between the crest of the

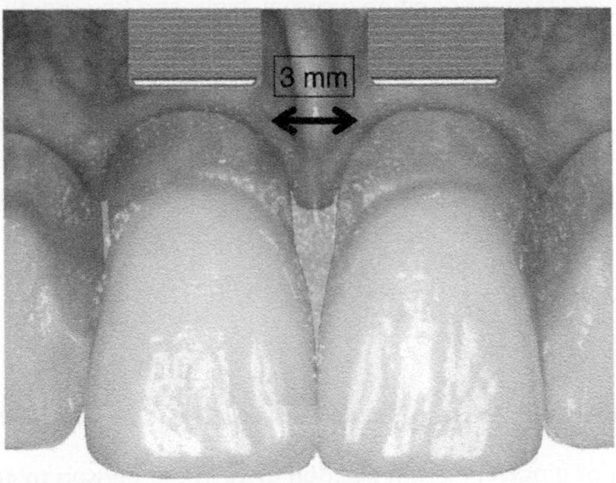

Fig. 11. Horizontal space between 2 adjacent implants.

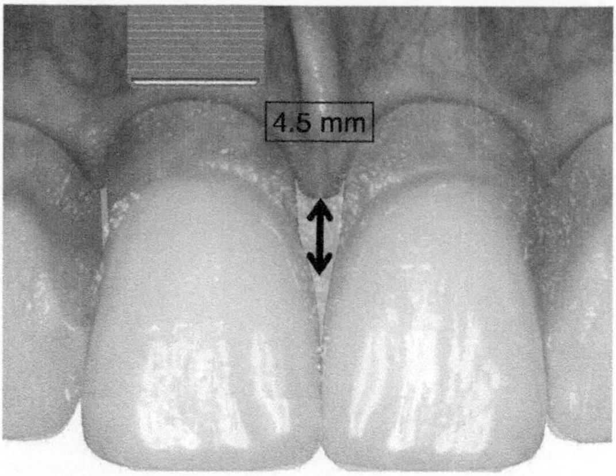

Fig. 12. Vertical distance from the alveolar crest to the restorative contact position between a tooth and an implant.

alveolar bone surrounding a tooth, the connective tissue attachment, the epithelial attachment, and the sulcus depth was defined as shown in **Table 1**.

The most constant dimension was the distance from the base of the epithelial attachment to the crest of the alveolar ridge, with an average measurement of 1.07 mm. The most variable dimension was the length of epithelial attachment, with an average measurement of 0.97 mm. The combination of epithelial attachment and connective tissue was termed "biologic width" by Cohen.[30] In another study, Vacek and colleagues[31] found the following measurements for the sulcus depth to be 1.34 mm, 1.14 for epithelial attachment, and 0.77 mm for connective tissue attachment. The connective tissue attachment was the most consistent measurement.

Restorative Margin Location and Periodontal-Restorative Interface

Understanding the interaction between the restorative margin position and the dentogingival complex[32] allows the provider the ability to deliver esthetic restorations that are harmonious with biology. Restorative margin location is influenced by biological and esthetic principles and is ideally located slightly coronal to the CEJ.

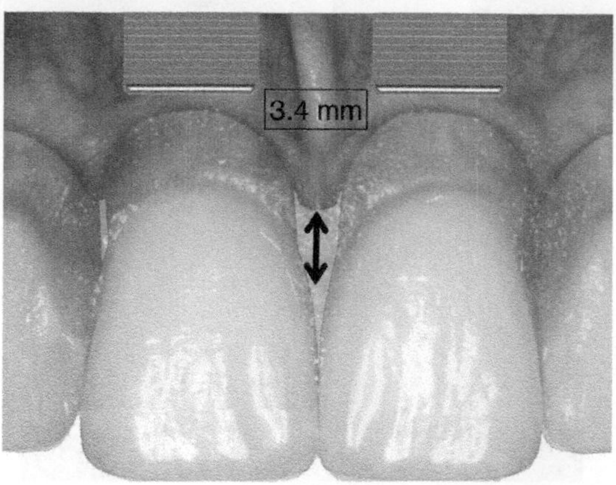

Fig. 13. Vertical distance from the alveolar crest to the restorative contact position between 2 adjacent implants.

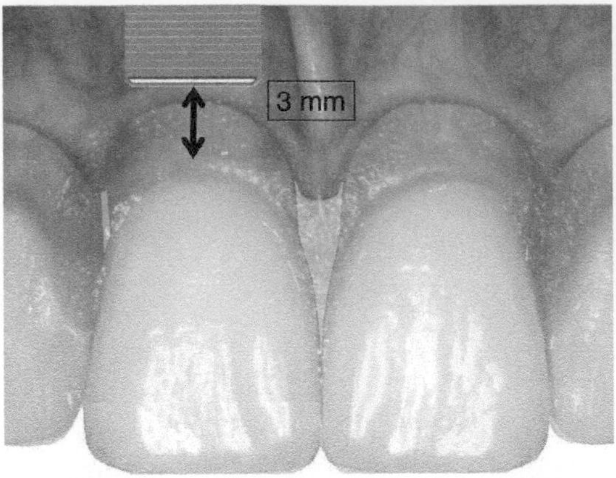

Fig. 14. Apical distance from the planned gingival margin to the implant platform.

Restorative margin location is influenced by myriad of factors, including esthetics, mechanical principles (retentive and resistant form), root caries, position of the CEJ, and existing gingival recession. Although supragingival margin placement is preferred to maintain periodontal health, many other factors dictate an equal-gingival or subgingival margin location. It has been demonstrated that in time (5 years), many subgingival margins (68%) become equal-gingival or supragingival margins due to gingival recession.[33] Subgingival margin placement is also associated with greater attachment loss (1.2 mm) when compared with supragingival margin placement (0.6 mm).[33]

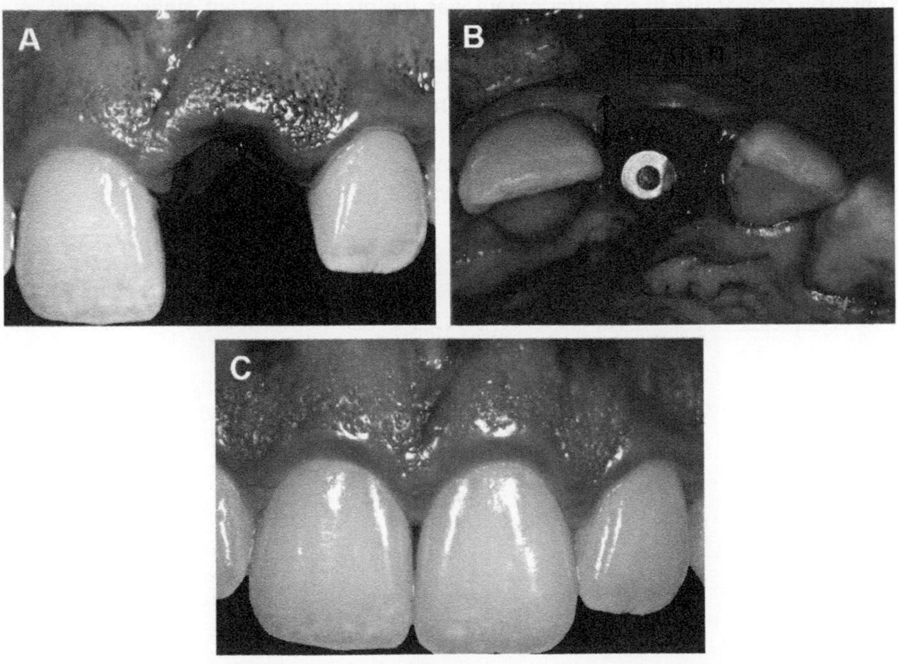

Fig. 15. Labial-Palatal Distance of 2 mm. (*A*) Atraumatic Extraction. (*B*) Implant Placement. (*C*) Final Implant Restoration.

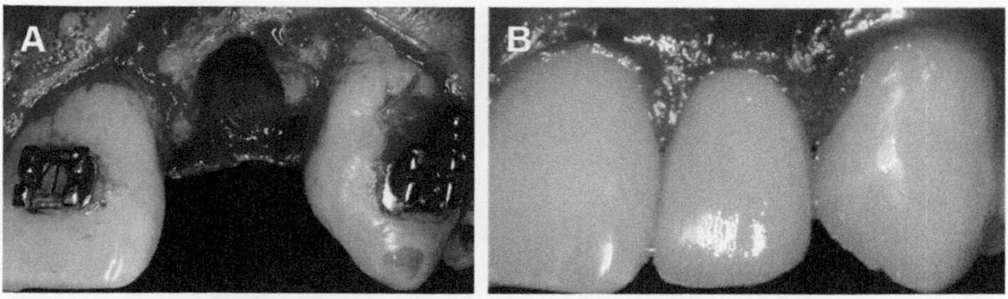

Fig. 16. Hard and Soft Tissue Contours Supporting Implant Restoration. (*A*) Hard Tissue Contour. (*B*) Soft Tissue Contour.

When determining margin location, it is important to individualize the approach due to the variance in biology encountered from one patient to the other. Bone sounding will aid in this individualized approach because it allows locating the position of the alveolar crest in relationship to gingival margin and CEJ. As previously mentioned, in a thick/average periodontal biotype, since the alveolar crest is located closer to the CEJ,[7] a subgingival margin location may pose an increased risk for biologic width impingement (**Fig. 17**). To preserve biologic width in patients with altered passive eruption, crown lengthening and establishing a new restorative margin will prevent the exposure of adjacent CEJ (**Fig. 18**). In the absence of altered passive eruption, orthodontic extrusion followed by crown lengthening and establishing a new restorative margin will prevent the exposure of adjacent CEJ preserving biologic width (**Fig. 19**). In a thin periodontal biotype, because the alveolar crest position is more apically positioned to the CEJ, the placement of a subgingival margin may result in postoperative recession. As the distance from a normal crest position (**Fig. 20**A) increases (**Fig. 20**B), as seen in a thin periodontal biotype, there may be an increase in chance of gingival recession with the placement of a subgingival margin. As the distance from a normal crest position (see **Fig. 20**A) decreases (**Fig. 20**C), as seen in a thick/average periodontal biotype, there may be an increase in chance of biologic width impingement with the placement of a subgingival margin.

A new restorative margin can be established through surgical crown lengthening by surgically repositioning the alveolar crest in relation to the gingival margin. Changes in gingival margin can be affected by surgical technique and gingival biotype. Bragger and colleagues[34] showed minimal changes in gingival margin placement from the time of surgery when the surgical flap was repositioned 3 mm coronal to the newly

Table 1
Relationship between the crest of the alveolar bone surrounding a tooth, the connective tissue attachment, the epithelial attachment, and the sulcus depth

Dentogingival Component	Location	Dimension	Clinical Significance
Histologic sulcus	Gingival margin to the epithelial attachment	0.69 mm	May differ from the clinical sulcus depth
Epithelial attachment	Distance from coronal to apical portion of the attachment	0.97 mm	The most variable component
Connective tissue attachment	Distance from epithelial attachment to crest of alveolar bone	1.07 mm	The most consistent component

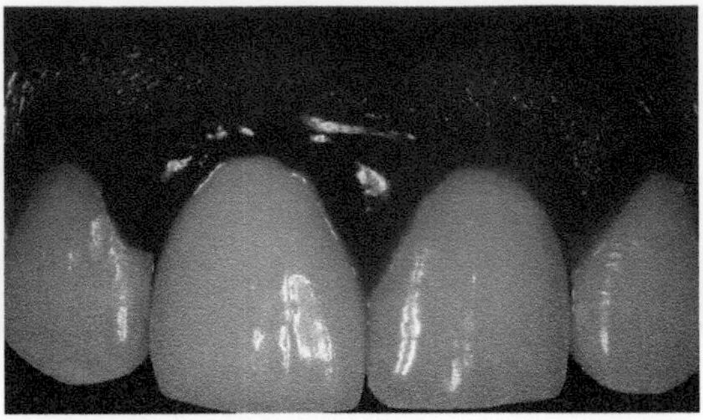

Fig. 17. Biologic width impingement.

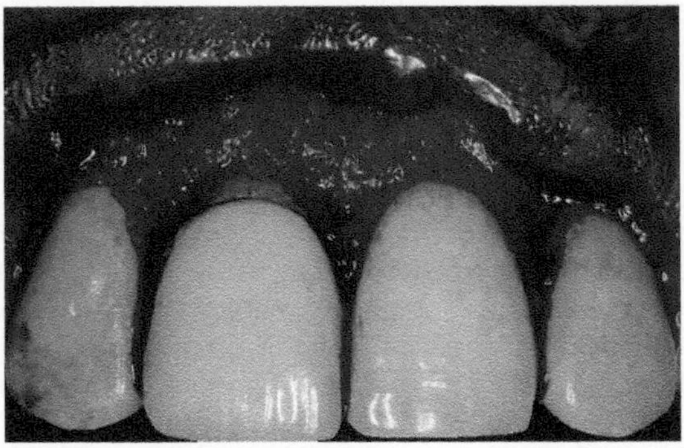

Fig. 18. Crown lengthening of adjacent teeth with altered passive eruption.

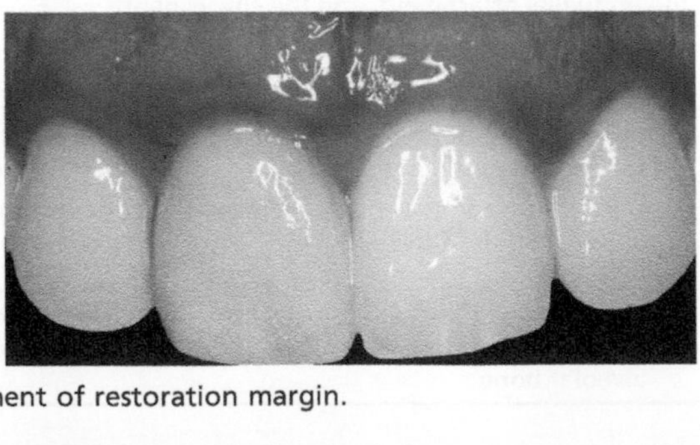

Fig. 19. Establishment of restoration margin.

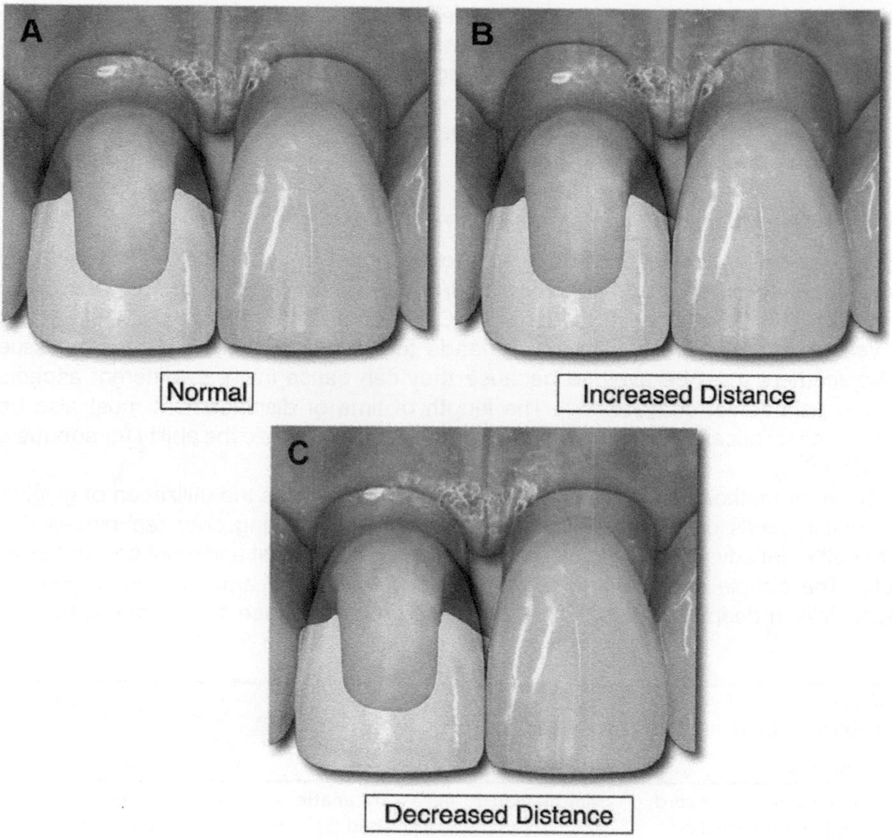

Fig. 20. (*A*) Normal crest to restorative margin position. (*B*) Increased distance—crest to restorative margin position. (*C*) Decreased distance—crest to restorative margin position.

established alveolar crest. When the surgical flap was positioned below or at the level of the alveolar crest, the postsurgical soft tissue regrowth continued even after a year.[35] Furthermore, patients with thick tissue biotype demonstrated significantly more coronal soft tissue regrowth than patients with thin tissue biotype.[35]

Inflammation and Periodontal-Restorative Interface

Controlling inflammation is detrimental in regard to the periodontal restorative interface and fixed dental restorations. Before the start of any prosthetic treatment, the periodontium must be kept in a healthy state to optimize the intrasulcular environment.[36] Inflamed gingivae are more susceptible to bleeding, making it difficult to obtain an accurate impression of the margins.[37] Inflammation and recession of the free gingival margin is a common occurrence associated with provisional restorations.[38–41] Donaldson[38] showed that provisional restorations contributed to some recession in 80% of the free gingival margin sites evaluated and the degree of recession was time dependent. The placement of the definitive restoration would often lead to gingival recovery, but in the presence of gingival recession only one-third was reversible. These undesirable results are related to the poor contour, marginal adaptation, and surface roughness of the provisional restoration, irrespective of the material selection, because they contribute to plaque accumulation decreasing periodontal health.[40] Instead provisional restorations should be smooth, well-fitting, and properly contoured.[42–45] Garvin and colleagues[41] concluded that periodontal inflammation associated with provisional treatment could be expected to be a reversible process provided that the amount of gingival irritation is minimal and provisional treatment occurs over a short time span.

Gingival Retraction and Periodontal-Restorative Interface

Proper consideration should be given to the gingival retraction technique used because they all result in mechanical and/or chemical trauma to the gingival tissue triggering the inflammatory response.[46] Often times the injury is self-limited and reversible.[46,47] Other times the injury leads to recession.[48] Heavy forces in tissue displacement must be avoided because they can cause injury to different aspects of the periodontal complex.[36,49] The length of time of displacement must also be kept minimal because prolonged displacement may jeopardize the ability for adequate healing.[50]

Different methods exist for gingival displacement such as the utilization of gingival retraction cords or cordless displacement materials. Varying cord techniques that offer different advantages and disadvantages (**Table 2**)[51] exist and must be used carefully. The double cord technique, for example, is favored amongst prosthodontist especially in deep finish lines, but has the potential to induce more gingival trauma,

Table 2
Retraction procedures for anterior region

Technique	Indication	Advantages	Disadvantages
Single Cord—single cord beginning encircling prep from mesial, lingual, distal, and facial surface; continuing the same cord on to mesial, lingual, and distal allows double packing at these surfaces, avoiding double packing on the facial gingival	Healthy tissues	Least traumatic Decreased postoperative gingival recession	Inadequate impression material due to lack of tissue displacement
Selective Double Cord—extra thin cord placed in the regions prone to bleeding; a second cord is placed as described for single-string technique; the initial cord remains in the crevice during impression	Healthy tissues with localized inflammation	Control of bleeding Good lateral displacement	Increased treatment time
Double Cord—extra thin cord is placed in the entire crevice; a second cord is placed as described for single-string technique; the initial cord remains in during the impression	Inflamed tissues	Control of bleeding Excellent lateral displacement	Increased treatment time Potential trauma Unpredictable gingival response

especially in a thin biotype.[52] Cordless displacement materials have the potential to cause less damage because they generate less pressure (37.7 times less)[53] at placement than retraction cord, but the amount and duration of gingival displacement may be less than in retraction cord.[54] The aim in soft tissue management of tooth-borne restorations is the production of acceptable restorative margins that can be captured in a good impression without irreparable damage to the periodontal tissues.[55]

Material Selection and Periodontal-Restorative Interface

Differing gingival response exists within the assortment of materials present for fixed dental restorations that can be attributed to their variations in plaque accumulation.[56,57] Clinical studies have shown that patient compliance with personal oral home care and periodontal maintenance are more detrimental in regard to periodontal health than restorative material selection.[56,58] In fact, in motivated patients who adhered to self-performed plaque control, there was no statistical difference in plaque and gingival inflammation levels between nontreated teeth and teeth with full-coverage restorations.[59] In patients with true allergic reactions, material selection may be of more importance. Despite very limited evidence, zirconia-based restorations can be an option for patients with true metal allergies.[60] For most patients, it is often the quality of the fit and finish of the restoration rather than the material itself, even if placed subgingivally, which is more important in gingival health.[61]

REFERENCES

1. Hirschfield I. A study of skulls in the American Museum of Natural History in relation to periodontal disease. J Dent Res 1923;5:251–65.
2. Ochsenbein C, Ross S. A re-evaluation of osseous surgery. Dent Clin North Am 1969;13(1):87–102.
3. Weisgold AS. Contours of the full crown restoration. Alpha Omegan 1977;70: 77–89.
4. Olsson M, Lindhe J. Periodontal characteristics in individuals with varying form of the upper central incisors. J Clin Periodontol 1991;18:78–82.
5. Olsson M, Lindhe J, Marinello CP. On the relationship between crown form and clinical features of the gingiva in adolescents. J Clin Periodontol 1993;20: 570–7.
6. De Rouck TD, Eghbali R, Collys K, et al. The gingival biotype revisited: transparency of the periodontal probe through the gingival margin as a method to discriminate thin from thick gingiva. J Clin Periodontol 2009;36:428–33.
7. Cook DR, Mealey BL, Verrett RG, et al. Relationship between clinical periodontal biotype and labial plate thickness: an in vivo study. Int J Periodontics Restorative Dent 2011;31:344–54.
8. Becker W, Ochsenbein C, Tibbetts L, et al. Alveolar bone anatomic profiles as measured from dry skulls. J Clin Periodontol 1997;24:727–31.
9. Kois J. The restorative-periodontal interface: biological parameters. Periodontol 2000 1996;11:29–38.
10. Machado AW. 10 commandments of smile esthetics. Dental Press J Orthod 2014; 19:136–57.
11. Sonick M. Esthetic crown lengthening for maxillary anterior teeth. Compend Contin Educ Dent 1997;18:814–9.
12. Chu SJ, Tan JH, Stappert CF, et al. Gingival zenith positions and levels of the maxillary anterior dentition. J Esthet Restor Dent 2009;21:113–20.

13. Khzam N. Systematic review of soft tissue alterations and esthetic outcomes following immediate implant placement and restoration of single implants in the anterior maxilla. J Periodontol 2015;86:1321–30.
14. Kan JY, Rungcharassaeng K, Lozada JL, et al. Facial gingival tissue stability following immediate placement and provisionalization of maxillary anterior single implants: a 2- to 8-year follow-up. Int J Oral Maxillofac Implants 2011;26:179–87.
15. Buser D, Martin W, Belser UC. Optimizing esthetics for implant restorations in the anterior maxilla: anatomic and surgical considerations. Int J Oral Maxillofac Implants 2004;19:43–61.
16. Springer NC, Chang C, Fields HW, et al. Smile esthetics from the layperson's perspective. Am J Orthod Dentofacial Orthop 2011;139:91–101.
17. Berglundh T, Lindhe J. Dimension of the periimplant mucosa. Biologic width revisited. J Clin Periodontol 1996;23:971–3.
18. Esposito M, Ekestubbe A, Gröndahl K. Radiological evaluation of marginal bone loss at tooth surfaces facing single Brånemark implants. Clin Oral Implants Res 1993;4:151–7.
19. Tarnow DP, Cho SC, Wallace SS. The effect of inter-implant distance on the height of inter-implant bone crest. J Periodontol 2000;71:546–9.
20. Grunder U. Stability of the mucosal topography around single-tooth implants and adjacent teeth: 1-year results. Int J Periodontics Restorative Dent 2000;20:11–7.
21. Tarnow DP. Vertical distance from the crest of bone to the height of the interproximal papilla between adjacent implants. J Periodontol 2003;74(12):1785–8.
22. Cooper LF, Pin-Harry OC. "Rules of six"- diagnostic and therapeutic guidelines for single- tooth implant success. Compend Contin Educ Dent 2013;34:94–8.
23. Rojas-Vizcaya F. Biological aspects as a rule for single implant placement. The 3A-2B rule: a clinical report. J Prosthodont 2013;22:575–80.
24. Kois JC. Predictable single-tooth peri-implant esthetics: five diagnostic keys. Compend Contin Educ Dent 2004;25:895–900.
25. Kois JC. Altering gingival levels: the restorative connection. Part 1: biologic variables. J Esthet Dent 1994;6:1 3–9.
26. Dolt AH III, Robbins JW. Altered passive eruption: an etiology of short clinical crowns. Quintessence Int 1997;28:363–72.
27. Tarnow DP, Magner AW, Fletcher P. The effect of the distance from the contact point to the crest of bone on the presence or absence of the interproximal dental papilla. J Periodontol 1992;63:995–6.
28. Sicher H. Changing concept of the supporting dental structures. Oral Surg Oral Med Oral Pathol 1959;12:31–5.
29. Gargiulo AW, Wentz FM, Orban B. Dimensions and relations of the dentogingival junction in humans. J Periodontol 1961;32(3):261–7.
30. Cohen DW. Lecture. Walter Reed Army Medical Center; 1962.
31. Vacek JS, Gher ME, Assad DA, et al. The dimensions of the human dentogingival junction. Int J Periodontics Restorative Dent 1994;14:154–65.
32. Nevins M, Skurow HM. Periodontics and restorative dentistry: the clinical interrelationship. CDA J 1984;12:101–5.
33. Valderhaugw J, Birkeland JM. Periodontal conditions in patients 5 years following insertion of fixed prostheses. J Oral Rehabil 1976;3:237–43.
34. Brägger U, Lauchenauer D, Lang NP. Surgical lengthening of the clinical crown. J Clin Periodontol 1992;191:58–63.
35. Pontoriero R, Carnevale G. Surgical crown lengthening: a 12-month clinical wound healing study. J Periodontol 2001;72:841–8.

36. Wilson RD, Maynard G. Intracrevicular restorative dentistry. Int J Periodontics Restorative Dent 1981;1:34–49.
37. Sorensen JA, Doherty FM, Newman MG, et al. Gingival enhancement in fixed prosthodontics: Part I. Clinical findings. J Prosthet Dent 1991;65:100–7.
38. Donaldson D. Gingival recession associated with temporary crowns. J Periodontol 1973;44:691–6.
39. Donaldson D. The etiology of gingival recession associated with temporary crowns. J Periodontol 1974;45:468–71.
40. Waerhaug J, Zander HA. Reaction of gingival tissues to self-curing acrylic restorations. J Am Dent Assoc 1957;54:760–8.
41. Garvin PH, Malone WP, Toto PD, et al. Effect of self-curing acrylic resin treatment restorations on the crevicular fluid volume. J Prosthet Dent 1982;47:284–9.
42. Waerhaug J. Effect of rough surfaces upon gingival tissue. J Dent Res 1956;35:323–5.
43. Chiche G. Improving marginal adaptation of provisional restorations. Quintessence Int 1990;21:325–9.
44. Orkin DA, Reddy J, Bradshaw D. The relationship of the position of crown margins to gingival health. J Prosthet Dent 1987;57:421–4.
45. Dragoo MR, Williams GB. Periodontal tissue reactions to restorative procedures, part II. Int J Periodontics Restorative Dent 1982;2:34–45.
46. de Gennaro GG, Landesman HM, Calhoun JE, et al. A comparison of gingival inflammation related to retraction cords. J Prosthet Dent 1982;47:384–9.
47. Harrison JD. Effect of retraction materials on the gingival sulcus epithelium. J Prosthet Dent 1961;11:514–21.
48. Ruel J, Schuessler PJ, Malament K, et al. Effect of retraction procedures on the periodontium in humans. J Prosthet Dent 1980;44:508–15.
49. Xhonga FA. Gingival retraction techniques and their healing effect on the gingiva. J Prosthet Dent 1971;26:640–8.
50. Ramadan FA, El-Sadeek M, Hassanein ES. Histopathologic response of gingival tissues to hemodent and aluminum chloride solutions as tissue displacement materials. Egypt Dent J 1972;18:337–52.
51. Chiche GJ, Pinault A. Impressions for the anterior dentition. Esthetics of anterior fixed prosthodontics. Chicago: Quintessence Publishing Co.; 1994. p. 161–75.
52. Baba N, Goodacre CJ, Jekki R, et al. Gingival displacement for impression making in fixed prosthodontics contemporary principles, materials, and techniques. Dent Clin North Am 2014;58:45–68.
53. Bennani V, Aarts JM, He LH. A comparison of pressure generated by cordless gingival displacement techniques. J Prosthet Dent 2012;107:388–92.
54. Chandra S, Singh A, Gupta KK, et al. Effect of gingival displacement cord and cordless systems on the closure, displacement, and inflammation of the gingival crevice. J Prosthet Dent 2016;115(2):177–82.
55. Benson BW, Bonberg TJ, Hatch RA, et al. Tissue displacement methods in fixed prosthodontics. J Prosthet Dent 1986;55:175–81.
56. Litonjua LA, Cabanilla LL, Abbott LJ. Plaque formation and marginal gingivitis associated with restorative materials. Compend Contin Educ Dent 2012;33:6–10.
57. Heschl A, Haas M, Haas J, et al. Maxillary rehabilitation of periodontally compromised patients with extensive one-piece fixed prostheses supported by natural teeth: a retrospective longitudinal study. Clin Oral Investig 2013;17:45–53.
58. Konradsson K, Claesson R, van Dijken JW. Dental biofilm, gingivitis and interleukin-1 adjacent to approximal sites of a bonded ceramic. J Clin Periodontol 2007;34:1062–7.

59. Morris HF. Veterans Administration Cooperative Studies Project No 147. Part VIII: plaque accumulation on metal ceramic resto- rations cast from noble and nickel-based alloys. A five-year report. J Prosthet Dent 1989;61:543–9.
60. Gokcen-Rohlig B, Saruhanoglu A, Cifter ED, et al. Applicability of zirconia dental prostheses for metal allergy patients. Int J Prosthodont 2010;23:562–5.
61. Richter WA, Ueno H. Relationship of crown margin placement to gingival inflammation. J Prosthet Dent 1973;30:156–61.

The Current State of Chairside Digital Dentistry and Materials

Markus B. Blatz, DMD, PhD*, Julian Conejo, DDS, MSc

KEYWORDS

• Chairside • CAD/CAM • Digital dentistry • Ceramics • Dental materials

KEY POINTS

- Chairside computer-aided design (CAD) computer-aided manufacturing (CAM) technologies have emerged into user-friendly and patient-friendly, versatile, and accurate clinical assets.
- Current intraoral scanning technologies are as accurate as, or even more accurate than, conventional impression techniques, at least for single-span and short-span multiunit restorations.
- Design software has been simplified with excellent features to produce natural esthetics and function.
- Milling machines have become smaller, more accurate, and more versatile for a large variety of materials.
- Most modern materials fabricated in the laboratory can also be fabricated chairside in a single visit: composite resins and various types of ceramics, even zirconia.

INTRODUCTION

Computer-aided design (CAD) computer-aided manufacturing (CAM) systems were initially developed in 1950 by the defense arm of the United States Air Force for use in aircraft and automotive manufacturing. It took 3 decades until such technologies were applied in dentistry, when Francois Duret developed a dental CAD/CAM device that included an optical impression of the abutment tooth and a numerically controlled milling machine.[1] The first restoration was milled in 1983 and the system demonstrated at the French Dental Association's International congress in November 1985. Werner Mormann is known as the developer of the first commercial CAD/CAM

Disclosure: The authors have nothing to disclose.
Department of Preventive and Restorative Sciences, University of Pennsylvania School of Dental Medicine, 240 South 40th Street, Philadelphia, PA 19104, USA
* Corresponding author.
E-mail address: mblatz@upenn.edu

Dent Clin N Am 63 (2019) 175–197
https://doi.org/10.1016/j.cden.2018.11.002
dental.theclinics.com

system: CEREC (Dentsply Sirona), an acronym for ceramic reconstruction or chairside economical restoration of esthetic ceramics. The first CEREC chairside treatment was performed in 1985 at University of Zurich Dental School. That this system could, based on an optical scan, fabricate indirect same-day ceramic dental restorations in the dental office was revolutionary.[2–6]

Laboratory-based CAD/CAM systems that included an optical or mechanical scan of a master cast, digital restoration design, and a CAM system either in the dental laboratory or a centralized milling center followed shortly. In the meantime, digital planning, design, and manufacturing technologies have been the common standard in dental laboratory technology for many years now. The digital work flow and its manufacturing components provide high accuracy and precision, predictability, efficiency, cost-effectiveness, and a wide range of restorative and prosthetic materials with physical, optical, and biological properties that often exceed those fabricated conventionally. Digital tooth design and treatment planning have changed fundamentally. Independent of the wax-up skills of the practitioner or the dental technician, so-called digital wax-ups allow the use of scan files of natural teeth and smiles and, therefore, the ability to mimic nature. Combined with current face-scanning technologies, artificial intelligence and machine learning tools will allow automated generation of individual digital smile designs and treatment plans in the near future.

Early CAD/CAM systems were limited to fabricating inlays, onlays, and single crowns. Now, with the plethora of CAD/CAM technologies, systems, milling machines, and other tools available, there is virtually no limit to the type of dental restoration that can be fabricated, from single-unit inlays, onlays, crowns, veneers, implant abutments, and restorations to fixed and removable dental prostheses for partially and completely edentulous patients. Although currently the most prominent method of fabrication is subtractive through milling processes, additive technologies such as three-dimensional (3D) printing are becoming increasingly popular and are already applied for printing models, impression trays, night guards, surgical guides, orthodontics aligners, dentures, provisionals, and other devices. With the development of better printers and additional restorative materials in the future, 3D printing may well become the manufacturing process of choice.

The spectrum of restorations that can be fabricated with a chairside system depends on the size of the milling machine, the size of the material block, and the properties of the selected material. However, the lines between chairside digital manufacturing and laboratory-based CAD/CAM technologies have become blurred. Most chairside systems provide the possibility to send a scan file to any manufacturing site with the option to either produce a restoration in the office, often within minutes, or delegate this responsibility to the dental laboratory. The material choices for both options are increasing steadily, ranging from composite resins and polymethyl methacrylates (PMMAs) to silica-based and high-strength ceramics such as zirconia. Many laboratories mill wax or acrylic pattern resin copings and frameworks for casting metal alloys.

Despite its advantages, common application of chairside CAD/CAM technology has not yet been fully embraced by the dental community. The main reasons cited for that are related to high initial and maintenance cost, a steep learning curve, and the need to change procedures that practitioners have learned in dental school and become used to.

CHAIRSIDE COMPUTER-AIDED DESIGN COMPUTER-AIDED MANUFACTURING SYSTEMS

The list of intraoral scanners, milling machines, sintering furnaces, 3D printers, and other CAD/CAM equipment available on the market is growing exponentially at an unexpected rate.[7] At present, the 2 most popular systems that offer the entire range of equipment from scanning to in-house milling are CEREC (Dentsply Sirona, York, PA) and Planmeca (Planmeca Oy, Helsinki, Finland). The current portfolio of the CEREC system includes the CEREC Omnicam scanner and CEREC MC, X, and XL 4-axis milling units. These milling units can accommodate material blocks of up to 20 mm (MC), 40 mm (MCX), or 85 mm (MCXL) and mill either wet or dry. The Planmeca chairside work flow offers the Emerald camera and the PlanScan intraoral scanner in combination with the PlanMill 40s or the smaller PlanMill 30s milling machine. Other manufacturers that offer total chairside solutions are Carestream Dental (Atlanta, GA) with the CS 3600 intraoral scanner and the CS 3000 milling machine, Dental Wings (Montreal, Canada) with its DW IntraOral scanner and the DW Lasermill, and Zfx (Dachau, Germany) with the IntraScan scanner and the Inhouse5x milling unit.

Several manufacturers offer various components of the chairside digital workflow; for example, 3Shape (Copenhagen, Denmark) with its popular Trios 3 Wireless scanner or Ivoclar Vivadent (Schaan, Liechtenstein), which recently introduced the PrograMill One chairside milling machine.

TOOTH PREPARATION

Keeping in mind the type of restoration material used, mostly brittle ceramics, and that different milling parameters, such as size of bur, greatly affect the internal fit of the ultimate restoration, any abutment tooth preparations intended for CAD/CAM restorations should provide adequate space and be rounded. Sharp corners and edges are not likely to be properly represented in intaglio surfaces of the restoration. Inadequate space and thin margins may lead to fractures. The preferred preparation finish line design is an internally rounded shoulder or a chamfer.[8] It was shown that the preparation quality has a direct effect on the marginal fit of chairside CAD/CAM crowns.[9]

A provisional restoration becomes unnecessary when the complete chairside approach is applied and the definitive restoration is fabricated and inserted in 1 visit. The clinician may choose to immediately seal the prepared dentin tooth surfaces with a bonding agent (immediate dentin sealing technique), even before scanning.

INTRAORAL SCANNERS

Different technologies are used to obtain a digital impression of teeth and surrounding intraoral tissues.[10] These technologies are constantly updated and refined, and so are the actual scanners to make them smaller, user and patient friendly, as well as easy to navigate and handle in the oral cavity. A strategic scanning technique that subsequently captures all areas and angles has to be used and become routine for maximum scanning efficiency and quality outcomes. Current intraoral scanners do not require the once-necessary antireflective powder and have the ability to scan colors as well as determining tooth shades. Besides eliminating uncomfortable aspects of a conventional impression, one of the great advantages of intraoral scanning is that select areas that may not have been adequately captured can simply be rescanned without having to retake the entire impression.

Intraoral scanners function by projecting structured light (white, red, or blue), which is recorded as individual images or video and compiled by the software after recognition of specific points of interest. Different coordinates are used, the first 2 (x and y) of each point are evaluated on the image, and the third coordinate (z) is then calculated depending on the distance of each object to the camera. A 3D model is then generated by matching the points of interest taken under different angles. Extreme points can also be statistically eliminated to reduce noise.

The accuracy of the restorations is independent of the impression technique, analog or digital.[11,12] However, the time needed for taking a digital impression is less than that for a conventional impression.[13] In addition, patients clearly prefer the digital scan. It is also interesting that dental students favored the scans rather than traditional impressions, whereas trained clinicians were split evenly regarding their preferences.[14] This finding may be related to habits and experience with a technique they were familiar with since dental school.

Digital full-arch impressions taken with an intraoral scanner seem to have slight deviations in respect to cross-arch accuracy.[15] Other researchers found similar accuracy levels for full-arch scans between scanners.[16] A recent literature review concluded that, currently, the literature does not support the use of intraoral scanners for long-span restorations on teeth or implants[17] and that there are still areas in respect to digital impressions of dental implants that need further investigation.[18] However, new intraoral scanning technologies, such as photogrammetric imaging, allow high accuracy even for full-arch implant restorations.[19]

Because chairside-fabricated CAD/CAM restorations are typically limited to single-span or short-span units, the questions related to long-span restorations on multiple teeth and implants may not be critical. However, scanning technique and sequence also play a major role in the accuracy of the scan. When properly applied, the digital impression technique seems to be more accurate than a conventional impression.[20,21] **Fig. 1** depicts the clinical application of an intraoral scanner.

In the past, intraoral scanners were connected to mobile carts as a complete unit with the computer and monitor. More recent versions of scanners are connected directly or wirelessly to a laptop computer. Companies that produce scanners as well as dental chairs offer the option of incorporating the scanner into the dental chair.

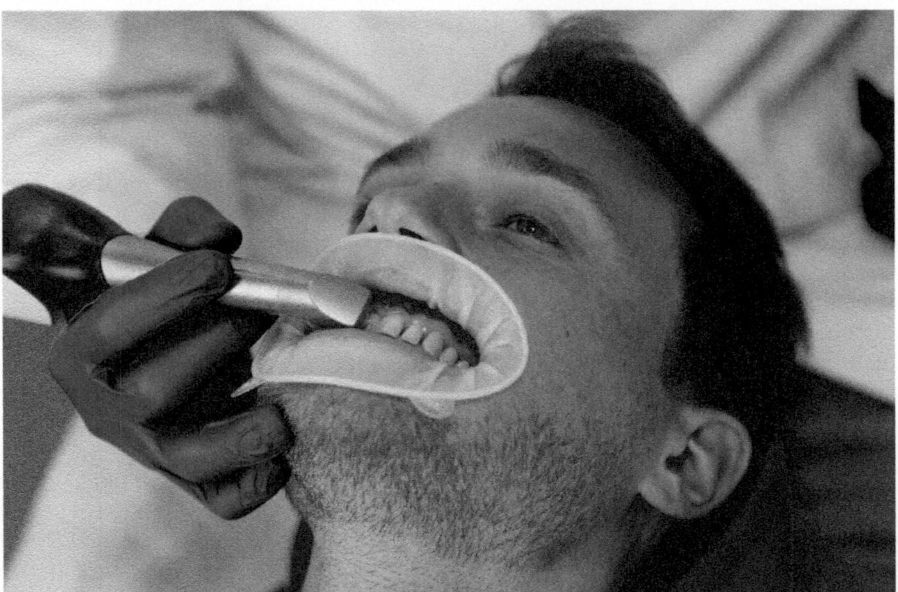

Fig. 1. Intraoral scanners have become significantly smaller as well as user and patient friendly.

COMPUTER-AIDED DESIGN COMPUTER-AIDED MANUFACTURING DESIGN SOFTWARE

The ability to visualize and analyze digital impressions immediately after scanning is one of the key advantages of the chairside work flow (**Fig. 2**).[7] Unlike conventional impressions, where errors are often only detected after fabricating the mastercast, an erroneous or deficient digital impression can be analyzed and corrected immediately. Specific software (eg, PrepCheck, Dentsply Sirona) is available to detect errors in the tooth preparation, such as inadequate occlusal clearance, undercuts, unclear preparation margin, sharp corners, and rough surfaces. These features are specifically useful in a teaching environment.

Different software is available for each type and intended use of CAD/CAM systems: clinical or laboratory. The reason is that restorations and materials for chairside CAD/CAM are more limited because of time restrictions. The main objective of the chairside work flow is to complete a definitive restoration in 1 visit, avoiding the need for a temporary restoration and a second patient appointment for final restoration delivery. With the developments in high-strength ceramic materials and implant prosthetic solutions, the latest chairside CAD/CAM software versions are able to design and produce fixed dental prostheses and implant-supported restorations. Dental restoration design software has become increasingly user friendly, with many features like preparation finish line detection and tooth digital wax-up now automated. Clinicians can select from digital libraries of natural tooth shapes and morphologies or create a mirror image of an existing tooth in the patient's mouth. With these features, esthetic and natural tooth shapes that are not hand made by a dental technician can be applied based on the individual esthetic needs and desires of the specific patient. STL or other files and tooth libraries can be imported from other sources. Advanced options include digital smile design features and face scan technology to optimize esthetic outcomes.

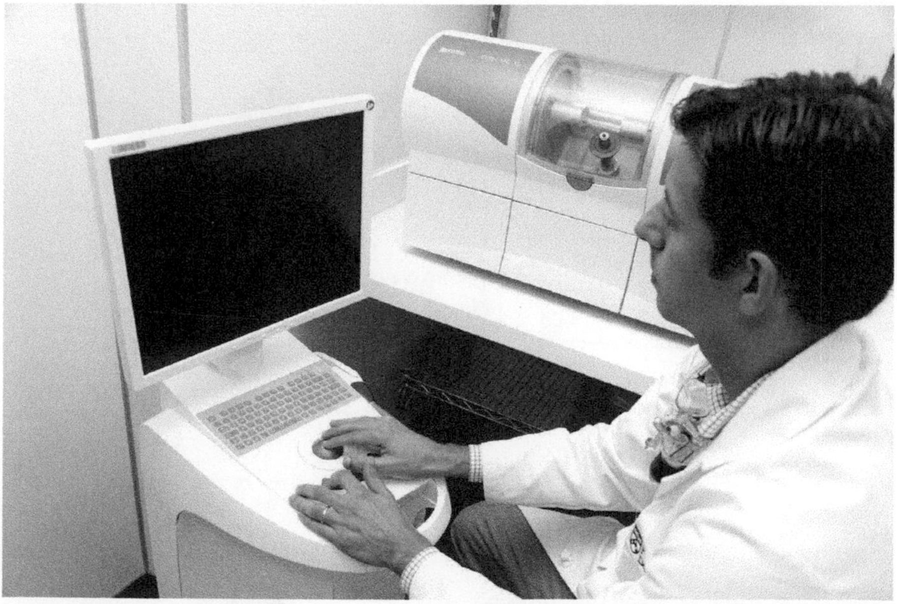

Fig. 2. The quality of the tooth preparation and the digital impression can be evaluated immediately. Files of natural teeth and smiles can be applied to digitally designed esthetic and functional restorations.

Clinicians who want to incorporate digital impressions in their practices but do not want to mill and finish the restorations in house select a semichairside workflow, which includes the intraoral scan without the design and milling of restorations. After review of the scan images and definition of the preparation margins, the digital impression is sent electronically to the dental laboratory where the restorations are fabricated. System-specific software is available for that feature (eg, Sirona connect, Dentsply Sirona). The laboratory can then use compatible laboratory-specific software for the design and manufacturing (eg, exocad, exocad GmbH, Darmstadt, Germany).

Archiving stone study models and mastercasts requires ample space. Digital scans and data sets can be stored and archived virtually on a designated server. However, it is important to understand and follow patient data privacy rules and regulations when deciding where and how to store patient data and scan files. With most systems, CAD data are handled and transmitted in an STL format, which has become the standard file format in 3D printing and rapid prototyping. Other formats that are currently used are PLY, DCM, and UDX. To communicate with a milling machine, these file formats are translated into millable data file formats (CNC [computer numerical control]). STL files describe only the surface geometry of a 3D object without any representation of color, texture, or other common CAD model attributes.

CHAIRSIDE MILLING MACHINES

A large number of milling machines with a small footprint, intended for use in the dental office, have entered the market in recent years and are geared toward the ability to mill all different kinds of restorative material blocks (**Fig. 3**).[22] Compact milling units are indicated for dental offices that want to scan, mill, and deliver restorations in 1 appointment. This type of milling unit is typically a 4-axis mill, which means that the milling bur moves in the 3 axes, x, y, and z, and the material block can rotate in 1 additional axis (also termed 3 + 1 axis milling machine). Some units use 2 burs on 2

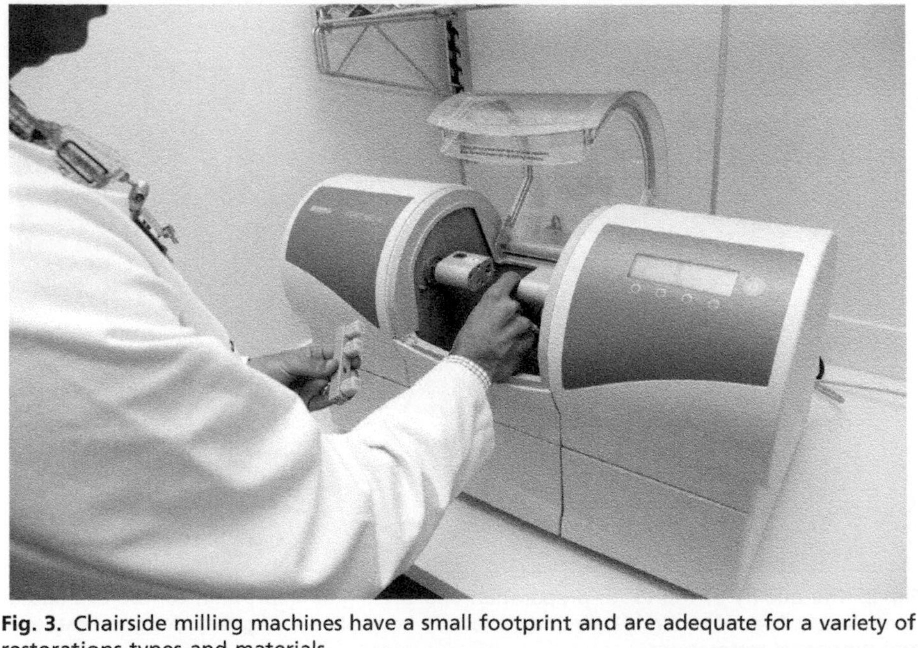

Fig. 3. Chairside milling machines have a small footprint and are adequate for a variety of restorations types and materials.

separate motors to mill the material block at the same time, making the process faster, with an average milling time of 8 minutes for a single crown and with an accuracy of 25 μm.[22]

Accuracy and milling time are determined by various factors, such as number of axes and spindles, bur size and abrasiveness, milling speed, and the material. Silica-based ceramics are typically milled in a wet environment, whereas composite and zirconia blanks are dry milled. Not all milling machines offer both wet and dry milling. It is therefore critical to carefully consider specific material needs and preferences before selecting a milling machine.

Four-axis (3 + 1) milling machines have long been the standard for small in-office milling and are perfectly adequate for most clinical applications, such as veneers, inlays/onlays, crowns, and fixed dental prostheses. Milling machines with 5 or more axes can rotate the material block in additional axes, which enable milling of more complex designs, even with undercuts such as implant superstructure where the implant screw access opening may be angulated in different directions. They also seem to provide greater accuracy.[23] Rotary cutting instruments with a smaller diameter lead to greater accuracy but require longer milling times.[23]

The more compact chairside milling units can accommodate material blocks of up to 20 mm, 40 mm, and 85 mm. Five-axis milling units are able to process polymer, hybrid ceramic, glass ceramic, silicate ceramic, and zirconium oxide from discs of 98.5 mm in diameter and up to 30 mm in thickness. With a multiblock holder, they can also mill up to 6 blocks at the same time for maximum productivity and efficiency.

Laser milling of dental restorations uses millions of short, high-intensity laser pulses to remove small amounts of material from a standard block to complete the restoration. The extremely small laser spot size allows a high resolution, resulting in improved morphology and microtexture on the restorations. The advantages of laser milling are the cost reduction of in-office production of restorations by eliminating cutting tools and coolants. The integrated 3D scanner has the ability to perform in-process quality control before the restoration is finished.

SINTER FURNACES

A furnace is needed for materials that require sintering or ceramic glazing. The CEREC Speedfire (Dentsply Sirona) and the Programat CS4 (Ivoclar Vivadent) are chairside furnaces with a small footprint that can be used for sintering zirconia, glazing ceramics, and crystallization/processing of lithium disilicates. They feature specific speed sintering cycles for timely finalization and delivery of all-ceramic restorations.

CHAIRSIDE COMPUTER-AIDED DESIGN COMPUTER-AIDED MANUFACTURING MATERIALS

One of the key benefits of chairside CAD/CAM technologies is the ability to fabricate indirect restorations in the dental office without the involvement of an external laboratory and within a short period of time. Various factors limit these restorations to single-span or short-span multiple units. The material range includes acrylics, indirect resin-based composites, and various ceramics. Proper selection of these materials based on indication as well as specific esthetic and functional needs is essential for clinical longevity. Several clinical studies indicate very high long-term success rates of chairside CAD/CAM restorations.[24,25] **Table 1** gives examples of popular commercial products in each material group. After milling, the sprue has to be removed from the restoration (**Fig. 4**) with adequate rotating instruments. Some materials, like composite

Table 1
Examples of dental materials for chairside digital dentistry

		Resin Matrix Ceramics		Silicate Ceramics				Oxide Ceramics
				Feldspathic Ceramics		Lithium Silicate Ceramics		
PMMA-Based Materials	Composite Resins	Resin-based Ceramics	Hybrid Ceramics	Traditional Feldspathic Ceramics	Leucite-Reinforced Glass Ceramics	Lithium Disilicate Ceramics	Zirconia-reinforced Lithium Silicate Ceramics	Zirconium Dioxide Ceramics
Telio CAD (Ivoclar Vivadent) VITA CAD-Temp MonoColors/ MultiColor Blocks (VITA Zahnfabrik) VITA CAD-Waxx Blocks (VITA North America) CEREC Guide Bloc/ inCoris PMMA (Densply Sirona) artBloc Temp (Merz Dental)	Paradigm MZ100 (3M ESPE). Tetric CAD (Ivoclar Vivadent) BRILLIANT Crios (Coltene)	Cerasmart (GC) Lava Ultimate (3M ESPE) Grandio Blocs (VOCO) HC Block CAD/ CAM Ceramic-Based Restorative (Shofu) KATANA AVENCIA Block (Kuraray Noritake Dental, Inc) BRILLIANT Crios (Coltene)	VITA ENAMIC (VITA Zahnfabrik)	VITABLOCS Mark II (VITA Zahnfabrik) VITABLOCS RealLife ceramic blocks (VITA) VITABLOC TriLux Forte (VITA) CEREC Blocs (Densply Sirona) CEREC Blocs C/C In/C PC (Densply Sirona)	IPS Empress CAD (Ivoclar Vivadent)	IPS e.max CAD (Ivoclar Vivadent)	VITA SUPRINITY PC (VITA Zahnfabrik) Celtra Duo (Densply Sirona)	CEREC Zirconia/ Zirconia meso (Densply Sirona) inCoris TZI/TZI/C/ ZI/ZI meso (Densply Sirona) KATANA Zirconia Block (Kuraray Noritake Dental, Inc) VITA YZ XT/ST/ $HT^{White}/HT^{Color}/T$ (VITA Zahnfabrik) Lava Zirconia Blocks (3M ESPE) IPS e.max ZirCAD (Ivoclar Vivadent)

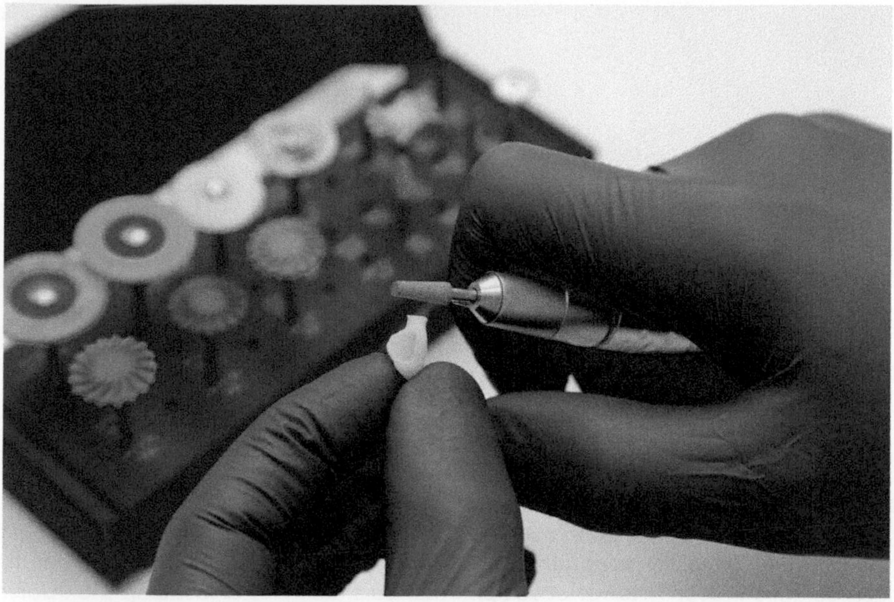

Fig. 4. The sprue is removed after the milling process with rotating instruments.

resins and resin matrix ceramics, only need polishing (**Fig. 5**) or application of light-cure stains and glaze. Silicate and oxide-based ceramics need to be crystallized or sintered either with or before staining and glazing (**Fig. 6**). Both of these steps require a special sinter furnace (**Fig. 7**).

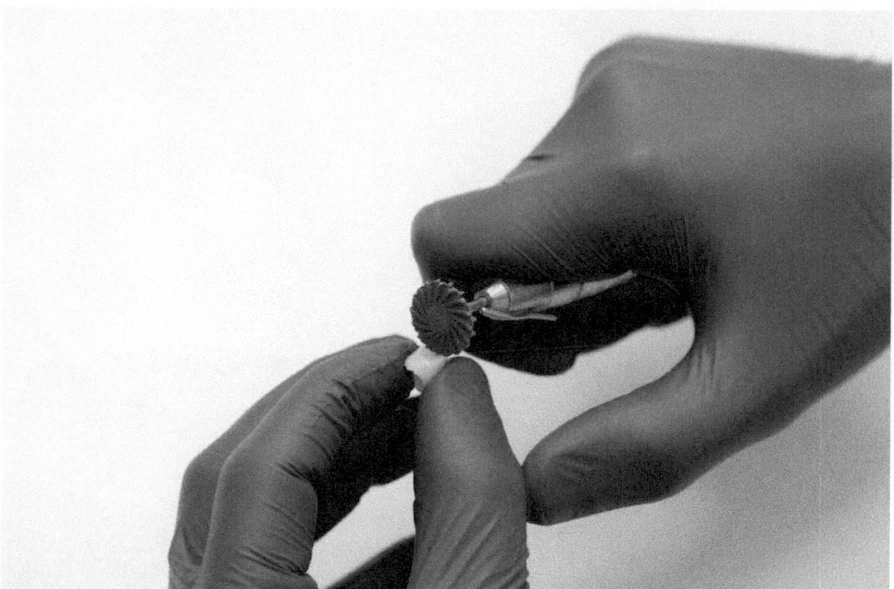

Fig. 5. The polishing protocol depends on the restorative material. Composite resins and resin matrix ceramics only require polishing or application of a light-cure glaze.

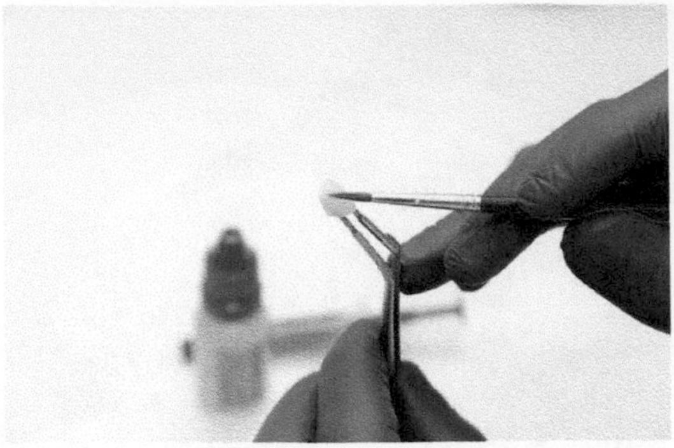

Fig. 6. Application of external stains and glaze.

POLYMETHYL METHACRYLATE–BASED MATERIALS

Crossed-linked PMMA CAD/CAM blocks (eg, Telio CAD, Ivoclar Vivadent) are typically used for provisional restorations. Laboratory studies suggest that polymeric inlays have a marginal adaptation and fracture load values that are similar to glass-ceramic inlays.[26] Newer developments, such as VITA CAD-Temp MultiColor Blocks (VITA Zahnfabrik, Bad Säckingen, Germany) offer increased physical and, through polychromatic layers of different shades and translucency levels, optical properties.

Some manufacturers offer acrylic blocks for milling copings, frameworks, and restorations that burn out without any residue for subsequent casting with metal alloys (eg, VITA CAD-Waxx Blocks, VITA North America, Yorba Linda, CA).

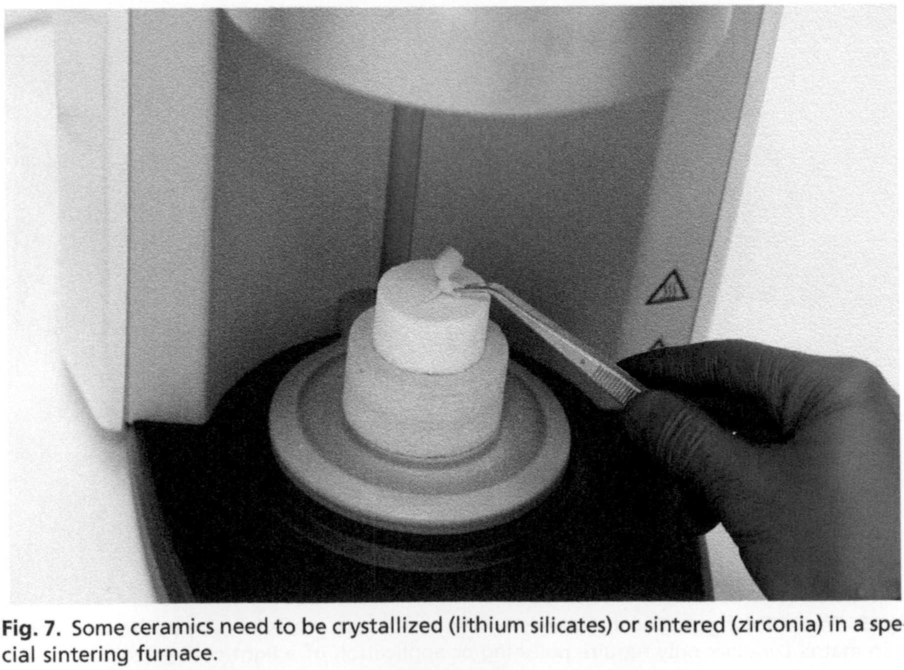

Fig. 7. Some ceramics need to be crystallized (lithium silicates) or sintered (zirconia) in a special sintering furnace.

COMPOSITE RESINS

Restorations milled from composite resin blocks have several advantages and are easy to use clinically. Polishing and, if needed, application of a light-cure stain is all that is necessary for finishing. Examples include Paradigm MZ100 (3M ESPE, Maplewood, MN). It was shown that such CAD/CAM composite resin materials have a higher fatigue resistance than some ceramics.[27,28] However, overall properties may not reach those of ceramic materials.[29,30]

CERAMICS

Dental ceramics are classified into 3 groups: resin matrix ceramics (RMCs), silicate ceramics, and oxide ceramics.[31] **Fig. 8** details a popular ceramic classification.[31]

Resin Matrix Ceramics

RMCs were classified as ceramics based on the 2013 version of the American Dental Association Code on Dental Procedures and Nomenclature, which defines the term porcelain/ceramic as pressed, fired, polished, or milled materials containing predominantly inorganic refractory compounds that may include porcelains, glasses, ceramics, and glass ceramics. RMCs are divided into 2 subgroups: resin-based ceramics and hybrid ceramics. Among their advantages compared with silica-based ceramics are higher load capacity, better modulus of elasticity, and favorable milling properties.[32,33] VITA ENAMIC Hybrid ceramic block (VITA Zahnfabrik) is a hybrid ceramic for chairside applications. It contains a ceramic network that is infiltrated with a polymer. Representatives of the resin-based ceramics subgroup, which contain a polymer matrix with at least 80% nanosized ceramic filler particles, include Katana Avencia Block (Kuraray Noritake, Inc, Tokyo, Japan), Cerasmart (GC International AG, Luzern, Switzerland), Lava Ultimate (3M ESPE), Grandio Blocs (VOCO, Cuxhaven, Germany), and HC Block CAD/CAM Ceramic-Based Restorative (Shofu, San Marcos, CA). Because of their recent introduction to the market, long-term clinical studies on these materials are not available. However, several laboratory studies confirm favorable physical properties.[34,35] Similar to composite resins, RMC restorations only require polishing. They can be glazed and customized with light-cure stains, making finishing simple and fast without the need for firing in a furnace. A key difference between hybrid and resin-based ceramics is the suggested bonding method.[36] The ceramic structure of the hybrid ceramic requires hydrofluoric (HF) acid etching, ideally for 60 seconds, and silane application. In contrast, resin-based ceramics should not be acid etched and must be pretreated with aluminum oxide air-particle abrasion and then silanized.[36]

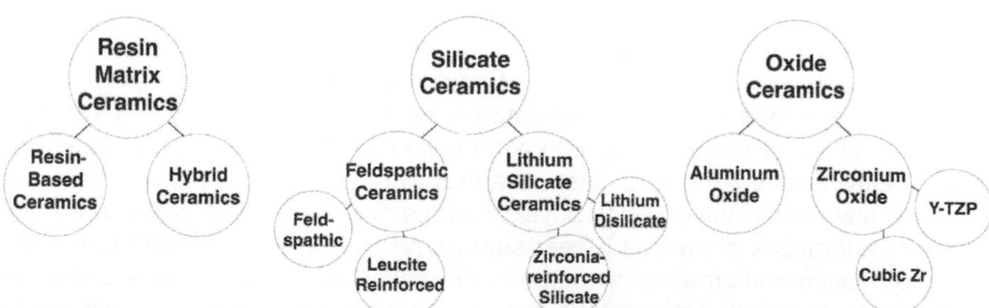

Fig. 8. Classification of current ceramic materials. Y-TZP, yttria-stabilized tetragonal zirconia polycrystal.

Silicate Ceramics

Silica-based ceramics are divided into feldspathic and silicate ceramics and are defined as mainly nonmetallic inorganic ceramic materials that contain a glass phase. The glass offers high translucency, optimal esthetics, and a natural appearance. However, because of their brittleness and low fracture strength, they must be adhesively bonded.[37] Long-term durable bond strengths to silica-based ceramics are established through HF acid etching and application of a silane coupling agent.[38,39] The etching time and concentration of the etchant depends on the crystalline content of the ceramic. For example, conventional feldspathic ceramics are acid etched with 9.8% HF acid for 2 minutes, leucite-reinforced feldspathic ceramics with the same concentration for 1 minute, and lithium disilicates should be etched with a lower-concentration HF (eg, 4.6%) for only 20 seconds. A silane coupling agent is applied after cleaning of any precipitates from the etched surface in an ultrasonic cleaning unit. After proper pretreatment and bonding of the tooth surfaces, a composite resin luting agent is applied. In a 10-year prospective evaluation of ceramic inlays, self-cure composite resin luting agents provided greater success than dual-cure materials with 100% versus 77% estimated survival rates.[24]

Traditional feldspathic ceramics

Traditional feldspathic ceramics are described as the most translucent and esthetic materials and are typically used as veneering porcelains for metal and ceramic frameworks or for bonded laminate veneers or inlays and onlays. They have remained popular in chairside CAD/CAM dentistry even for full-coverage crowns. Popular representatives are VITABLOCS Mark II (VITA Zahnfabrik), VITABLOCS RealLife Ceramic Blocks (VITA), and VITABLOC TriLux Forte (VITA). Some of these are now also available in polychromatic, multilayer blocks for enhanced esthetics to simulate the different shade and translucency layers of natural teeth.

Despite the low physical properties of feldspathic ceramic (porcelain), several clinical studies indicate excellent success. A 95% survival rate was found for chairside CAD/CAM feldspathic ceramic (VITABLOCS Mark II) shoulder crowns on molars and premolars after up to 12 years.[40] CAD/CAM porcelain laminate veneers had a survival rate of 94% after 9 years.[41] CEREC inlays and onlays showed a survival probability of 88.7% after up to 17 years of clinical service.[42] Of the 11% failures, 62% were ceramic fractures, 14% tooth fractures, 19% caries, and 5% endodontic problems. Reiss[43] followed CEREC inlays in a dental practice for more than 18 years. Probability of success was 84.4% after 16.7 years. Survival rate for restorations still in place was higher, with 89% at 18.3 years. Prognosis was influenced by restoration size, tooth location (premolars had greater success), and vitality (vital teeth had greater success).

Leucite-reinforced glass ceramics

With increased strength compared with traditional feldspathic ceramics and high translucency, this material group is indicated especially for anterior crowns and posterior inlays/onlays. Resin bonding with composite resin luting agents is a necessity. More recently, leucite-reinforced glass ceramics were largely replaced by lithium silicate ceramics, which have better physical properties. CAD/CAM partial-coverage posterior restorations showed a 5-year survival rate of 96% for CEREC Blocs and 94.6% for leucite-reinforced glass-ceramic Empress CAD Blocs.[44] Restorations on nonvital teeth revealed significantly higher ceramic fracture rates. In a split-mouth design study, Guess and colleagues[45] reported survival rates of 100% for partial-coverage restorations made from pressed lithium disilicate (IPS e.max, Ivoclar

Vivadent) and 97% for CAD/CAM partial-coverage restorations made from leucite-reinforced glass ceramics (ProCAD, Karlsruhe, Germany) after 3 years.

Lithium silicate ceramics

Lithium silicate ceramics have become popular for several indications, especially monolithic crowns, inlays, and onlays. With a biaxial flexural strength of around 407 MPa, they are considered the strongest silica-based ceramics in dentistry.[31] Lithium silicate ceramics have a crystalline phase consisting of lithium disilicate and lithium orthophosphate, which increases fracture resistance without negatively influencing translucency. These materials must be crystalized in a sintering furnace after milling. They can also be stained and glazed. Excellent success rates are well documented in the recent literature, especially for single-unit restorations.[31] In this group, the extremely popular IPS e.max CAD (Ivoclar Vivadent) was recently joined by novel zirconia-reinforced lithium silicate ceramics: VITA Suprinity PC (VITA Zahnfabrik) and Celtra Duo (Dentsply Sirona). In combination with a titanium base, these materials can be used for monolithic implant-supported crowns. The special blocks for this indication have an appropriately sized hole to accommodate the Ti bases, which are resin bonded into the block.[46] However, clinical data are missing.[47] Neves and colleagues[48] reported that heat-pressed and CEREC chairside CAD/CAM system–fabricated lithium disilicate crowns have minimal marginal misfit, and others confirmed that the accuracy of fit is uniform and consistent.[49] Crowns fabricated with the E4D laser scanner CAD/CAM system revealed greater gaps. A 30-μm or 60-μm virtual die spacer thickness was recommended for that system.[50] Others found that both analog and chairside CAD/CAM-fabricated lithium disilicate onlays have clinically acceptable fracture strength values.[51] Short-term and medium-term survival of respective crowns are very high.[52–54]

Oxide Ceramics

High-strength polycrystalline metal oxide–based CAD/CAM ceramics such as zirconium dioxide (zirconia) are characterized by excellent mechanical properties, which are significantly greater than those of silica-based ceramics. Flexural strength values of conventional yttria-stabilized tetragonal zirconia polycrystal ranges between 1000 and 1500 MPa.[31] Their inherent strength allows for conventional cementation of adequately dimensioned full-coverage restorations.[55] The first generations of zirconia had only limited translucency and were, therefore, used for copings and frameworks that had to be veneered with a feldspathic veneering porcelain. Success rates were similar to porcelain-fused-to-metal restorations.[56,57] However, recent trends favor monolithic ceramic restorations.[58] The latest zirconia generations offer significantly greater light transmission. Pre-shaded multilayer high-translucent zirconia materials in particular offer more esthetic treatment options and can even be applied for anterior teeth. The higher translucency is achieved by slight changes of the Y_2O_3 content (5 mol% or more instead of 3 mol%), resulting in a higher amount of cubic-phase particles. More cubic zirconia offers significantly higher light transmission but lower flexural strength values than conventional zirconia, between 550 and 800 MPa.[59,60] Although early reports and in vitro studies seem favorable,[58] there are currently very few scientific data available.

High-translucent zirconia blocks for chairside CAD/CAM systems[61] have recently entered the marketplace, such as CEREC Zirconia (Dentsply Sirona), Katana Zirconia Block (Kuraray Noritake Dental, Inc), VITA YZ (VITA Zahnfabrik), Lava Zirconia Block (3M ESPE), and IPS e.max ZirCAD (Ivoclar Vivadent). The restorations are milled from presintered blocks with slightly enlarged dimensions, compensating for the 20% to 25% material shrinkage during the final sinter step after milling. With a special chairside furnace (eg, CEREC Speedfire, Dentsply Sirona) and speed sintering program, the sintering of a single crown can be accomplished within 19 minutes (after dry milling) to 30 minutes (after wet milling).

Given the great popularity of zirconia restorations, clinical application and cementation protocols are widely debated. In general, these restorations are typically considered cementable because of their high inherent flexural strength, which exceeds natural chewing forces.[62] Therefore, zirconia-based crowns and bridges with adequate retention and ceramic material thickness can be cemented conventionally. Resin-modified glass-ionomer or self-adhesive resin cements are preferred and provide at least a certain level of adhesion to both teeth and ceramic without additional time-consuming and technique-sensitive bonding and priming steps.[62] However, zirconia restorations that are less strong, thin, lack retention, or rely on resin bonding, such as resin-bonded fixed prostheses or bonded laminate veneers, require resin bonding with composite resin luting agents. To achieve the high and long-term durable resin bond strengths to zirconia in a practical manner, a 3-step approach is recommended. The authors have termed it the APC-zirconia–bonding concept:[62]

1. Air-particle abrade the bonding surface with aluminum oxide (A)
2. Apply special zirconia primer (P)
3. Use dual-cure or self-cure composite resin cement (C)

After restoration cleaning, zirconia should be air-particle abraded with alumina or silica-coated alumina particles. Small particles (50–60 μm) at a low pressure (<200 kPa [2 bar]) are sufficient. The subsequent step includes application of a special ceramic primer (eg, Clearfil Ceramic Primer Plus, Kuraray Noritake), which contains special adhesive phosphate monomers. The monomer MDP (10-methacryloyloxydecyl dihydrogen phosphate) has been shown to be particularly effective to bond to metal oxides. Dual-cure or self-cure composite resins should be used to ensure adequate polymerization/conversion (eg, Panavia V5, Kuraray Noritake). Long-term success rates of certain resin-bonded zirconia restorations are excellent.[55]

THREE-DIMENSIONAL PRINTING

In combination with 3D printers, chairside CAD/CAM systems can provide an even greater range of clinical applications and appliances, including night guards, occlusal splints, orthodontic appliances, surgical guides, provisional restorations, and study models. In light of current developments in metal and ceramic printing, 3D printing may become the manufacturing method of choice in the future.

CHAIRSIDE DIGITAL WORK FLOW CASE REPORT

An example of the chairside digital work flow is provided by a clinical case. A 25-year-old female patient presented to our clinics with concerns about the esthetic appearance of her 2 upper central incisors (**Figs. 9** and **10**). After thorough clinical and radiographic evaluation, the final treatment plan included a full-coverage crown on the endodontically treated tooth 8 and a direct composite resin restoration because of a chipped incisal edge on tooth 9. After determining the shade (**Fig. 11**), the composite resin restoration was made (**Fig. 12**) and finalized with an optimized contour, shape, and morphology. Tooth 8 was prepared for a full-

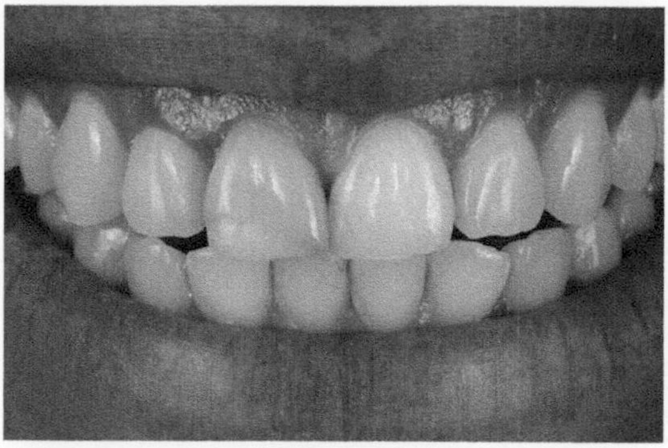

Fig. 9. Preoperative extraoral view of patient smile.

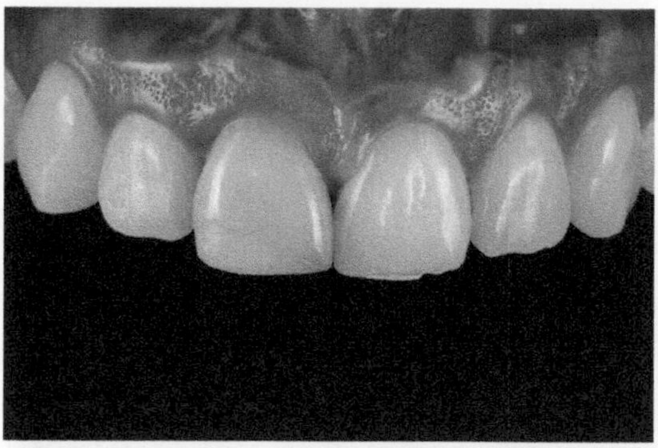

Fig. 10. Preoperative intraoral view of maxillary anterior teeth. The endodontically treated tooth 8 required a full-coverage crown and tooth 9 a composite resin restoration because of chipped incisal edge.

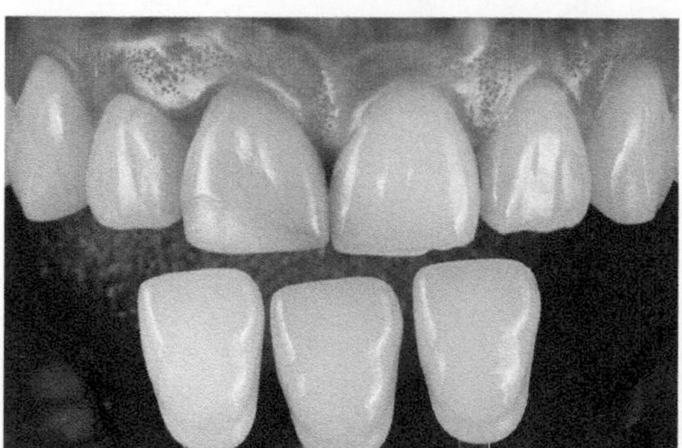

Fig. 11. Shade evaluation with classic shade guide.

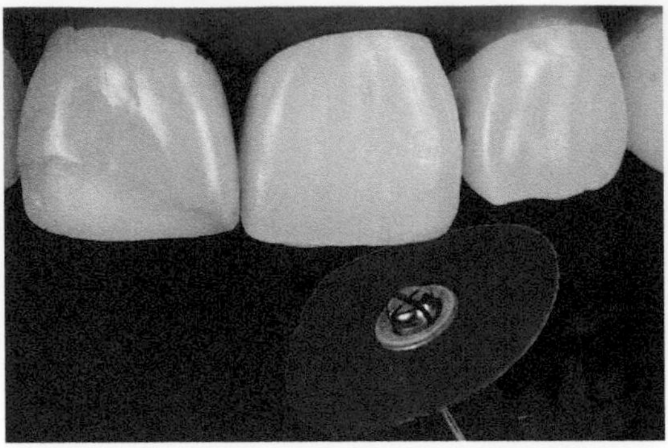

Fig. 12. Contouring and finishing of composite resin restoration on tooth 9.

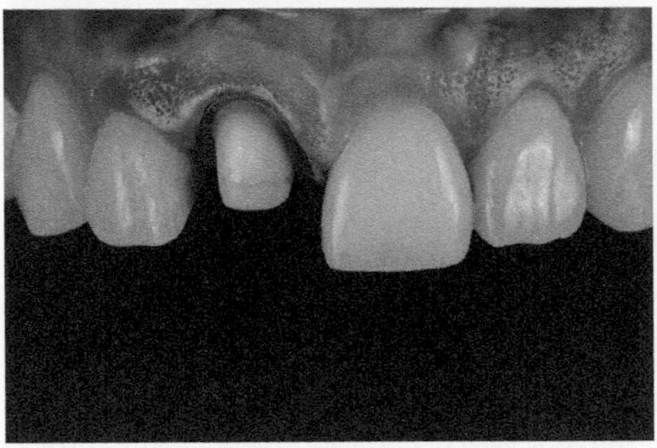

Fig. 13. Intraoral anterior view of crown preparation of tooth 8. Sharp edges and line angles should be rounded.

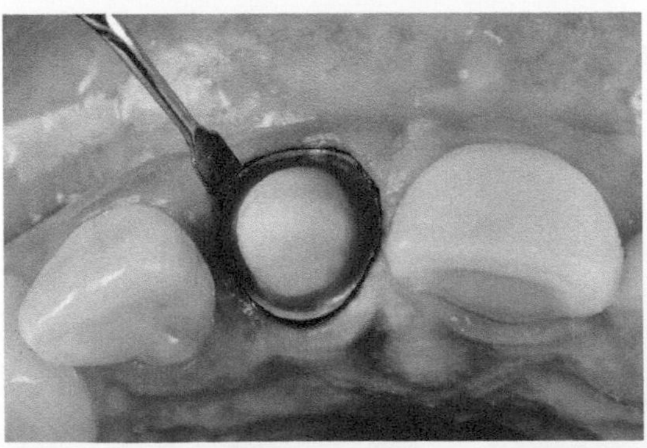

Fig. 14. Proper soft tissue control and retraction is critical for an accurate optical scan. Placement of retraction cord around prepared tooth 8.

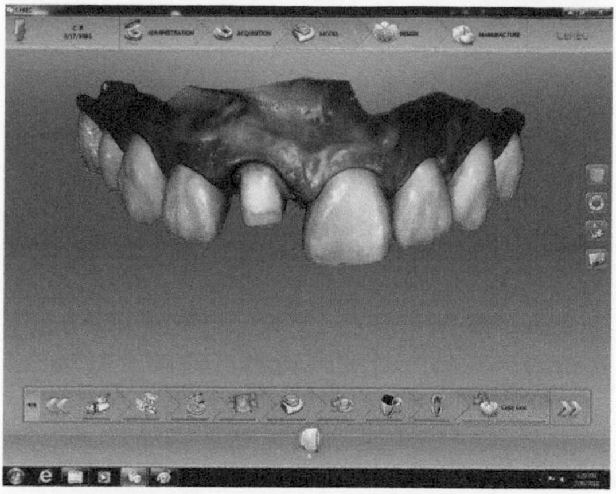

Fig. 15. Screenshot of intraoral scan of maxillary anterior teeth.

coverage crown. Sharp edges and line angles should be avoided and were rounded (**Fig. 13**). Proper soft tissue control and retraction are critical for an accurate optical scan. A retraction cord was carefully placed around the prepared tooth (**Fig. 14**). Intraoral digital impressions of both jaws as well as an optical interocclusal record were obtained. **Fig. 15** shows a screenshot of the scan of the maxillary anterior teeth. The preparation finish line was identified and defined on the computer screen (**Fig. 16**). The outline for the reference of tooth 9 was determined (**Fig. 17**) and an exact mirror image of the tooth was created, which was placed on abutment tooth 8 (**Fig. 18**). A polychromatic hybrid ceramic block was selected. Proper placement of the restoration in the block is key to simulating natural teeth as closely as possible (**Fig. 19**). The polished hybrid ceramic crown was tried in and proper fit, contour, morphology, esthetics, and function were verified (**Fig. 20**). **Figs. 21–23** show the postoperative intraoral views of the completed composite resin restoration on tooth 9 and chairside CAD/CAM-fabricated crown 8.

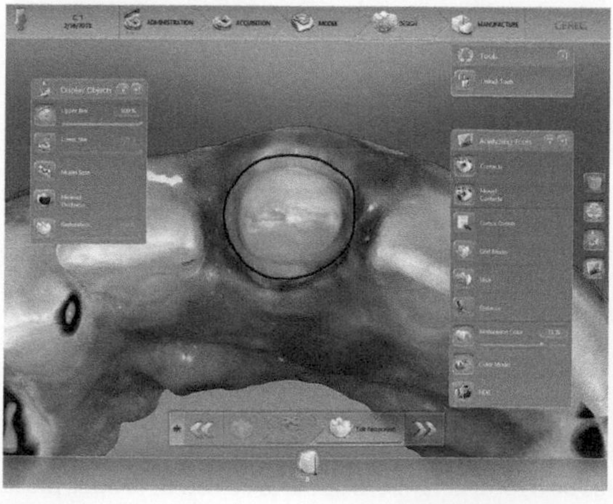

Fig. 16. Identification and definition of preparation finish line.

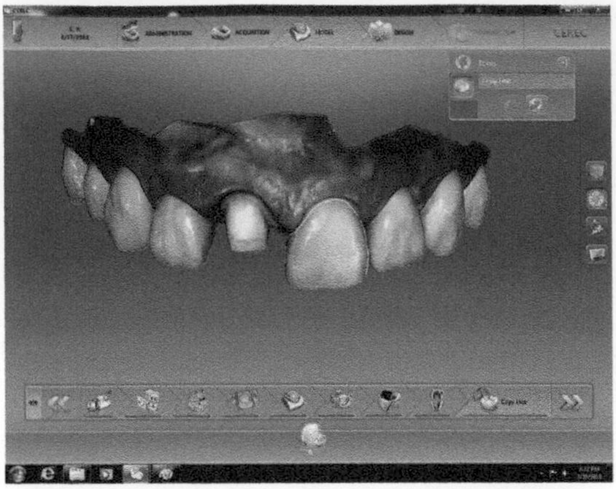

Fig. 17. The outline for the reference of tooth 9 is defined.

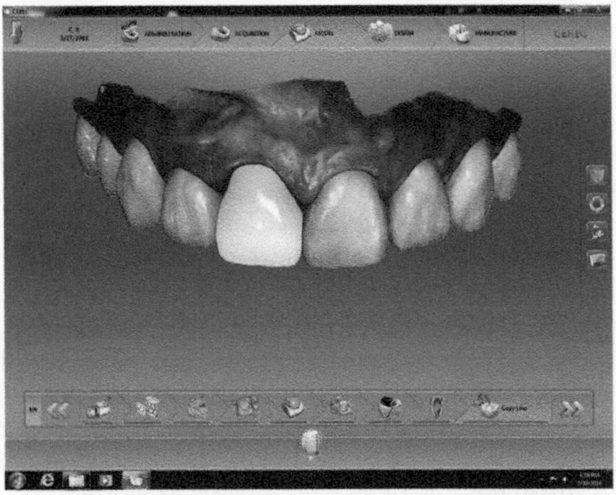

Fig. 18. Crown design: a mirror image of tooth 9 is created and placed on abutment tooth 8.

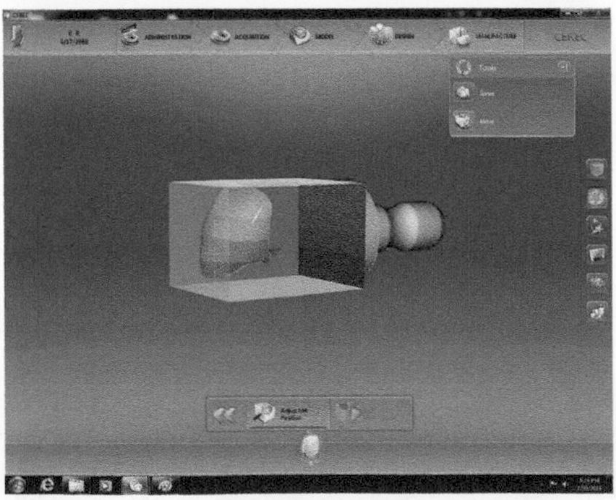

Fig. 19. A polychromatic hybrid ceramic block was selected. Proper placement of the restoration in the block is key to simulating natural teeth as closely as possible.

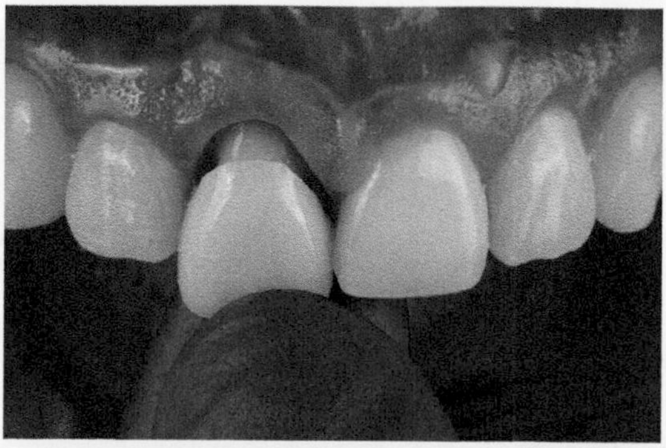

Fig. 20. Try-in of polished hybrid ceramic crown.

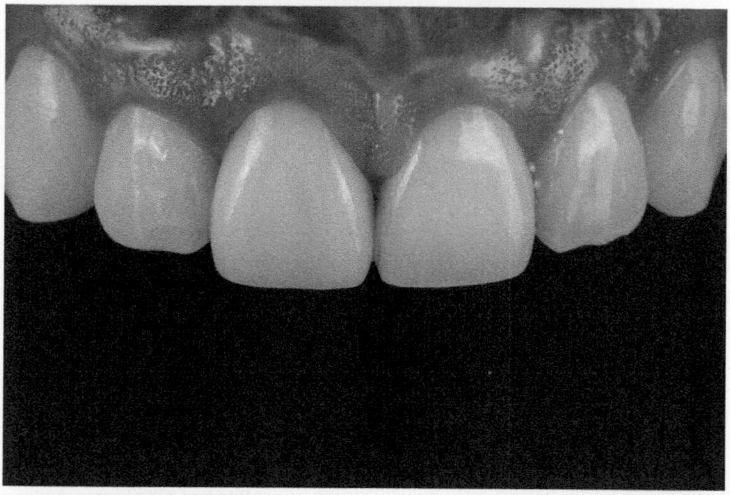

Fig. 21. Postoperative intraoral view of composite resin restoration on tooth 9 and chairside CAD/CAM-fabricated crown 8.

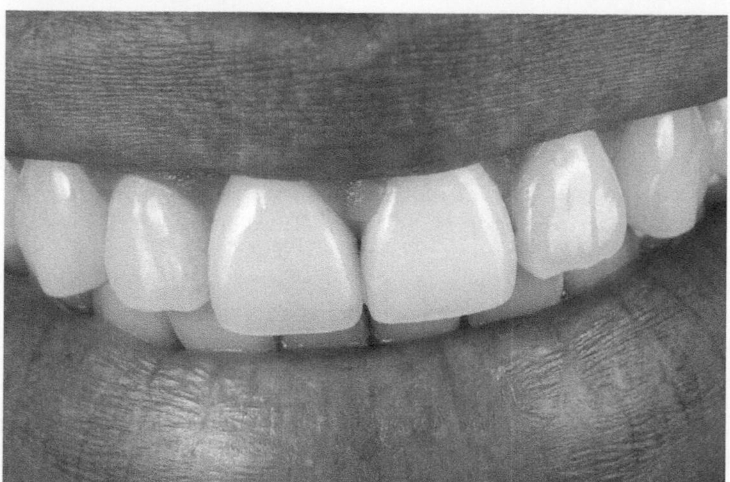

Fig. 22. Postoperative extraoral view.

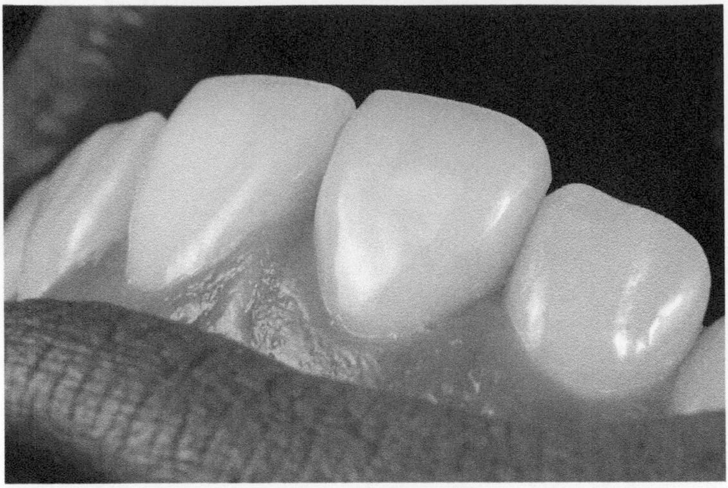

Fig. 23. Detailed postoperative view of final restorations.

SUMMARY

Chairside CAD/CAM technologies have emerged into user-friendly and patient-friendly, versatile, effective, predictable, and accurate clinical assets. Current intraoral scanning technologies are as accurate as, or even more accurate than, conventional impression techniques, at least for single or short multiunit restorations, and more comfortable for the patient. Design software has been simplified with excellent features to produce natural esthetics and function by applying files and shapes of natural teeth and smile designs. Milling machines have become smaller, more accurate, and more versatile for a large variety of materials. Most of the modern materials fabricated in the laboratory can also be fabricated chairside in a single visit, from PMMAs to composite resins and various types of ceramics with excellent clinical long-term success.

ACKNOWLEDGMENTS

The authors wish to thank Dr Andre Hausner, Munich, Germany, for his contributions to this article.

REFERENCES

1. Duret F, Blouin JL, Duret B. CAD-CAM in dentistry. J Am Dent Assoc 1988;117(6):715–20.
2. Mörmann WH. The evolution of the CEREC system. J Am Dent Assoc 2006;137(Suppl):7S–13S.
3. Miyazaki T, Hotta Y, Kunii J, et al. A review of dental CAD/CAM: current status and future perspectives from 20 years of experience. Dent Mater J 2009;28(1):44–56.
4. Miyazaki T, Hotta Y. CAD/CAM systems available for the fabrication of crown and bridge restorations. Aust Dent J 2011;56(Suppl 1):97–106.
5. Van Noort R. The future of dental devices is digital. Dent Mater 2012;28(1):3–12.
6. Davidowitz G, Kotick PG. The use of CAD/CAM in dentistry. Dent Clin North Am 2011;55(3):559–70.
7. Zaruba M, Mehl A. Chairside systems: a current review. Int J Comput Dent 2017;20(2):123–49.

8. Souza RO, Özcan M, Pavanelli CA, et al. Marginal and internal discrepancies related to margin design of ceramic crowns fabricated by a CAD/CAM system. J Prosthodont 2012;21(2):94–100.
9. Renne W, McGill ST, Forshee KV, et al. Predicting marginal fit of CAD/CAM crowns based on the presence or absence of common preparation errors. J Prosthet Dent 2012;108(5):310–5.
10. Richert R, Goujat A, Venet L, et al. Intraoral scanner technologies: a review to make a successful impression. J Healthc Eng 2017;2017:8427595.
11. Galhano GÁ, Pellizzer EP, Mazaro JV. Optical impression systems for CAD-CAM restorations. J Craniofac Surg 2012;23(6):e575–9.
12. Seelbach P, Brueckel C, Wöstmann B. Accuracy of digital and conventional impression techniques and workflow. Clin Oral Investig 2013;17(7):1759–64.
13. Yuzbasioglu E, Kurt H, Turunc R, et al. Comparison of digital and conventional impression techniques: evaluation of patients' perception, treatment comfort, effectiveness and clinical outcomes. BMC Oral Health 2014;14:10.
14. Lee SJ, Macarthur RX 4th, Gallucci GO, et al. An evaluation of student and clinician perception of digital and conventional implant impressions. J Prosthet Dent 2013;110(5):420–3.
15. Ender A, Mehl A. *In-vitro* evaluation of the accuracy of conventional and digital methods of obtaining full-arch dental impressions. Quintessence Int 2015;46(1): 9–17.
16. Patzelt SB, Emmanouilidi A, Stampf S, et al. Accuracy of full-arch scans using intraoral scanners. Clin Oral Investig 2014;18(6):1687–94.
17. Mangano F, Gandolfi A, Luongo G, et al. Intraoral scanners in dentistry: a review of the current literature. BMC Oral Health 2017;17(1):149.
18. Rutkūnas V, Gečiauskaitė A, Jegelevičius D, et al. Accuracy of digital implant impressions with intraoral scanners. A systematic review. Eur J Oral Implantol 2017; 10(Suppl 1):101–20.
19. Bratos M, Bergin JM, Rubenstein JE, et al. Effect of simulated intraoral variables on the accuracy of a photogrammetric imaging technique for complete-arch implant prostheses. J Prosthet Dent 2018;120(2):232–41.
20. Svanborg P, Skjerven H, Carlsson P, et al. Marginal and internal fit of cobalt-chromium fixed dental prostheses generated from digital and conventional impressions. Int J Dent 2014;2014:534382.
21. Chochlidakis KM, Papaspyridakos P, Geminiani A, et al. Digital versus conventional impressions for fixed prosthodontics: a systematic review and meta-analysis. J Prosthet Dent 2016;16:184–90.
22. Lebon N, Tapie L, Duret F, et al. Understanding dental CAD/CAM for restorations - dental milling machines from a mechanical engineering viewpoint. Part A: chairside milling machines. Int J Comput Dent 2016;19(1):45–62.
23. Bosch G, Ender A, Mehl A. A 3-dimensional accuracy analysis of chairside CAD/CAM milling processes. J Prosthet Dent 2014;112(6):1425–31.
24. Sjögren G, Molin M, van Dijken JW. A 10-year prospective evaluation of CAD/CAM-manufactured (Cerec) ceramic inlays cemented with a chemically cured or dual-cured resin composite. Int J Prosthodont 2004;17(2):241–6.
25. Morimoto S, Rebello de Sampaio FB, Braga MM, et al. Survival rate of resin and ceramic inlays, onlays, and overlays: a systematic review and meta-analysis. J Dent Res 2016;95(9):985–94.
26. Ender A, Bienz S, Mörmann W, et al. Marginal adaptation, fracture load and macroscopic failure mode of adhesively luted PMMA-based CAD/CAM inlays. Dent Mater 2016;32(2):e22–9.

27. Magne P, Schlichting LH, Maia HP, et al. *In vitro* fatigue resistance of CAD/CAM composite resin and ceramic posterior occlusal veneers. J Prosthet Dent 2010; 104(3):149–57.
28. Schlichting LH, Maia HP, Baratieri LN, et al. Novel-design ultra-thin CAD/CAM composite resin and ceramic occlusal veneers for the treatment of severe dental erosion. J Prosthet Dent 2011;105(4):217–26.
29. Ruse ND, Sadoun MJ. Resin-composite blocks for dental CAD/CAM applications. J Dent Res 2014;93(12):1232–4.
30. Mörmann WH, Stawarczyk B, Ender A, et al. Wear characteristics of current aesthetic dental restorative CAD/CAM materials: two-body wear, gloss retention, roughness and Martens hardness. J Mech Behav Biomed Mater 2013;20:113–25.
31. Conejo J, Nueesch R, Vonderheide M, et al. Clinical performance of all-ceramic restorations. Curr Oral Health Rep 2017;4(2):112–23.
32. Rohr N, Coldea A, Zitzmann NU, et al. Loading capacity of zirconia implant supported hybrid ceramic crowns. Dent Mater 2015;31:e279–88.
33. Awada A, Nathanson D. Mechanical properties of resin-ceramic CAD/CAM restorative materials. J Prosthet Dent 2015;114:587–93.
34. Chen C, Trindade FZ, de Jager N, et al. The fracture resistance of a CAD/CAM resin nano ceramic (RNC) and a CAD ceramic at different thicknesses. Dent Mater 2014;30(9):954–62.
35. Batson ER, Cooper LF, Duqum I, et al. Clinical outcomes of three different crown systems with CAD/CAM technology. J Prosthet Dent 2014;112(4):770–7.
36. Spitznagel FA, Horvath SD, Guess PC, et al. Resin bond to indirect composite and new ceramic/polymer materials: a review of the literature. J Esthet Restor Dent 2014;26(6):382–93.
37. Beier US, Dumfahrt H. Longevity of silicate ceramic restorations. Quintessence Int 2014;45:637–44.
38. Blatz MB, Sadan A, Kern M. Resin-ceramic bonding – a review of the literature. J Prosthet Dent 2003;89(3):268–74.
39. Blatz MB, Sadan A, Maltezos C, et al. In-vitro durability of the resin bond to feldspathic ceramics. Am J Dent 2004;17:169–72.
40. Otto T, Mormann WH. Clinical performance of chairside CAD/CAM feldspathic ceramic posterior shoulder crowns and endocrowns up to 12 years. Int J Comput Dent 2015;18:147–61.
41. Wiedhahn K, Kerschbaum T, Fasbinder DF. Clinical long-term results with 617 Cerec veneers: a nine-year report. Int J Comput Dent 2005;8(3):233–46.
42. Otto T, Schneider D. Long-term clinical results of chairside Cerec CAD/CAM inlays and onlays: a case series. Int J Prosthodont 2008;21(1):53–9.
43. Reiss B. Clinical results of Cerec inlays in a dental practice over a period of 18 years. Int J Comput Dent 2006;9(1):11–22.
44. Nejatidanesh F, Amjadi M, Akouchekian M, et al. Clinical performance of CEREC AC Bluecam conservative ceramic restorations after five years–a retrospective study. J Dent 2015;43(9):1076–82.
45. Guess PC, Strub JR, Steinhart N, et al. All-ceramic partial coverage restorations – midterm results of a 5-year prospective clinical splitmouth study. J Dent 2009; 37(8):627–37.
46. Conejo J, Blatz MB. Simplified fabrication of an esthetic implant-supported crown with a novel CAD/CAM glass ceramic. Compend Contin Educ Dent 2016;37(6): 396–9.

47. Conejo J, Kobayashi T, Anadioti E, et al. Performance of CAD/CAM monolithic ceramic implant-supported restorations bonded to titanium inserts: a systematic review. Eur J Oral Implantol 2017;10(Suppl 1):139–46.
48. Neves FD, Prado CJ, Prudente MS, et al. Micro-computed tomography evaluation of marginal fit of lithium disilicate crowns fabricated by using chairside CAD/CAM systems or the heat-pressing technique. J Prosthet Dent 2014;112(5):1134–40.
49. Mously HA, Finkelman M, Zandparsa R, et al. Marginal and internal adaptation of ceramic crown restorations fabricated with CAD/CAM technology and the heat-press technique. J Prosthet Dent 2014;112(2):249–56.
50. D'Arcy BL, Omer OE, Byrne DA, et al. The reproducibility and accuracy of internal fit of Cerec 3D CAD/CAM all ceramic crowns. Eur J Prosthodont Restor Dent 2009;17(2):73–7.
51. Yildiz C, Vanlıoğlu BA, Evren B, et al. Fracture resistance of manually and CAD/CAM manufactured ceramic onlays. J Prosthodont 2013;22(7):537–42.
52. Reich S, Fischer S, Sobotta B, et al. A preliminary study on the short-term efficacy of chairside computer-aided design/computer-assisted manufacturing–generated posterior lithium disilicate crowns. Int J Prosthodont 2010;23(3):214–6.
53. Reich S, Endres L, Weber C, et al. Three-unit CAD/CAM-generated lithium disilicate FDPs after a mean observation time of 46 months. Clin Oral Investig 2014;18(9):2171–8.
54. Reich S, Schierz O. Chair-side generated posterior lithium disilicate crowns after 4 years. Clin Oral Investig 2013;17(7):1765–72.
55. Blatz MB, Vonderheide M, Conejo J. The effect of resin bonding on long-term success of high-strength ceramics. J Dent Res 2018;97(2):132–9.
56. Takeichi T, Katsoulis J, Blatz MB. Clinical outcome of single porcelain-fused-to-zirconium dioxide crowns: a systematic review. J Prosthet Dent 2013;110(6):455–61.
57. Ozer F, Mante FK, Chiche G, et al. A retrospective survey on long-term survival of posterior zirconia and porcelain-fused-to-metal crowns in private practice. Quintessence Int 2014;45:31–8.
58. Sorrentino R, Triulzio C, Tricarico MG, et al. In vitro analysis of the fracture resistance of CAD-CAM monolithic zirconia molar crowns with different occlusal thickness. J Mech Behav Biomed Mater 2016;61:328–33.
59. Zhang F, Inokoshi M, Batuk M, et al. Strength, toughness and aging stability of highly-translucent Y-TZP ceramics for dental restorations. Dent Mater 2016;32(12):e327–37.
60. Zhang Y. Making yttria-stabilized tetragonal zirconia translucent. Dent Mater 2014;30(10):1195–203.
61. Skramstad M, DiTolla MC. Single-visit chairside zirconia. Dent Today 2016;35(8):84, 86-87.
62. Blatz MB, Alvarez M, Sawyer K, et al. How to bond to zirconia: the APC concept. Compend Contin Educ Dent 2016;37(9):611–8.

Prosthodontic Management of Implant Therapy

Esthetic Complications

Lyndon F. Cooper, DDS, PhD[a,*], Ingeborg J. De Kok, DDS, MS[b], Ghadeer Thalji, DDS, PhD[c], Matthew S. Bryington, DMD, MS[d]

KEYWORDS

• Implant dentistry • Esthetics • Implant complications • Implant failure • Esthetic complications • Implant esthetic complications • Implant removal

KEY POINTS

- Esthetic complications are often the result of inadequate or absent planning that leads to implant malposition, which may or may not be overcome by prosthetic means.
- Esthetic complications associated with relative discoloration of the crown and peri-implant tissues may be managed by use of alternative materials or enhancement of tissue thickness by surgical intervention.
- The unfortunate decision to remove an implant to solve major esthetic complications requires extreme caution and estimation of the resulting tissue deficiency that must be compensated for before replacement of a dental implant in the proper position.

Esthetic complications regarding implant therapy depend on the observations and the observer. This subjective reality requires careful consideration of implant complications within clinical practice. Patient preferences, visual display (low lip line), and superimposed disease (peri-implantitis) must be considered differentially among various scenarios.

Esthetic complications related to implant therapy can broadly be characterized under 3 categories of origin (**Table 1**): biological, prosthetic, and iatrogenic.

Identifying the biological and tissue architectural defect associated with esthetically failed implants requires consideration of the objective criteria for dental esthetics.

Disclosure Statement: The authors have nothing to disclose.

[a] Department of Oral Biology, University of Illinois at Chicago, 801 South Paulina Street, 402E, Chicago, IL 60612, USA; [b] Department of Restorative Sciences, University of North Carolina, CB #7450, Chapel Hill, NC 27599-7450, USA; [c] Department of Restorative Sciences, University of Illinois at Chicago, 801 South Paulina Street, Room 365B, Chicago, IL 60612, USA; [d] Department of Restorative Dentistry, West Virginia University, School of Dentistry, PO Box 9495, One Medical Center Drive, Morgantown, WV 26506-9495, USA

* Corresponding author.

E-mail address: cooperlf@uic.edu

Dent Clin N Am 63 (2019) 199–216

https://doi.org/10.1016/j.cden.2018.11.003

dental.theclinics.com

Table 1
Classification of implant esthetic complications

Biological		Prosthetic		Iatrogenic
Resorptive	Mucosal recession	Fracture	Implant, abutment, crown, prosthesis	Implant misplacement
Inflammatory	Mucosal hypertrophy, implant loss	Attrition	Crown, prosthesis	Cement retention
Positional change	Relative tooth intrusion	Color	Abutment, crown, prosthesis	Inappropriate prosthetic contours

Data from Chu SJ, Tarnow DP. Managing esthetic challenges with anterior implants. Part 1: midfacial recession defects from etiology to resolution. Compend Contin Educ Dent 2013;34(Spec No 7):26–31.

The treatment of unesthetic implants may require removal of the implant. Implant explantation can be an aggressive procedure, and complications in healing and complementary regenerative procedures may be needed (**Table 2**). Therefore, each decision to remove an implant should be carefully measured. Different causes of implant esthetic deficits must be considered separately.

The inappropriate depth of implant placement creates esthetic challenges. The unesthetic result of shallow implant placement leads to inappropriately short restorations, the use of unhygienic flanges, or inappropriately contoured restorations. Shallow implant placement could be addressed by (1) using a short abutment with violation of the biological width, (2) use of a ridge lap design to mask the error, and/or (3) removal of the implant and replacement at the appropriate depth. In **Fig. 1**, shallow (and buccal) implant placement precluded the planned and desired use of a fixed prosthesis. A more complex overdenture solution using custom conical abutments and locator attachments provided an esthetic solution. The motivated patient may choose to follow the route of implant replacement.

Depth of implant placement begins at the planning phase of treatment. In more complex scenarios, whereby tooth dimensions may change with (**Fig. 2**A), for example, crown lengthening, the location of the zenith must be defined before implant placement (**Fig. 2**B). When implants are positioned 3 to 4 mm apically from this position (**Fig. 2**C), implant esthetic harmony can be achieved with the surrounding teeth (**Fig. 2**D).

The unesthetic implant resulting from excessive depth of placement is challenged by the long-term continued facial tissue resorption to a point of biological stability

Table 2
Essential biological and tissue architectural features of the implant retreatment site

Buccal	Interproximal
Facial implant position	Loss of connective tissue attachment at adjacent teeth
Depth of implant placement	Implant proximity to adjacent tooth
Existing implant diameter	Existing implant diameter
Mucosal thickness	Mucosal thickness
Presence of keratinized tissue	Presence of keratinized tissue
Peri-implant mucosal inflammation	Peri-implant mucosal inflammation
Obvious infection	Obvious infection

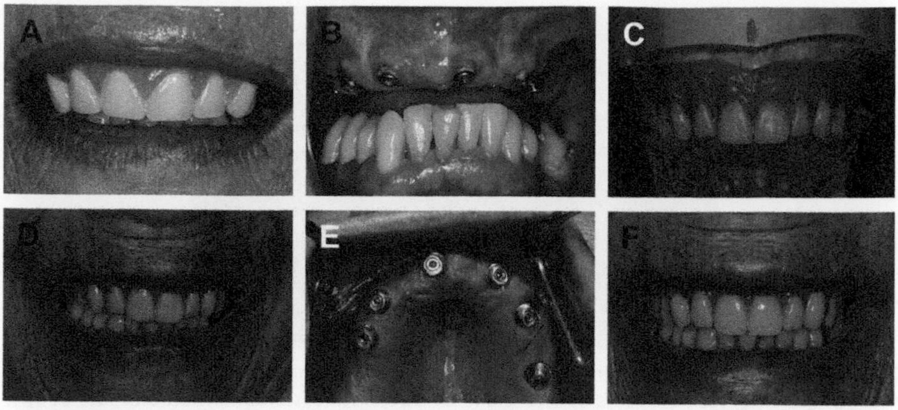

Fig. 1. Shallow implant placement diverts original treatment plans. (*A*) Patient presentation with implants placed and attempt to provide an interim complete denture revealed implant interference. No alveolectomy was performed to create required space. (*B*) Additional complications caused by buccal placement of implants is revealed. (*C*) New tooth position identified by diagnostic denture tooth arrangement to define space available for overdenture attachments. (*D*) Facial view affirming improved esthetics of prosthesis. (*E*) Custom cast abutments for overdenture conical retention were produced. (*F*) Definitive overdenture prosthesis provided improved esthetics, phonetics, and function. Case performed in collaboration with Dr Carolina Vera, UNC Chapel Hill School of Dentistry Graduate Prosthodontics.

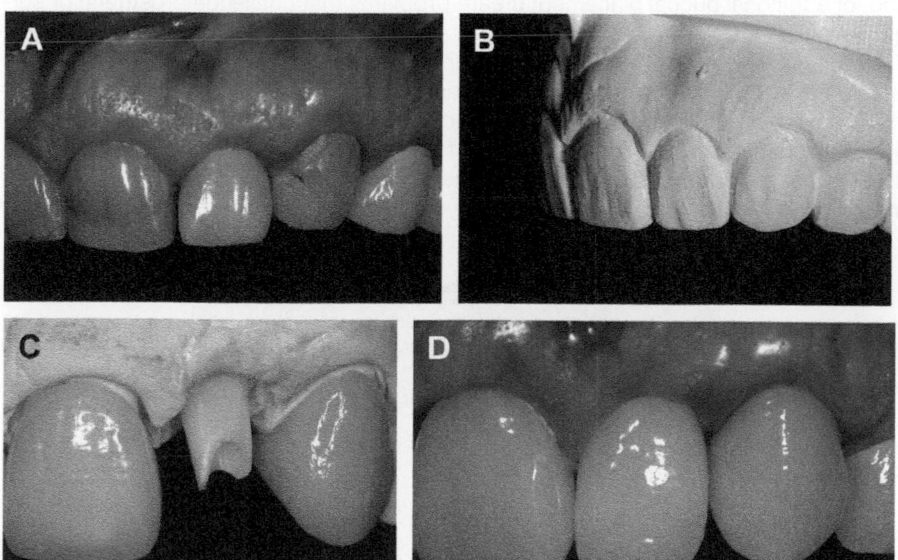

Fig. 2. Anticipating depth of placement using esthetic guidelines. (*A*) Patient presentation reveals failed maxillary left lateral incisor at time of request for enhanced anterior tooth esthetics requiring crown lengthening. (*B*) Diagnostic cast reveals waxed position of the gingival zeniths, indicating apical movement relative to existing maxillary left lateral incisor. (*C*) Postsurgical photograph reveals abutment in place surrounded by properly formed mucosa at position dictated by diagnostic wax-up and directed depth of implant placement. (*D*) Delivery of tooth and implant crowns displaying esthetic harmony.

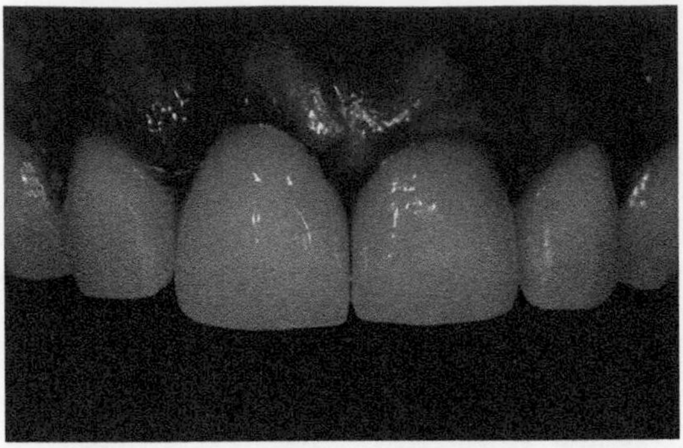

Fig. 3. Deep implant placement, here associated with reduced volume of alveolar bone without grafting, results in loss of 1 to 2 mm of buccal mucosal dimension and loss of symmetry. Some situations may be resolved by soft-tissue enhancement at this time.

(approximately 3 mm beyond the facial bone crest). The long crown associated with excessive depth of implant placement may benefit from a combination of prosthetic and surgical retreatment (**Fig. 3**). Minor discrepancies in crown length may be successfully addressed by altering the facial contour of the abutment and crown. Providing sufficient thickness of facial tissue and an appropriately contoured (narrow) abutment may enable abutment coverage and development of suitable implant-crown cementoenamel junction location relative to adjacent teeth. However, deep implant placement aggravated by other factors such as adjacent implants, the loss of soft tissue, or additional buccal placement create problems that challenge prosthetic or surgical resolution (**Fig. 4**).

Severe loss of vertical tissues can occur around implants (**Fig. 5**). In the scenario illustrated in **Fig. 5**, implant failure and associated bone loss was addressed by implant removal and immediate implant placement at an extremely deep location relative to adjacent teeth. Subsequently, loss of attachment at the adjacent teeth doomed the ultimate restoration despite the successful implant healing. This patient accepted treatment as the final result.

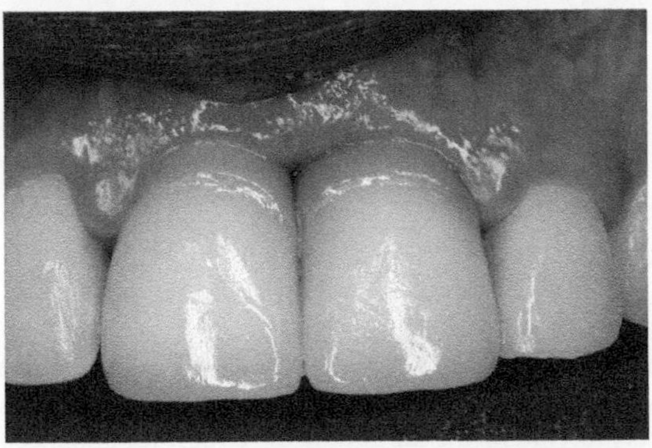

Fig. 4. Complex scenarios resulting from implant placement without grafting, subsequent bone loss, and tissue recession during the provisionalization phase created a situation that was not satisfactorily restored using 2 single-implant crowns with pink ceramic. These challenging situations require careful resolution, perhaps involving conventional prosthodontics.

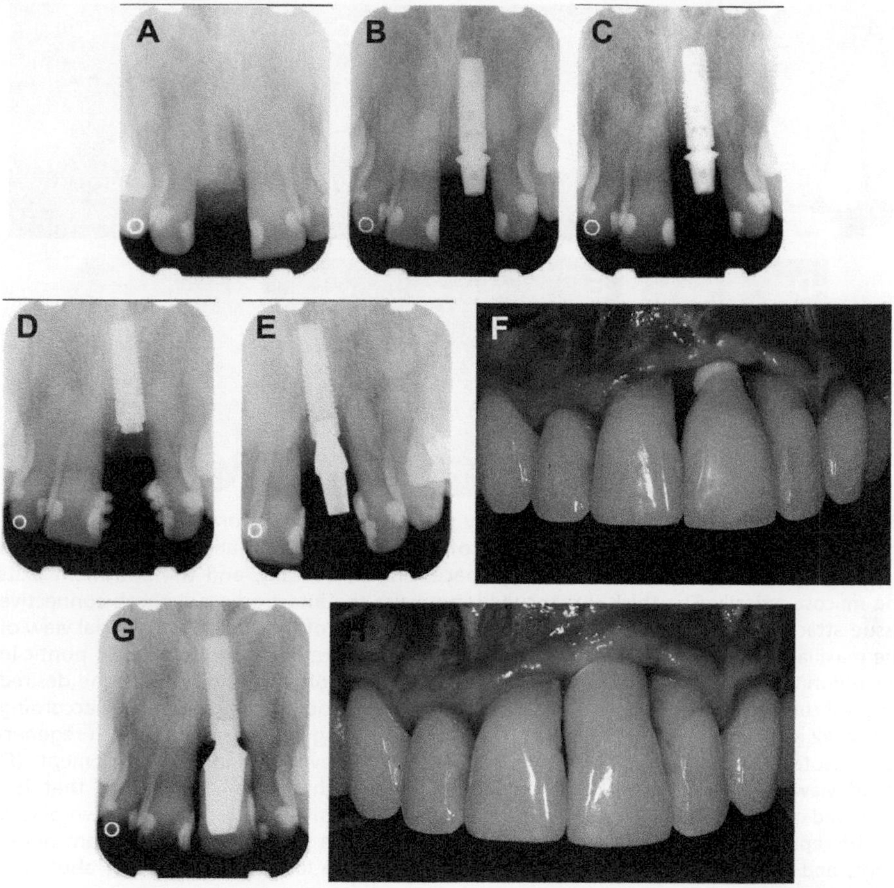

Fig. 5. Severe esthetic complications resulting from excessive depth of implant placement. (*A*) Radiograph illustrating satisfactory alveolar condition before implant placement, (*B*) radiograph illustrating deep position of implant placement before failure. (*C*) Radiograph at time of implant failure demonstrating crestal bone resorption. (*D*) Radiograph illustrating extreme depth of implant placement on erroneous simultaneous removal and replacement of the failed implant. (*E*) Radiograph illustrating position of a stock zirconia abutment after successful integration. (*F*) Facial photograph reveals marked tissue loss during the healing phase of the replaced implant. (*G*) Radiograph illustrating position of the definitive patient-specific zirconia abutment. (*H*) Facial photograph of the definitive implant crown that was accepted by this patient.

The unesthetic implant resulting from facial displacement of angulation often requires implant removal to secure success (**Fig. 6**). The actual facial displacement should be distinguished from dehiscence that results from the deficiency of alveolar bone and loss of the buccal plate of bone (**Fig. 7**). **Box 1** demonstrates the differences between facial displacement of an implant and dehiscence of the buccal plate of bone. When there is loss of the buccal plate of bone, the regeneration of bone and mucosa may be attempted without removal of the dental implant. However, it is the authors' opinion that this procedure be conducted following removal of the implant crown and abutment to permit spontaneous gingival regeneration to occur. This increases the volume of soft tissue and reduces the advancing of the flap and disruption of

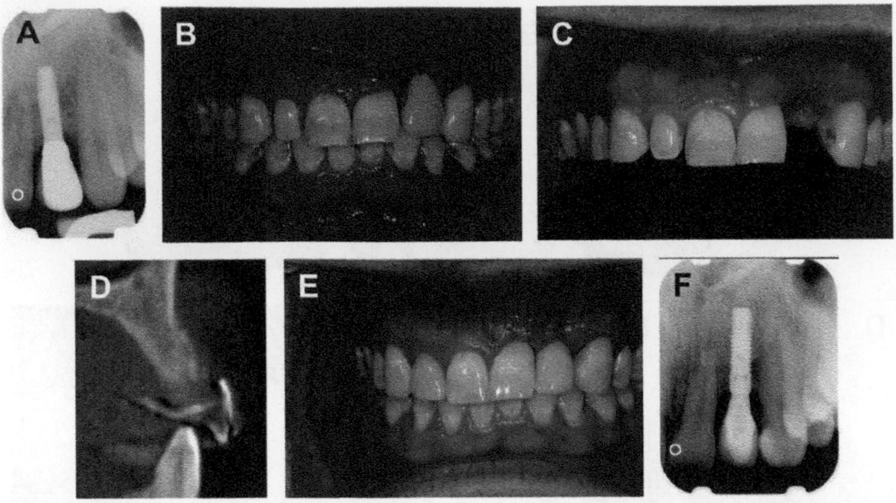

Fig. 6. Buccal angulation of an implant may preclude esthetic restoration. (*A*) Radiograph indicating the successful osseointegration of this misplaced implant. (*B*) The implant is placed distally in the bound edentulous space, angled buccally, and the abutment exits the mucosa apically. The thick soft-tissue biotype and the intact adjacent tooth connective tissue attachments favor careful removal and replacement of this implant. (*C*) Facial view of the maxillary left lateral incisor region following implant removal with a bonded pontic in place during healing. Note that we have organized the soft tissue to identify the desired gingival contour of the definitive restoration, and this guides implant placement according to the 3/2 rule. (*D*) CBCT sagittal image of the site following implant removal with regeneration. Note that there is sufficient bone volume to achieve ideal implant placement. (*E*) Facial view of the replaced implant with definitive lithium disilicate crown that has improved contours and color. (*F*) Radiograph of the definitive abutment and crown placed on the replaced implant. The modest remodeling of bone occurred before implant placement, and the thick tissue biotype permitted use of the longer transmucosal abutment dimension.

the mucogingival junction to accommodate grafting material volumes in the subsequent required procedures. When the implant must be removed, the resulting defect is typically a 3-walled defect. A flapless approach is not readily accommodated here. Furthermore, the impact of implant removal on the adjacent tooth connective tissue attachments must be predicted and minimized. Selecting the appropriate method of implant removal can influence the future outcome of therapy, and the least traumatic method should be selected. Four methods for implant removal are commonly reported and used (**Table 3**). Each method has the potential to create additional tissue damage, particularly the trephine drill. The main advantage of reverse high-torque instrumentation is that the implant may be removed without significant architectural change to the surrounding bone. Other methods such as heating the implant (using electrocautery instrumentation) are not endorsed with enthusiasm.

FACTORS INFLUENCING THE DECISION TO REMOVE A DENTAL IMPLANT

When the implant must be removed, considerable time and many appointments will be required. Provisionalization becomes a central and important part of planning excellent care.

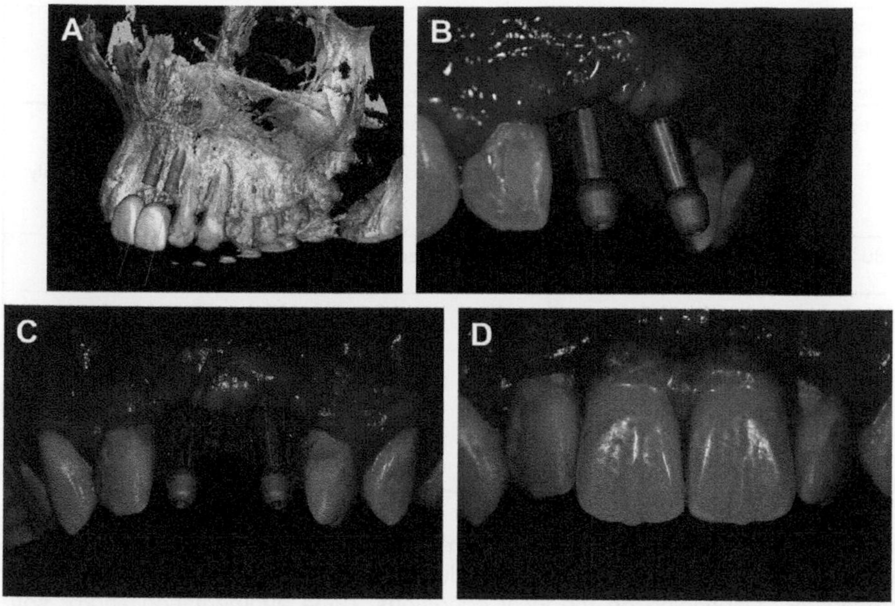

Fig. 7. Anterior maxillary implant esthetics can be negatively affected by excessive buccal implant angulation. (*A*) Simplant planning for ideal implant placement. (*B*) Placement of impression copings reveals the buccal orientation of the implant/abutment long axis. (*C*) Facial view of the impression copings reveals the accompanying axial displacement of the gingival zenith positions (far superior to the adjacent teeth). The surprising loss of adjacent tooth connective tissue attachment is unexplained, but complicates treatment. (*D*) The 2 implants were restored with a splinted prosthesis to prevent a vertical line disrupting the gingival ceramics (compare with **Fig. 4**). The quality of gingival ceramics is ever increasing and can be an alternative solution to tissue loss around implants, provided access for hygiene is maintained.

Steps in managing resorptive esthetic complications cannot be well managed prosthetically, but require prosthetic strategies in provisionalization and tissue management, Chu and Tarnow[1] outline a stepwise retreatment approach advocated here. When soft-tissue architecture surrounding the implant abutment must be altered, it is essential that sufficient tissue is available locally to (1) permit minor alterations or (2) enable grafting of remote tissues (eg, submucosal connective tissue graft). The removal of the crown and abutment from the implant followed by the placement of a cover-screw and soft-tissue healing over the implant is the first step. This acknowledges the decoronation (spontaneous gingival augmentation) approach in periodontal

Box 1
Factors influencing the dehiscence-type defect of dental implants

- Facial implant position or excessive implant angulation
- Extreme depth of implant placement or shallow implant placement
- Excessive implant diameter
- Incorrect abutment dimension or contour
- Thin mucosa

Table 3
Methods of dental implant removal

Method	Advantages	Disadvantages
Trephine drill	Widely applicable Effective	Requires full-thickness flap Potential to destroy adjacent bone/teeth Additional bone removed circumferentially Contraindicated when interimplant-tooth distance is small
Bur/elevator	Simple Familiar instrumentation	Requires full-thickness flap
Bur/forceps	Simple Familiar instrumentation	Requires full-thickness flap More bone reduction than elevator method
High-torque instrument	Simple No/small flap required Useful when interimplant-tooth distance is small	Limited use if coronal aspect of implant is fractured Added instrumentation

regeneration.[1] Subsequent surgical augmentation may be required and can be approached by tunneling (VISTA[2]) procedures or conventional mucoperiosteal flap procedures. Depending on the local conditions, bone augmentation and/or soft-tissue augmentation may be required. Irrespective of the approach, prosthodontic management is essential during these initial steps. Provisionalization will be required for the 6- to 8-week period of spontaneous gingival augmentation and 3 to 6 months will be required for the period of surgical augmentation. Thus, the provisionalization scheme must achieve the following goals: (1) an esthetic and functional replacement of the missing crown, (2) reversibility for ease of multiple subsequent interventions, (3) it adjusts to the changing soft-tissue contours, (4) is cleansable, and (5) is cost efficient. Fortunately, there exist several different methods for provisional replacement of the missing tooth during retreatment (**Table 4**). Given that they possess unique advantages and disadvantages, the chosen method must match the capabilities of both the surgical and restorative dentists and fit the needs of the patient. The use of a fixed provisional solution, though technically more challenging and more costly, offers several advantages in terms of soft-tissue contouring and management.

Materials-based complications are common in dental implant therapy. Chipping of ceramic veneered single crown restorations is reported to occur in 4.5% of the cases at the 5-year time point.[3] In a prospective clinical study, the extent of chipping was correlated with the presence and severity of attrition of the dentition. In that report, 10% chipping was reported for dentitions with attrition while 21.9% and 26.9% chipping was observed for dentitions with localized or generalized attrition, respectively.[2] Anterior and posterior tooth chipping rates were similar. Although chipping or wear of the veneering of restorations represent only some of the esthetic complications in implant therapy, comparison of accumulating data indicates a trend toward reduced esthetic complications associated with single crowns (15.9% published through 2000, 5.4% published after 2000).[4] Higher incidence for ceramic chipping for anterior crowns is also associated with lack of posterior support.

The type of material may influence the rate of chipping of ceramic implant prostheses. A 2008 report of 251 patients with 350 various implant prostheses revealed a 6.7% overall ceramic facture rate within 3 years. Importantly, this work suggests that fracture rate increases with the complexity of the reconstruction (1.3% single crown, 6.7% fixed dental prosthesis, 38.1% full arch). The authors suggested that

Table 4
Provisionalization schemes for managing single tooth implant complications

Technique	Application	Advantages	Disadvantages
Removable partial denture	All scenarios	Reversible, low cost	Mobile Negatively affects speech, psychology Affects healing tissues
Essick Retainer	All scenarios	Reversible, low cost, office manufacture	Mobile Can affect healing tissues Limited durability
Fixed dental prosthesis	Adjacent prepared tooth exists	Simple technology Excellent tissue management potential Relatively simple to remove and replace	Invasive Cost
Resin-bonded prosthesis	Adjacent teeth intact	Reversible Excellent tissue management potential	Requires occlusal clearance Time-intensive removal and replacement Risk of debonding Cost
Bonded ceramic pontic	Adjacent teeth intact	Reversible Excellent tissue management	Risk of debonding Time intensive

eccentric contacts contribute to ceramic fracture.[5] A comprehensive systematic review including 73 articles revealed that single crown and fixed partial prostheses of screw-retained design present more technical complications than cemented prostheses. For full arch prosthesis, the resin and ceramic chipping rates were 10.04 and 8.95 per 100 years, respectively. Again, complications increased with the complexity or extent of the prosthesis.[6] Although earlier studies indicated that the risk of ceramic facture was greater for implant-supported restorations than for tooth-supported restorations, a recent systematic review of the clinical success of tooth and implant-supported zirconia-based fixed prosthesis demonstrated similar cumulative 5-year complication rates of 27.6% and 30.5% for tooth- and implant-supported fixed dental prostheses, respectively. Recent reports of monolithic zirconia prostheses indicate a nearly absolute absence of chipping complications in the near term.[7,8] However, even moderate esthetic veneering of a monolithic Zr prosthesis can result in chipping. Clearly the risk of veneered ceramic prosthesis chipping suggests that long-term management of implant esthetics must address chipping of implant prostheses (**Fig. 8**).

Acrylic prostheses also require management for tooth fracture, tooth loss, or wear (**Fig. 9**). Concerning wear, although there are no defined lifetimes for acrylic tooth longevity for implant prostheses, a 2016 report indicated that the mean time between delivery of the prosthesis and replacement of the teeth caused by wear/attrition was 7.8 years (1.1–22.9 years). Individuals requiring multiple tooth replacement sought this re-veneering treatment earlier. The nature of the opposing dentition also influenced the duration of service before re-veneering; implant- and tooth-supported ceramometal fixed prostheses opposing the acrylic/metal hybrid resulted in the earliest retreatment, whereas acrylic/metal hybrid prostheses opposing natural teeth, a complete denture, or a transitioned denture were in service longest before re-veneering.[9] A comprehensive estimate of complications associated with implant-supported fixed

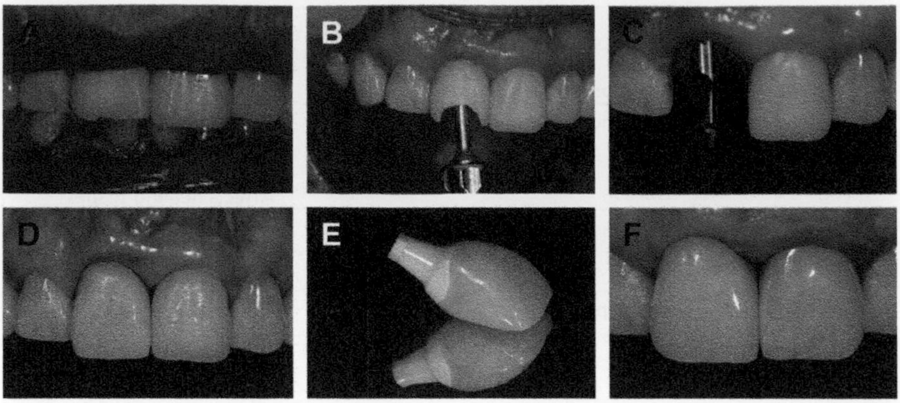

Fig. 8. Chipping of implant crowns occurs and can be managed by crown replacement. (*A*) Facial extraoral photograph reveals chipping of a layered lithium disilicate crown 9 years after placement. (*B*) Rapid access to the abutment and abutment screw is created, and the abutment and cemented crown is removed. (*C*) An abutment-level impression is made. (*D*) A temporary abutment and bis-acryl provisional crown is placed. (*E*) A new abutment and a new monolithic crown are produced by a digital work flow. (*F*) Facial intraoral photograph of the new implant crown (right central incisor) and replacement left central incisor crown.

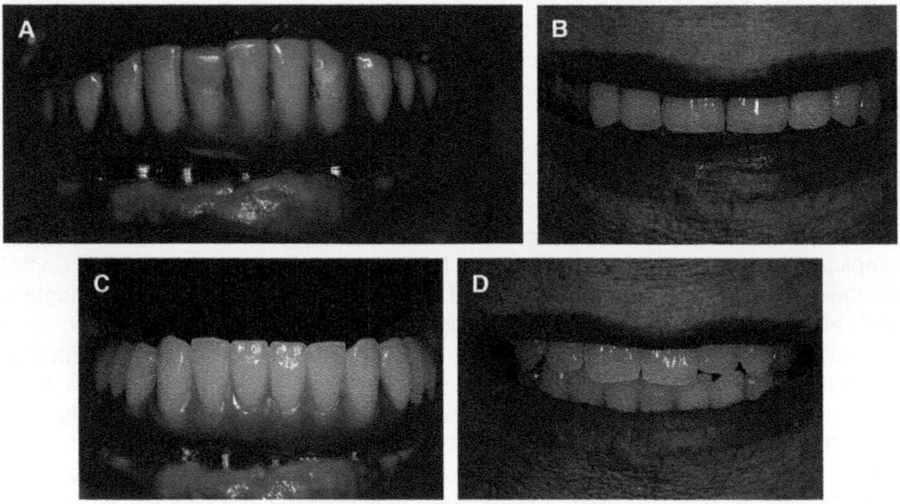

Fig. 9. Wear and chipping of acrylic implant prosthesis is common. The replacement of such prostheses must be part of every implant practice. (*A*) Intraoral photograph reveals mandibular implant-supported hybrid prosthesis demonstrating marked tooth wear and historical repair of incisor chipping. The accumulation of plaque and staining is also revealed. (*B*) The extraoral facial photograph illustrates the esthetic value of the opposing maxillary complete denture. (*C*) Intraoral photograph reveals the condition of the mandibular prosthesis after replacement of the denture teeth and veneering acrylic resin. Note the restoration of vertical dimension by increasing the dimension of the teeth. (*D*) Extraoral facial photograph illustrates the esthetic value of the new opposing maxillary complete denture.

dental prosthesis indicates that the complication of resin tooth and veneer fracture and wear is progressive over a 15-year period. This systematic review indicates that within 10 to 15 years nearly one-half of all such prostheses demonstrate tooth and veneer wear and fracture.[10] Examples of prospective and retrospective analyses of metal acrylic hybrid complications illustrate these findings.[11,12] Importantly, loss of anterior acrylic teeth from maxillary prostheses is commonly reported in the literature. It is essential that the observation of posterior tooth wear be addressed early to prevent anterior tooth fracture or dislodgment. It is concluded here that all acrylic/metal hybrid prostheses require continued surveillance and attendant maintenance.

The long-term management of implant prostheses requires consideration for lasting esthetics. Managing chipping or wear of teeth is an important factor for single-unit, multiple-unit, and full arch restorations (**Table 5**). Screw-retained restorations clearly assist the clinician in managing these complications. This may be of limited consequence for a chipped single-unit crown because the fractured/chipped crown can be easily retrieved and repaired.

Esthetic complications with implant abutments include both discoloration of the peri-implant mucosa and unesthetic display associated with midfacial resorption. The mechanical complications of screw loosening, screw fracture, and abutment fracture are not the focus of this review. However, unattended abutment screw loosening can lead to marked inflammation that results in mucosal redness, hypertrophy, and marginal bone loss.

The clinical appearance of the definitive implant restoration is affected by the potential translucency of the peri-implant mucosa, and the color of the transmucosal abutment affects the optical properties of this peri-implant soft-tissue color. One of the drawbacks of using a silver-colored titanium abutment is the potential for gray discoloration of the surrounding mucosa (**Fig. 10**).[13–15] This is exacerbated by the presence of a thin biotype, because the mucosa is unable to block the reflective light from the metallic abutment.[16] To improve the esthetic results other materials have been advocated, including alumina and anodized titanium alloy (gold-shaded), as well as a variety of colors in zirconia (different shades and translucencies in white). These

Table 5
Factors influencing the management of prosthesis wear and chipping

Material Factor	Significance
Abutment versus implant connection	Abutment connection simplifies retrieval
Cement versus screw retention	Screw retention simplifies retrieval May result in higher chipping/fracture rate for veneered ceramic
Resin materials	Enables direct, intraoral repair or in-office repair Subject to wear and staining
Veneered ceramic materials	Subject to chipping; Zr framework > metal framework
Monolithic $LiSi_2$/Zr prosthesis	May resist chipping of single-unit ($LiSi_2$) or multiunit (Zr) prosthesis May resist staining
Segmented reconstruction	Enables removal of only part of a reconstruction when chipping is repaired
Unit-constructed prosthesis	Permits removal of the chipped crown from the otherwise intact prosthesis May stain at the crown/superstructure interface

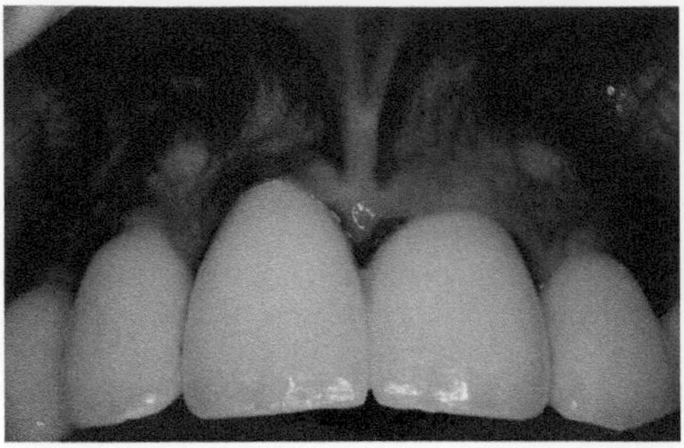

Fig. 10. Intraoral photograph of gray mucosa superficial to the maxillary right central incisor implant that is lacking buccal bone coverage. This negative outcome was not observed following initial implant placement and restoration, but was revealed several years later and is due to subsequent bone resorption that was a result of facial implant placement.

alternatively colored materials may reduce the discoloration of the peri-implant mucosa.[17,18] Titanium and zirconia have been advocated as materials to be used in the anterior region for good esthetic results.[19]

Discoloration of peri-implant mucosa represents a challenging prosthetic problem. The color of the soft tissues around the titanium implant is also significantly different to the gingiva around natural teeth.[20] Peri-implant tissues around zirconia abutments mimic the color of the natural gingiva.[21] However, zirconia abutments could increase the brightness of the peri-implant mucosa, affecting the final esthetic result. Thoma and colleagues[22] used spectrophotometric analysis to evaluate the esthetic difference between a fluorescent hybrid zirconia abutments cemented on titanium base compared with a nonfluorescent one-piece zirconia abutment. Twenty-four patients had single tooth implants restored with both types of prosthesis; the color of the peri-implant tissues was then measured with a spectrophotometer. The results showed no statistical difference with either of the materials; however, when thickness of the mucosa was considered, the one-piece zirconia abutment showed esthetic improvement in a thin mucosa (less than 2 mm).[22] Lops and colleagues[23] also measured the influence of abutment material on the peri-implant soft-tissue color. Fifteen patients received a single tooth implant and each one of them was restored with a gold alloy abutment, a zirconia computer-aided design and manufacture (CAD/CAM) abutment, and titanium CAD/CAM abutment. Tissue thickness was measured, and peri-implant soft-tissue color was obtained with a spectrophotometer. The results for the titanium abutment showed statistically greater discoloration when compared with the gold or zirconia abutment when soft tissues were less than 2 mm in thickness.[23] The use of zirconia abutments may enhance esthetics around the peri-implant mucosa.[17,24] Systematic review and meta-analysis have revealed that zirconia abutments provided appreciably better esthetic results when compared with titanium abutments.[25,26] The use of zirconia abutments may further enhance color control of implant crowns (**Fig. 11**).

The thickness of the mucosa is reported to have a significant influence on the discoloration of the peri-implant mucosa.[27] Therefore, connective tissue grafting to augment the thickness of the peri-implant mucosa has been advocated,[28–30] suggesting that through this procedure an additional 1.2 to 1.6 mm of soft-tissue thickness can be

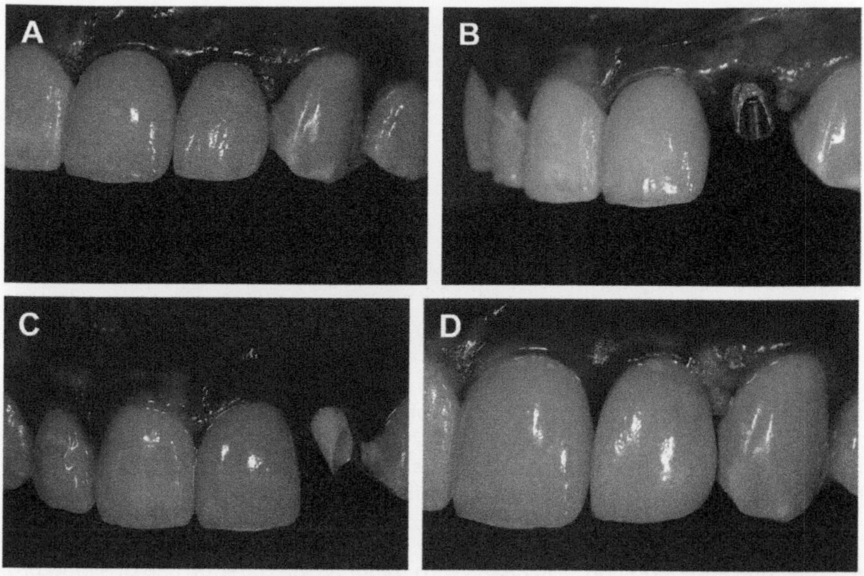

Fig. 11. Ceramic crown discoloration can be due to the color of the abutment substrate. (*A*) Maxillary left lateral incisor with a stock titanium abutment with modest buccal orientation. (*B*) The discoloration of the monolithic lithium disilicate crown does not harmonize with the veneer on the adjacent central incisor or the natural adjacent canine tooth. (*C*) Replacement of the titanium abutment with a stock zirconia abutment. (*D*) Milling, staining, and glazing of a monolithic lithium disilicate crown provides better color harmonization with the adjacent teeth.

obtained and maintained at 1 year. These results concluded with a perceived esthetic improvement around the implant restoration. In summary, when confronted with thin mucosa, esthetic improvement may be achieved by changing the abutment color/material.

Management of esthetics with dental implants can be more challenging when there are multiple missing teeth. Interimplant spacing, number of implants, and precise positioning to avoid embrasure sites are factors that should be carefully planned to provide optimum esthetic results. It is generally accepted that creation of a papilla between 2 adjacent implants is more challenging than between an implant and a natural tooth (**Figs. 12** and **13**). An interimplant distance of less than 3 mm was shown to have a nonfavorable effect on interproximal papilla height because of increased crestal bone loss.[31] For cases in which multiple teeth are to be replaced, it is more esthetically preferable to alternate implants with pontics sites. Salama and colleagues[32] demonstrated that papilla height is greater around a pontic-pontic (6 mm) and implant-pontic (5.5 mm) than between 2 implants. Loss of teeth may be associated with both hard- and soft-tissue defects horizontally and vertically. This could be due to: (1) lack of alveolar bone development in patients with congenitally missing teeth (eg, ectodermal dysplasia), (2) systemic diseases; (3) trauma; (4) local factors such as periodontitis, endodontic lesions, or tumor; or (5) iatrogenic conditions caused by traumatic tooth extractions.[33] Reconstruction of deficient tissues may be done via surgical and/or prosthetic treatment approaches. Techniques used to augment hard tissues include block bone graft, guided bone regeneration, orthodontic tooth extrusion, and distraction methods. Vertical gain of bone height is often less predictable

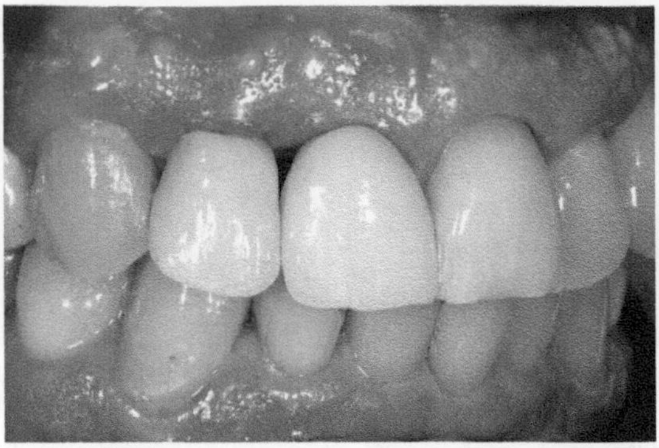

Fig. 12. Intraoral photograph of implant crowns supported by adjacent implants in the maxillary right central and lateral incisor positions. The lack of interproximal tissues creates a common esthetic deficit that occurs when 2 adjacent maxillary anterior implants are restored. Although it is often advocated to use only one implant and a pontic to restore to missing adjacent teeth, this remains a daunting clinical challenge.

than horizontal augmentation.[34] In cases with minor tissue defects, use of a long proximal contact area may hinder the unesthetic visualization of interproximal black triangle (see **Fig. 12**). Use of prosthetic gingiva with either pink ceramics or resins may be needed to compensate larger deficits in hard and soft tissues.[35] Prosthetic reconstitution of soft-tissue defects is less traumatic to the patients with reduced morbidity and shortened treatment time, and is less costly. However, it should be noted that use of gingiva-colored prosthetic materials requires high dental technical skills (see **Figs. 4** and **7**). Repositioning of transition zone (link between the prosthesis and natural gingiva) with alveoloplasty below the lip perimeter on maximum smile is critical for concealment of the unesthetic display of this juncture. This is particularly important in rehabilitation of the fully edentulous maxilla. In addition, alveoloplasty to establish a flat pontic design allows better hygiene. Achieving optimum esthetic results in fully edentulous patients requires meticulous planning. Diagnostic determination of future midline, occlusal plane, incisal edge position, and relationship of alveolar ridge to smile line are initial key points. Determination of incisal edge position based on esthetics and speech influences future prosthetic designs and the need for gingiva-colored prosthetic material.

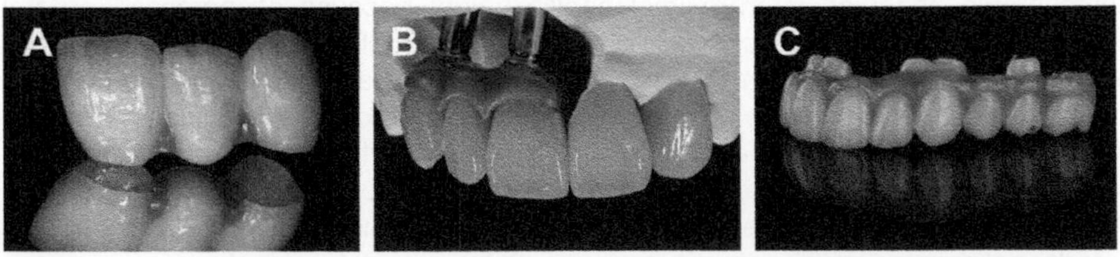

Fig. 13. Pink prosthetic materials may be artfully applied to replace missing peri-implant mucosa. (*A*) This exemplifies the addition of pink ceramic to accommodate missing papilla. (*B*) The creation of missing alveolar tissue (in this case for a cleft palate graft patient) can be achieved using composite resin materials. (*C*) More recently, the esthetic veneering of gingival tissues onto monolithic zirconia restorations has enabled clinicians to avoid significant grafting and rely on gingival restoration.

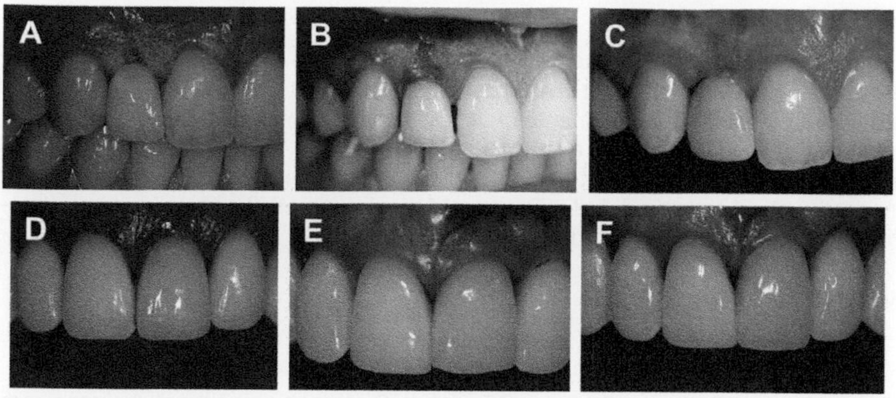

Fig. 14. Tooth movement relative to dental implants occurs over time in some individuals. (*A*) Intraoral photograph reveals a maxillary right lateral incisor implant crown shortly after restoration. (*B*) Intraoral photograph reveals the same implant crown with a mesial diastema and distal open contact several years afterward. (*C*) Intraoral photograph demonstrates the improved esthetic result following replacement of both the abutment and crown with a patient-specific CAD/CAM abutment and a monolithic lithium disilicate crown. (*D*) Intraoral photograph of a maxillary left central incisor implant crown shortly after restoration. (*E*) Photograph of the same implant crown after 10 years reveals relative implant intrusion. (*F*) Intraoral photograph of the same implant after retreatment placing both a zirconia abutment and a new monolithic lithium disilicate crown.

Improper placement of implants coronal to the smile line when soft-tissue replacement is needed with pink ceramic may lead to esthetic failure (see **Fig. 1**). In such cases, it may be required that the patient is restored with removable complete overdenture rather than a fixed prosthesis to help conceal the prosthesis tissue junction. Potential advantages for use of a maxillary overdenture versus an implant-supported fixed denture include facial scaffolding and ease of cleaning.[36] Other treatment options include removal of existing implants and alveoloplasty to move the transition zone apical to the smile line followed by fixed implant dental rehabilitation, or plastic surgery intervention with lip repositioning[37]

A long-term esthetic complication for dental implants is related to adjacent teeth movement, which may lead to spacing (mesiodistally) and infraposition of implant restorations (**Fig. 14**). This is a particularly significant problem with high prevalence (**Table 6**). The risk for infraposition of dental implant restorations is not limited to younger patients; it can also occur in mature adults. Remake of the implant restorations is needed in such cases. The relative risks for infraposition of implants remain undefined.

Table 6
Percentage of long-term implants in infraposition

Authors, Year	Type of Study	Percentage of Implant Restorations in Infraposition	Follow-up Years
Dierens et al,[38] 2013	Retrospective	71	16–22
Bernard et al,[39] 2004	Retrospective	100	4.2
Chang and Wennström,[40] 2012	Retrospective	58	8
Jemt et al,[41] 2007	Retrospective	60	>15

SUMMARY

Correct treatment planning and materials selection help to assure ideal dental implant esthetics. There exist sufficient clinical data to indicate that implant placement considerations are important determinants of dental implant esthetics. When implant placement is not ideal, abutment and prosthesis alterations can be made to improve esthetics. When possible, soft-tissue grafting can be used to augment buccal (and modest) vertical esthetic deficits. The use of gingival prosthetic techniques can provide acceptable solutions for mucosa-associated esthetic limitations.

REFERENCES

1. Langer B. Spontaneous in situ gingival augmentation. Int J Periodontics Restorative Dent 1994;14(6):524–35.
2. Wittneben JG, Buser D, Salvi GE, et al. Complication and failure rates with implant-supported fixed dental prostheses and single crowns: a 10-year retrospective study. Clin Implant Dent Relat Res 2014;16(3):356–64.
3. Jung RE, Pjetursson BE, Glauser R, et al. A systematic review of the 5-year survival and complication rates of implant-supported single crowns. Clin Oral Implants Res 2008;19(2):119–30.
4. Pjetursson BE, Asgeirsson AG, Zwahlen M, et al. Improvements in implant dentistry over the last decade: comparison of survival and complication rates in older and newer publications. Int J Oral Maxillofac Implants 2014;29(Suppl):308–24.
5. Linkevicius T, Vladimirovas E, Grybauskas S, et al. Veneer fracture in implant-supported metal-ceramic restorations. Part I: overall success rate and impact of occlusal guidance. Stomatologija 2008;10(4):133–9.
6. Millen C, Bragger U, Wittneben JG. Influence of prosthesis type and retention mechanism on complications with fixed implant-supported prostheses: a systematic review applying multivariate analyses. Int J Oral Maxillofac Implants 2015;30(1):110–24.
7. Bidra AS, Rungruanganunt P, Gauthier M. Clinical outcomes of full arch fixed implant-supported zirconia prostheses: a systematic review. Eur J Oral Implantol 2017;10(Suppl 1):35–45.
8. Abdulmajeed AA, Lim KG, Narhi TO, et al. Complete-arch implant-supported monolithic zirconia fixed dental prostheses: a systematic review. J Prosthet Dent 2016;115(6):672–677 e1.
9. Balshi TJ, Wolfinger GJ, Alfano SG, et al. The retread: a definition and retrospective analysis of 205 implant-supported fixed prostheses. Int J Prosthodont 2016;29(2):126–31.
10. Bozini T, Petridis H, Garefis K, et al. A meta-analysis of prosthodontic complication rates of implant-supported fixed dental prostheses in edentulous patients after an observation period of at least 5 years. Int J Oral Maxillofac Implants 2011;26(2):304–18.
11. Fischer K, Stenberg T. Prospective 10-year cohort study based on a randomized, controlled trial (RCT) on implant-supported full-arch maxillary prostheses. part II: prosthetic outcomes and maintenance. Clin Implant Dent Relat Res 2013;15(4):498–508.
12. Priest G, Smith J, Wilson MG. Implant survival and prosthetic complications of mandibular metal-acrylic resin implant complete fixed dental prostheses. J Prosthet Dent 2014;111(6):466–75.

13. Abduo J, Lyons K. Rationale for the use of CAD/CAM technology in implant prosthodontics. Int J Dent 2013;2013:768121.
14. Jemt T. Customized titanium single-implant abutments: 2-year follow-up pilot study. Int J Prosthodont 1998;11(4):312–6.
15. Heydecke G, Kohal R, Glaser R. Optimal esthetics in single-tooth replacement with the Re-Implant system: a case report. Int J Prosthodont 1999;12(2):184–9.
16. Yildirim M, Edelhoff D, Hanisch O, et al. Ceramic abutments—a new era in achieving optimal esthetics in implant dentistry. Int J Periodontics Restorative Dent 2000;20(1):81–91.
17. Bressan E, Paniz G, Lops D, et al. Influence of abutment material on the gingival color of implant-supported all-ceramic restorations: a prospective multicenter study. Clin Oral Implants Res 2011;22(6):631–7.
18. Jung RE, Sailer I, Hammerle CH, et al. In vitro color changes of soft tissues caused by restorative materials. Int J Periodontics Restorative Dent 2007;27(3): 251–7.
19. Bidra AS, Rungruanganunt P. Clinical outcomes of implant abutments in the anterior region: a systematic review. J Esthet Restor Dent 2013;25(3):159–76.
20. Park SE, Da Silva JD, Weber HP, et al. Optical phenomenon of peri-implant soft tissue. Part I. Spectrophotometric assessment of natural tooth gingiva and peri-implant mucosa. Clin Oral Implants Res 2007;18(5):569–74.
21. Happe A, Korner G. Biologic Interfaces in esthetic dentistry. Part II: the peri-implant/restorative interface. Eur J Esthet Dent 2011;6(2):226–51.
22. Thoma DS, Gamper FB, Sapata VM, et al. Spectrophotometric analysis of fluorescent zirconia abutments compared to "conventional" zirconia abutments: a within subject controlled clinical trial. Clin Implant Dent Relat Res 2017;19(4):760–6.
23. Lops D, Stellini E, Sbricoli L, et al. Influence of abutment material on peri-implant soft tissues in anterior areas with thin gingival biotype: a multicentric prospective study. Clin Oral Implants Res 2017;28(10):1263–8.
24. Zembic A, Sailer I, Jung RE, et al. Randomized-controlled clinical trial of customized zirconia and titanium implant abutments for single-tooth implants in canine and posterior regions: 3-year results. Clin Oral Implants Res 2009;20(8):802–8.
25. Cai H, Chen J, Li C, et al. Quantitative discoloration assessment of peri-implant soft tissue around zirconia and other abutments with different colours: a systematic review and meta-analysis. J Dent 2018;70:110–7.
26. Linkevicius T, Vaitelis J. The effect of zirconia or titanium as abutment material on soft peri-implant tissues: a systematic review and meta-analysis. Clin Oral Implants Res 2015;26(Suppl 11):139–47.
27. Jung RE, Holderegger C, Sailer I, et al. The effect of all-ceramic and porcelain-fused-to-metal restorations on marginal peri-implant soft tissue color: a randomized controlled clinical trial. Int J Periodontics Restorative Dent 2008;28(4): 357–65.
28. Sicilia A, Quirynen M, Fontolliet A, et al. Long-term stability of peri-implant tissues after bone or soft tissue augmentation. Effect of zirconia or titanium abutments on peri-implant soft tissues. Summary and consensus statements. The 4th EAO Consensus Conference 2015. Clin Oral Implants Res 2015;26(Suppl 11):148–52.
29. Wiesner G, Esposito M, Worthington H, et al. Connective tissue grafts for thickening peri-implant tissues at implant placement. One-year results from an explanatory split-mouth randomised controlled clinical trial. Eur J Oral Implantol 2010; 3(1):27–35.

30. Zucchelli G, Mazzotti C, Bentivogli V, et al. The connective tissue platform technique for soft tissue augmentation. Int J Periodontics Restorative Dent 2012; 32(6):665–75.
31. Tarnow DP, Magner AW, Fletcher P. The effect of the distance from the contact point to the crest of bone on the presence or absence of the interproximal dental papilla. J Periodontol 1992;63(12):995–6.
32. Salama M, Ishikawa T, Salama H, et al. Advantages of the root submergence technique for pontic site development in estheticimplant therapy. Int J Periodontics Restorative Dent 2007;27(6):521–7.
33. Hämmerle CHF, Tarnow D. J The etiology of hard- and soft-tissue deficiencies at dental implants: a narrative review. Periodontol 2018;89(Suppl 1):S291–303.
34. Esposito M, Grusovin MG, Felice P, et al. Interventions for replacing missing teeth: horizontal and vertical bone augmentation techniques for dental implant treatment. Cochrane Database Syst Rev 2009;(4):CD003607.
35. Coachman C, Salama M, Garber D, et al. Prosthetic gingival reconstruction in a fixed partial restoration. Part 1: introduction to artificial gingiva as an alternative therapy. Int J Periodontics Restorative Dent 2009;29(5):471–7.
36. Sadowsky SJ, Zitzmann NU. Protocols for the maxillary implant overdenture: a systematic review. Int J Oral Maxillofac Implants 2016;31(Suppl):s182–91.
37. Bidra AS. A technique for transferring a patient's smile line to a cone beam computed tomography (CBCT) image. J Prosthet Dent 2014;112(2):108–11.
38. Dierens M, de Bruecker E, Vandeweghe S, et al. Alterations in soft tissue levels and aesthetics over a 16-22 year period following single implant treatment in periodontally-healthy patients: a retrospective case series. J Clin Periodontol 2013;40(3):311–8.
39. Bernard JP, Schatz JP, Christou P, et al. Long-term vertical changes of the anterior maxillary teeth adjacent to single implants in young and mature adults. A retrospective study. J Clin Periodontol 2004;31(11):1024–8.
40. Chang M, Wennström JL. Longitudinal changes in tooth/single-implant relationship and bone topography: an 8-year retrospective analysis. Clin Implant Dent Relat Res 2012;14(3):388–94.
41. Jemt T, Ahlberg G, Henriksson K, et al. Tooth movements adjacent to single-implant restorations after more than 15 years of follow-up. Int J Prosthodont 2007;20(6):626–32.

Management of Implant/ Prosthodontic Complications

Ingeborg J. De Kok, DDS, MS[a,*], Ibrahim S. Duqum, DDS, MS[b],
Lauren H. Katz, DDS[a], Lyndon F. Cooper, DDS, PhD[c]

KEYWORDS

• Prosthetic complication • Prosthesis fracture • Dental implants
• Complication management

KEY POINTS

- Dental implant restorations have a high success rate but require careful planning and management to minimize complications.
- Most prosthetic complications occur after many years of the prosthesis being in place, and it is expected that the materials will fatigue.
- Frequent mechanical complications include abutment screw loosening, abutment fracture, and prosthesis fracture of both the veneer and the framework.

INTRODUCTION

The success rates for dental implants are very high, and have historically been measured by the presence of osseointegration and lack of periimplantitis. Nevertheless, every treatment can present complications. These complications are reported to involve implant components and prostheses at higher rates compared with implant loss. The cause of these complications is multifactorial and can be biological or mechanical. These types of complications increase in incidence over time, indicating that the risk of component and material complications increase with continued use.[1]

Prosthetic complications occur in dental implant therapies of all types, including single and multiple implants restored using fixed and removable prostheses. The cause-and-effect relationship of the complications has not been fully considered, and dynamics in the implant and component treatment result in a complex restoration

Disclosure: The authors have nothing to disclose.

[a] Department of Restorative Sciences, University of North Carolina, CB # 7450, Chapel Hill, NC 27599-7450, USA; [b] Division of Prosthodontics, Department of Restorative Sciences, University of North Carolina, CB # 7450, Chapel Hill, NC 27599-7450, USA; [c] Department of Oral Biology, University of Illinois at Chicago, College of Dentistry, Room 402E, 801 S Paulina Street, Chicago, IL 60612, USA
* Corresponding author.
E-mail address: ingeborg_dekok@unc.edu

Dent Clin N Am 63 (2019) 217–231
https://doi.org/10.1016/j.cden.2018.11.004 dental.theclinics.com
0011-8532/19/

that can experience mechanical complications with a tendency to become a cause of failure to the component selection, design, or manufacture. The most commonly reported implant mechanical complications include adjustment of overdentures because of loss of retention, relines, or clip/attachment fracture[2–5]; veneer fracture in fixed prostheses[6,7]; overdenture fracture[8,9]; acrylic resin fracture in hybrid prostheses[1,10,11]; screw loosening and screw fracture[12,13]; and metal framework fracture.[14,15] Many of these complications are related to poor planning, poor case selection, or even poor implementation of the treatment plan.

IMPLANT MALPOSITION

Implant malposition contributes to the increased risk of biomechanical complications with implants, components, and prostheses. Displacement of the implant axis from the imposed functional load creates or increases the bending moment acting on the implant restoration. This increase manifests itself in a variety of ways, the consequences of which include biological, mechanical, and esthetic complications and even implant failure.

Improper positioning of implants, whether it is in a buccolingual, mesiodistal, or occlusogingival location from the ideal position, may compromise the bony and soft tissue support necessary for long-term biological implant success. Mechanical complications arise from the increased forces being applied on the prosthesis, abutment, and/or implant body.[16,17] Esthetic parameters, such as emergence profile and contours of the prosthesis, may be considerably affected by implant malposition as well. The inability to clean the prosthesis may superimpose biofilm-mediated inflammatory challenges that lead to loss of bony support.[18,19] Although careful planning of the definitive restoration as the starting point for implant position is the ideal approach to ensuring proper implant position and related consequences of loading to limit biomechanical and biological risks, there are various methods to overcome misplacement-related complications. Some of those strategies include the use of customized abutment solutions and prosthetics enhancements using gingival-colored ceramics.

The ultimate goal in managing implant malposition is to create a restoration that is biologically, functionally, and esthetically synergistic with the patient's function and expectations. One problem that is often encountered is lack of the restorative space (occlusogingival dimension) required for the creation of a robust and properly formed dental prosthesis (**Fig. 1**). For a single-unit restoration in situations of occlusogingival dimensional limitations, a screw-retained option with crown and abutment fabricated as 1 piece reduces the required space to construct the restoration compared with a cement-retained restoration. In this situation, screw-retained restorations present less risk for prosthesis dislodgement because of lack of resistance and retention features in the implant abutment that a cement-retained restoration might have (**Fig. 2**). This point is also true for segmental fixed dental prostheses. Restorative space for full-arch restorations is critical to their success for both esthetic and structural reasons. This prosthetic solution has minimal dimensional requirements, based on the chosen restorative material, to meet the strength requirements and minimize potential risk for mechanical failure (**Fig. 3**). Another critical aspect for full-arch restorations is the length of the distal cantilever and how much leverage it adds to the abutments and implants.

When considering options for a multiunit prosthesis, a removable option may be fabricated instead of a fixed restoration. Although this may not meet an individual's initial expectations, it can provide a viable solution for a prosthesis that may otherwise be unaesthetic, unhygienic, and susceptible to further complications.

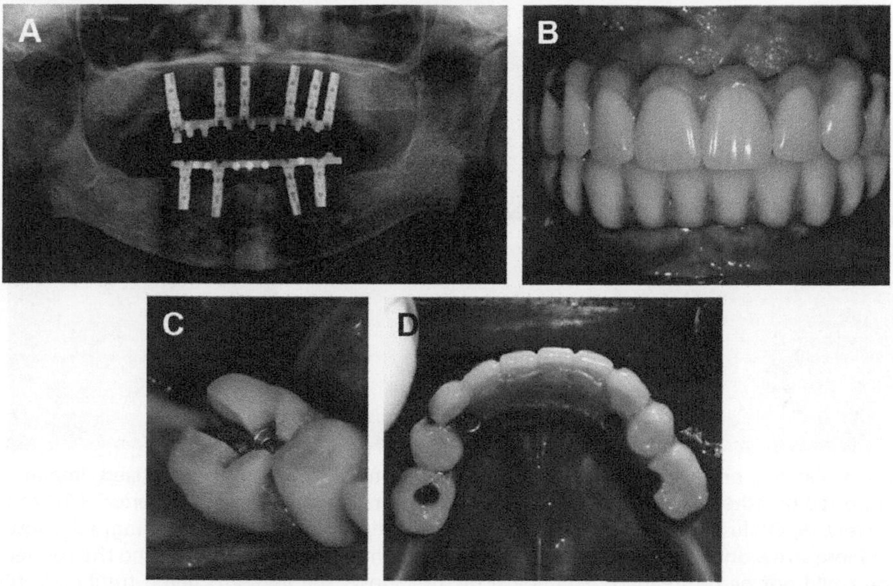

Fig. 1. Inadequate bone reduction to create prosthetic space for the final prosthesis resulting in prosthesis failure: (*A*) panoramic radiograph of the final prosthesis; (*B*) frontal view of the final prosthesis; (*C*) prosthetic tooth fracture as a consequence of lack of restorative space; (*D*) tooth was replaced in the prosthesis.

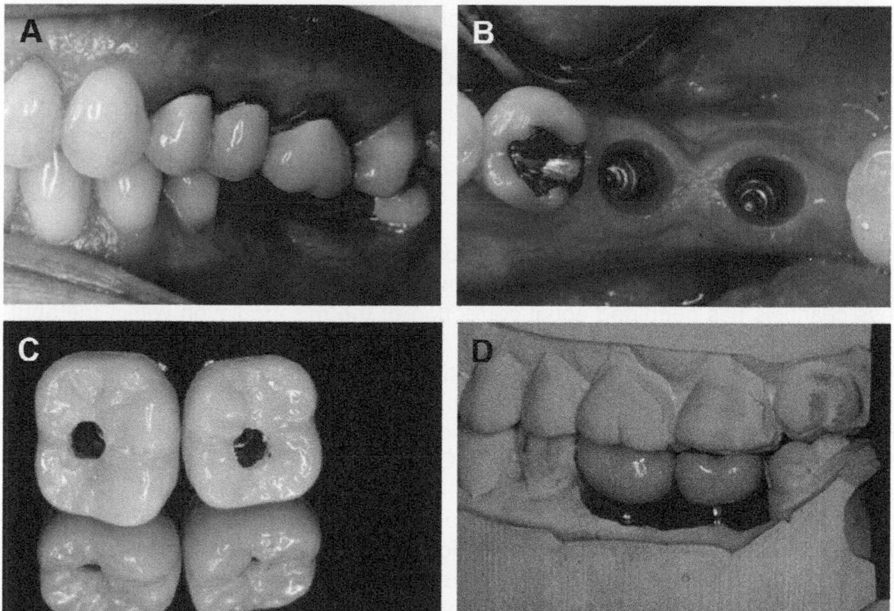

Fig. 2. Limited interarch space is present when replacing teeth 18 and 19. (*A*) Lateral view shows insufficient occlusal clearance for a prosthesis. (*B*) Occlusal view shows that implants were placed correctly in a mesiodistal and buccolingual position. (*C*) Zirconia crowns over computer-assisted design/computer-assisted manufacturing (CAD/CAM) abutments for screw-retained crowns were fabricated to gain space. (*D*) Lateral view of the restorations shows the short emergence profile of the restorations.

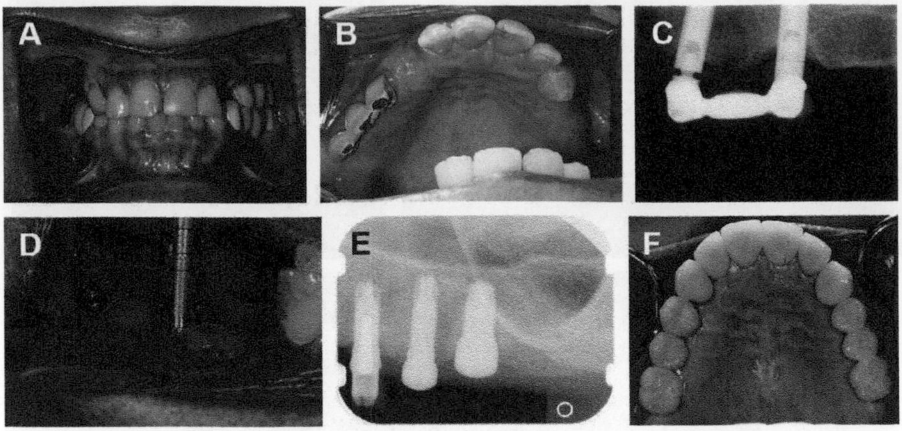

Fig. 3. Patient presents with fractured porcelain-fused-to-metal (PFM) fixed implant-supported prosthesis, reporting frequent screw loosening for an extended period. (*A*) Frontal view. (*B*) Occlusal view showing the fractured prosthesis. (*C*) Periapical radiograph shows the loose screw on an external hex connection; both implants were stripped and the connection could not be rethreaded. (*D*) Clinical picture shows the implants being trephined. (*E*) Periapical radiograph shows new implants placed after grafting. (*F*) Occlusal view shows the completed restoration with full-arch rehabilitation.

Improper implant placement resulting in inadequate volume and contour of the bony and/or gingival architecture has several options for management. Preemptively, hard or soft tissue grafting may be used to restore the appropriate tissue dimensions with varying degrees of success.[20,21] Creative prosthesis design incorporating gingival-colored ceramic or acrylic may also be used to replace absent or inadequate gingival architecture. This approach must be performed with caution, because an overcontoured or bulky prosthesis can lead to further biological consequences because of lack of cleanability.

Another complication commonly seen is a screw access channel exiting through a nonideal location, such as the incisal edge, an embrasure space, or even through the buccal surface. A viable option for correction is using an angled abutment, which can correct up to 25° of the misangulation.[22] Most recently, the use of angulated screw access channels has permitted equal correction of the misangulation within the abutment and crown (**Fig. 4**). This method is a remarkably effective way to overcome screw access channel limitations of esthetics and design and requires only specific screwdrivers to accommodate this design. If the restoration was initially planned to be screw retained, another solution can be found using computer-assisted design/computer-assisted manufacturing (CAD/CAM) custom abutments and cement-retained restorations (see **Fig. 4**).

Not all options to overcome implant malposition may be adequate to facilitate construction of prostheses with acceptable biological, functional, and esthetic parameters. Under such circumstances, implant removal may be considered. Although the time and cost to remove the implant, perform a bone graft, and place a new implant may be substantial, the long-term benefits are superior.

MANAGEMENT OF DENTAL IMPLANT COMPONENT COMPLICATIONS

A variety of implant and abutment designs and materials have been introduced to overcome perceived and real limitations found clinically. The mechanical integrity

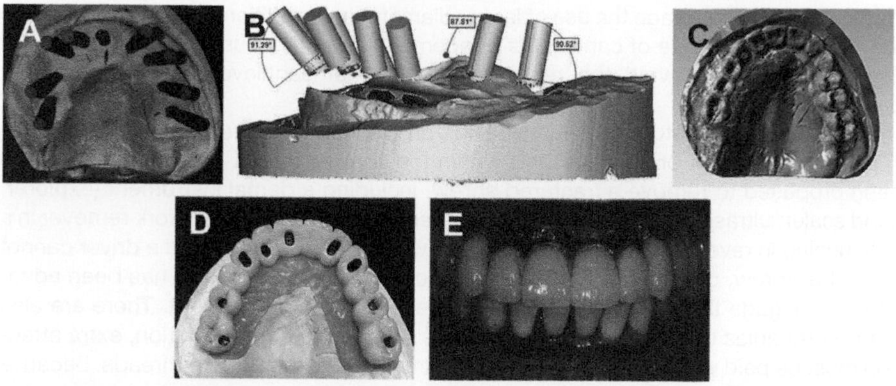

Fig. 4. Correction of the misangulation present in the implant through the use of an angulated screw access channel in the abutment. (*A*) Occlusal view of scanned cast shows misalignment of all implants present. (*B*) Lateral view shows number of degrees between the implants. (*C*) Digitized superimposition of proposed restorations. (*D*) Occlusal view of the completed prostheses with all access screw holes aligned in the lingual or occlusal surfaces of the teeth. (*E*) Frontal view of completed restoration. (*Courtesy of* Conrad Rensburg, ND, NHD, Absolute Dental Services, Durham, NC).

of these components is determined by the dimension, type of connection, type of material, and type of restoration.[23,24] The general categorization of abutments includes titanium versus zirconium and internal conus versus internal sliding fit or external hex connections. When internal connection abutments were compared with external connection abutments by systematic review, the abutment did not influence implant survival or complication rates, but internal conus connections showed less marginal bone loss.[25] Regarding the materials, no differences regarding the survival or failure of ceramic or metal abutments were observed in a review of single-tooth implants.[26] However, complications emerge in clinical practice.

Screw loosening or fracture is more common with prosthetic screws compared with abutment screws,[14] and this is the most common component complication. Screw complications are also more common in single-tooth implant restorations compared with multiple units.[27] Consistently, one of the most frequently reported complications is loosening of both the abutment screw and the prosthetic screw, with an incidence of 5.6% after 5 years, and it could be as high as 59.6% within 15 years.[28,29] The outcome is affected by design of the implant connection, with implants with external connections having a higher incidence, with a mean of 18.3% after 5 years,[30–33] whereas screw loosening associated with internal connection was 2.7% after 4.5 years.[28,34–37] It has always been proposed that abutment and prosthetic screws must be tightened with a torque instrument to achieve the required clamping force derived from the recommended torque.

Occlusion and cantilevers are considered important risk factors in the outcome of the implant restoration. Fracture of implants is a terminal failure for implant therapy and is associated with several factors, including material, implant diameter and length, presence of a cantilever, and bruxism.[38] Bruxism may significantly reduce implant survival.[39] The presence of a cantilever in implant prostheses is associated with increased incidence of complications such as veneer fracture and screw loosening.[40] These two factors of increased force and magnification of imposed force should be paramount concerns in treatment planning. Encountering bruxism or increased loading should encourage the use of larger diameter and additional implants as well as the absolute avoidance of cantilevers. Placement of implants using short implants or tilted implants can avoid the requirement of distal cantilevers in many implant prostheses.

Retrieval of the fractured screw depends on whether the screw is loose within the implant or abutment or tightly bound within the screw threads. Many methods have been proposed to remove a fractured screw, including a dental instrument (explorer, hand scaler, ultrasonic scalers) rotated counterclockwise as well as a fork remover in a drill running in reverse. If the head of the screw has been stripped and a driver cannot grasp the screw, drilling a horizontal groove cut into the screw head has been advocated to engage the instrument with a flat-head driver or instrument. There are also many companies that provide screw-retrieval kits; no matter the solution, extra attention must be paid when drilling so as to not damage the internal bore threads, because then the implant might need to be removed.

The prefabricated titanium-bonding base (Ti Base) is used to create a hybrid abutment or a screw-retained implant crown. Although this system offers several advantages, including low component cost, chair-side manufacture, titanium-titanium implant connection, and ability to lute extraorally, there are reports of fracture and Ti Base debonding. These complications may be caused by the small surface area and cross-sectional area of these components. However, clinical data are lacking. Management of the Ti Base debonding consists of using an abutment with a more robust base to support the restoration, including a cast-to abutment system or a CAD/CAM custom abutment (**Fig. 5**).

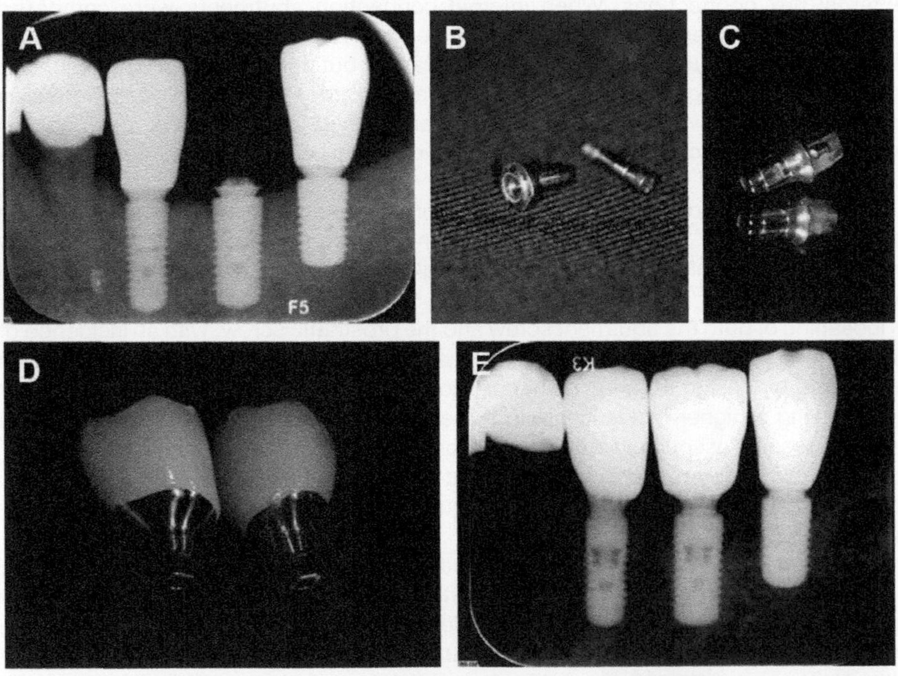

Fig. 5. (*A*) Periapical radiograph shows a restoration with Ti Base abutments, in which the middle abutment fractured. (*B*) Fractured abutment. (*C*) The adjacent crown debonded from the abutment. (*D*) Replacement CAD/CAM abutments with zirconia crowns were manufactured. (*E*) Periapical radiograph of the new prostheses inserted.

MANAGEMENT OF DENTAL IMPLANT PROSTHESIS COMPLICATIONS

Complications involving implant-supported or implant-retained prostheses are common occurrences in dental implant therapy. These complications can range from being minimal and easily managed to catastrophic requiring complex management and even complete replacement of the implant prosthesis.

Prosthetic implant complications for various types and prosthetic designs can be categorized as the following: prosthetic material wear and fracture, loss of retention of overdenture prosthesis, fracture or loss of overdenture attachments, fracture of prosthetic framework, prosthetic screw loosening or fracture, and esthetic complications.

Prosthetic Material Wear and Fracture

This complication can occur in all types of implant reconstructions but occurs in full-arch metal-acrylic resin complete implant fixed prostheses in particular (**Fig. 6**). Bozini and colleagues[1] documented in a meta-analysis that wear and fracture of the veneer material in full-arch metal-acrylic resin complete implant fixed prostheses was the most frequent complication. Sadid-Zadeh and colleagues[28] in a literature review reported an incidence of 3.4% for the fracture of the veneer ceramic and metal-ceramic restorations after 5 years.[29,33,41] Their investigation showed a higher incidence of the complication for posterior implants (3.1%) than for anterior implants (1.7%). It also revealed a higher incidence in external connection implants (5.4%) compared with internal connection implants (2.9%) after 4.7 years. The incidence of veneering material fracture increases to 12.4% in multiunit fixed implant-supported prostheses after 5 years.[37,42,43]

Priest and colleagues[15] documented the need for replacement of denture teeth caused by wear or fracture as the most common prosthetic complication for mandibular full-arch implant-supported prostheses. In addition, they observed that cantilevered frameworks had a high risk of fracture when opposed by fixed prostheses. In contrast, no fractures occurred for any of the frameworks opposed by complete dentures or removable implant prostheses.[15] For such prostheses, replacement of denture teeth and gingival-colored resin while maintaining the supporting metal substructure is a common practice (**Fig. 7**). This protocol is normally implemented to repair fractures or as a reconstruction protocol to address advanced wear of denture teeth and lack of occlusal functionality of prostheses (**Fig. 8**). In metal-ceramic–layered and full-ceramic–layered

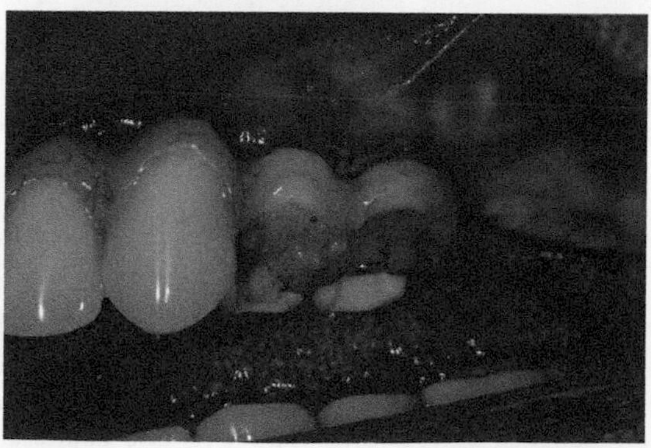

Fig. 6. Intraoral view of fractured prosthetic teeth in a full-arch metal-acrylic resin complete implant fixed prosthesis.

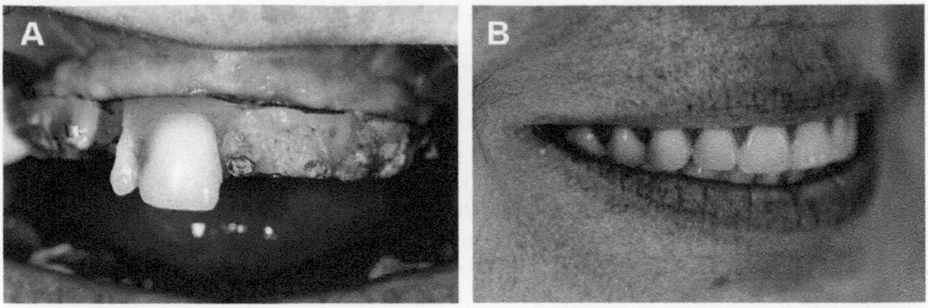

Fig. 7. (*A*) Intraoral frontal view of an extreme case of fractured teeth and acrylic resin in a maxillary full-arch metal-acrylic resin complete implant fixed prosthesis. New teeth were arranged, over existing metal bar, and prosthesis was processed. (*B*) Lateral view of final prosthesis at time of insertion.

full-arch reconstructions, fracture or chipping of the overlying ceramic may occur. The management of such complications may range from minor polishing adjustment of the restoration in cases of minor chipping to complete stripping and replacement of the overlying ceramic in cases of major fractures that significantly affect the esthetics and the functionality of the prosthesis. Protocols such as bonding milled ceramic restoration to existing restorations in a ceramic veneer–like fashion have been used.[44] Moreover, protocols to bond composite resin to repair fractured and chipped ceramic have been reported, although the predictability of this protocol remains questionable.[45] Veneering ceramic chipping and fracture can also occur in single-unit and multiunit partial-arch and short-span fixed implant restorations with rare occurrences of complete fracture of the entire restorative core.[14,46] In cases of major fracture that involves the core restorative material or fracture of the connector area of an implant-supported prosthesis, a complete remake of the prosthesis is normally indicated. **Fig. 9** shows an

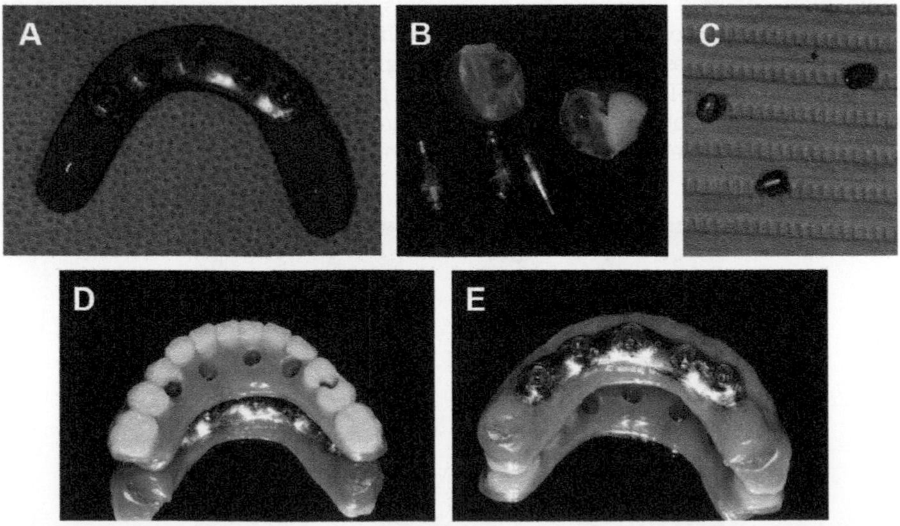

Fig. 8. (*A–E*) Fractured abutments and bridge screws in hybrid prosthesis caused by long cantilevers. Complication managed by replacing abutments and screws and shortening the cantilever. Prosthesis was rehabilitated by replacing prosthetic teeth and gingival-colored acrylic. Note shorter cantilever in new prosthesis.

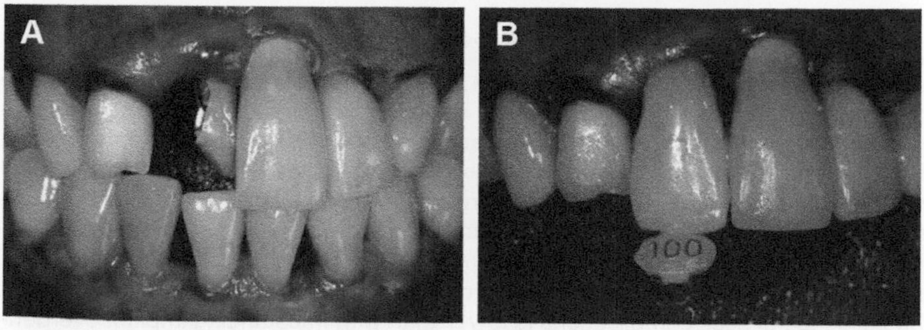

Fig. 9. (*A*) Fracture of a definitive crown. (*B*) Prosthetic failure was managed with a prefabricated polycarbonate provisional crown relined with composite resin–based provisional material.

example of a catastrophic fracture of an anterior implant crown; the fracture was immediately managed by the fabrication of interim restoration using a prefabricated polycarbonate provisional crown form that was relined with composite resin–based provisional material with a full ceramic or metal-ceramic crown as the definitive restoration. In fixed implant-supported prostheses, a common place for fracture is the connector area between pontics and retainers or between pontics. Studies using finite element analysis showed that this is the area of highest stress concentration, especially in cases with minimal interocclusal space and short connectors.[7] This finding reiterates the importance of restorative space in the construction of a robust implant prosthesis. Proper implant planning, design of the prosthesis, managing occlusal stress, choosing proper prosthetic materials, and number of implants are important factors in minimizing complications and material fracture in dental implant therapy[28,47–49] (**Fig. 10**).

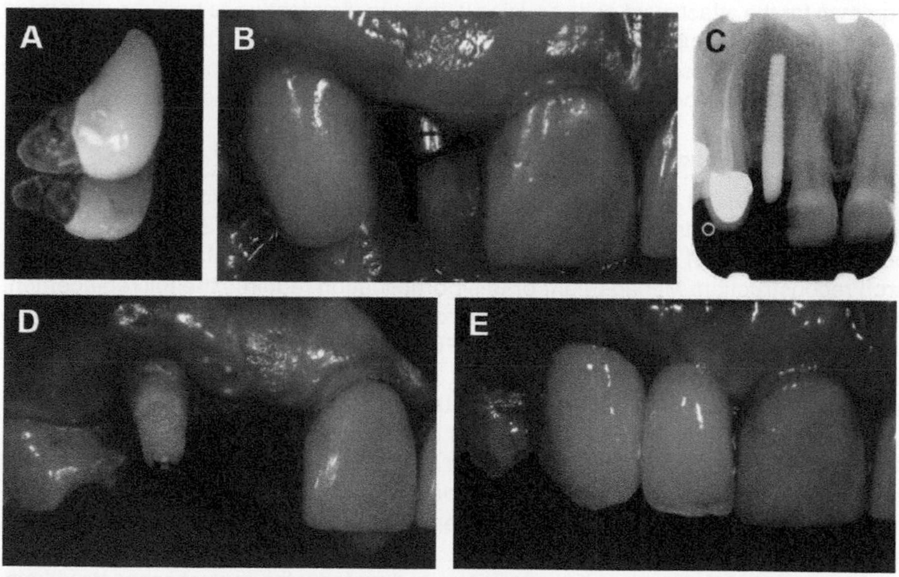

Fig. 10. (*A*) A fractured PFM crown. (*B*) Clinical examination reveals limited interocclusal clearance for the prosthesis. (*C*) Periapical radiograph shows a 1-piece implant system, in which the abutment cannot be changed. (*D*) Clinical view shows that the implant has been buried and adjacent canine prepared for a fixed partial denture. (*E*) Frontal view of definitive cantilever fixed partial denture.

Loss of Retention of Overdenture Prosthesis

Implant overdentures are a reliable option for edentulous patients, particularly in the mandibular arch. However, they require continuous maintenance.[50,51] One of the main complications associated with implant overdentures is loss of retention, which is normally attributed to the wear that occurs in the attachment male insert embedded in the denture base. This complication can be easily managed by replacing the male insert with a new one. However, a discussion with the patient about the need for long-term maintenance and follow-up is paramount for patient satisfaction. Similar complications can occur with bar-supported overdentures, although the literature shows that the incidence of such complications is lower than with freestanding implant overdentures.[14,50] Wear of the overdenture transmucosal abutment in the mouth is another complication that can occur over time, particularly with implants that are off axis and not parallel. To overcome this problem, a new abutment needs to be installed. Such complications are associated with significant treatment cost and need to be addressed with patients in the treatment planning stage. Another factor in the loss of retention in overdenture prostheses is the need for denture relines caused by continuous residual ridge resorption. This complication is common in mandibular 2-implant overdenture prostheses.[51,52] A laboratory or chair-side reline procedure is required to manage this complication.

Fracture or Loss of Overdenture Attachments

Another prosthetic complication related to implant-retained overdenture prostheses is the loss or fracture of the attachment.[14] Fracture of the abutment inside the implant requires the retrieval of the remaining abutment part that is still inside the implant connection. This retrieval has to be done carefully to avoid damaging the connection. Similar techniques for removal of broken abutments or fractured screws must be followed. It is common for the attachment or its housing within the overdenture to become debonded or lost. Intraoral pickup with either a fast-setting repair resin or a light cured composite resin material is necessary and should always be conducted in a closed-mouth position to ensure that this procedure does not alter the established occlusion of the prosthesis.

Fracture of Prosthetic Framework

Complete fracture of a prosthesis framework is a rare complication, but it can occur and present a catastrophic failure of the implant restoration. This complication can occur in all types of prosthetic reconstruction, from single-unit prosthesis to full-arch reconstruction. Management of this complication requires the full replacement of the prosthesis and most of the time a provisional restoration is required while the definitive restoration is being fabricated (**Fig. 11**). If the definitive prosthesis was a metal-ceramic restoration, the framework can be soldered or welded and reused as a framework for the replacement prosthesis. Common areas where fracture of framework occur are connector areas and cantilever segments that extend beyond the acceptable limits.[14,28,46,53] The advent of CAD/CAM frameworks has improved both the design and the manufacture of prostheses. The improved fit of these frameworks avoids the requirement of the soldering or laser welding that created at-risk sites for fracture.

More recently, zirconia has become a favored material for implant reconstructions, particularly large or full-arch prostheses. Systematic reviews favorably report fewer complications for monolithic zirconia restorations.[54,55] However, Ti Base debonding and rare catastrophic fracture are reported. When veneered, chipping of the veneering material is reported. For prostheses constructed using fully veneered zirconia

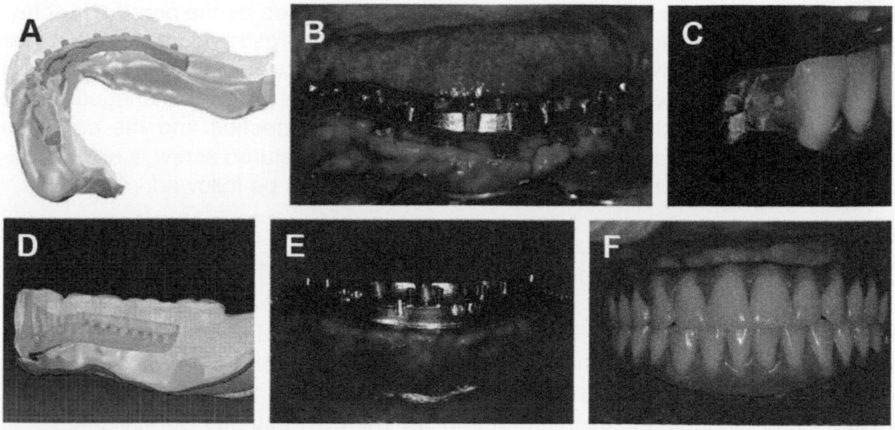

Fig. 11. (*A*) Original design of a titanium CAD/CAM bar for hybrid prosthesis. (*B*) Frontal view of the original titanium framework. (*C*) Fractured metal framework. (*D*) New titanium framework was designed, adding thickness to the structure. (*E*) New framework. (*F*) Intraoral frontal view of new prosthesis.

frameworks, veneer fracture and chipping are more commonly observed[56] and these is not recommended in light of the alternative use of monolithic designs (**Fig. 12**).

Prosthetic Screw Loosening or Fracture

This complication is similar to abutment screw loosening and fracture. Prosthetic (and abutment) screw loosening is more frequently reported than screw fracture.[57] In the

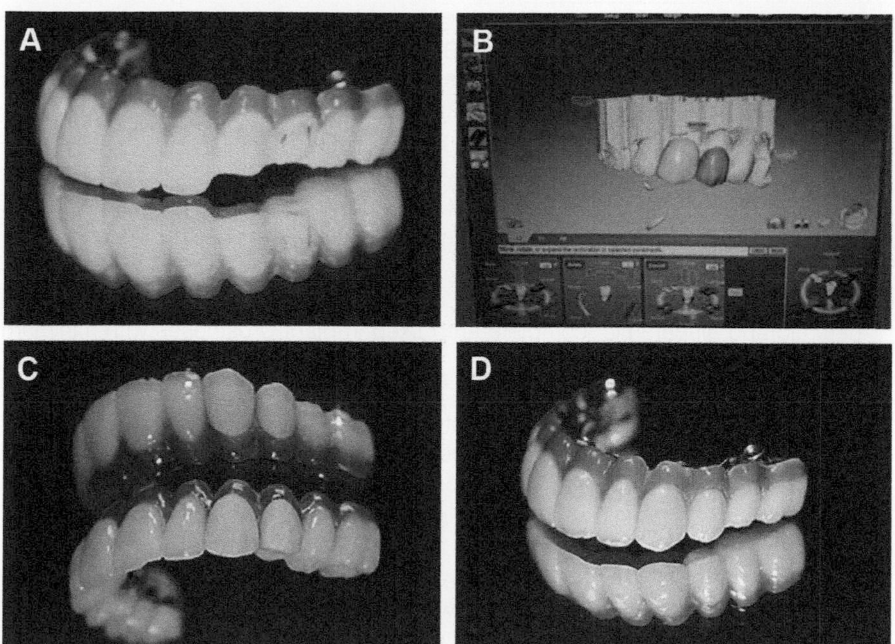

Fig. 12. (*A–D*) Repair of fractured ceramic on a full-arch metal-ceramic implant prosthesis using in-house CAD/CAM system milled lithium disilicate ceramic veneers bonded to the original prosthesis. (*Courtesy of* Dario Zuniga, CDT, Denver, CO).

case of screw-retained restorations, the prosthesis is fixated by the prosthetic screw and loosening or fracture of the screw results in the prosthesis being mobile or completely dislodged. Normally, such a complication can be addressed by tightening and torqueing the screw in case of loosening. The fracture screw is managed by the removal of the remaining screw inside the implant connection and the complete replacement of the prosthetic screw. For retrieving the fractured screw, a similar protocol to that of the fractured abutment screw retrieval can be followed.

Esthetic Complications

Esthetic complications are common in implant therapy. These complications can include shade and contour issues and problems with recession, abutment margin placement, and implant positioning in the occlusogingival or mesiodistal dimensions.[12,16] A detailed discussion of esthetic implant complications is beyond the scope of this article and is presented in detail (see Lyndon F. Cooper and colleagues' article, "Prosthodontic Management of Implant Therapy: Esthetic Complications," in this issue).

REFERENCES

1. Bozini T, Petridis H, Garefis K, et al. A meta-analysis of prosthodontic complication rates of implant-supported fixed dental prostheses in edentulous patients after an observation period of at least 5 years. Int J Oral Maxillofac Implants 2011;26(2):304–18.
2. Hemmings KW, Schmitt A, Zarb GA. Complications and maintenance requirements for fixed prostheses and overdentures in the edentulous mandible: a 5-year report. Int J Oral Maxillofac Implants 1994;9(2):191–6.
3. Jemt T, Book K, Linden B, et al. Failures and complications in 92 consecutively inserted overdentures supported by Branemark implants in severely resorbed edentulous maxillae: a study from prosthetic treatment to first annual check-up. Int J Oral Maxillofac Implants 1992;7(2):162–7.
4. Johns RB, Jemt T, Heath MR, et al. A multicenter study of overdentures supported by Branemark implants. Int J Oral Maxillofac Implants 1992;7(4):513–22.
5. Kiener P, Oetterli M, Mericske E, et al. Effectiveness of maxillary overdentures supported by implants: maintenance and prosthetic complications. Int J Prosthodont 2001;14(2):133–40.
6. Wong CKK, Narvekar U, Petridis H. Prosthodontic complications of metal-ceramic and all-ceramic, complete-arch fixed implant prostheses with minimum 5 years mean follow-up period. a systematic review and meta-analysis. J Prosthodont 2018. https://doi.org/10.1111/jopr.12797.
7. Wang JH, Judge R, Bailey D. A 5-year retrospective assay of implant treatments and complications in private practice: the restorative complications of single and short-span implant-supported fixed prostheses. Int J Prosthodont 2016;29(5):435–44.
8. Gonda T, Maeda Y, Walton JN, et al. Fracture incidence in mandibular overdentures retained by one or two implants. J Prosthet Dent 2010;103(3):178–81.
9. Walton JN, Glick N, Macentee MI. A randomized clinical trial comparing patient satisfaction and prosthetic outcomes with mandibular overdentures retained by one or two implants. Int J Prosthodont 2009;22(4):331–9.
10. Johansson G, Palmqvist S. Complications, supplementary treatment, and maintenance in edentulous arches with implant-supported fixed prostheses. Int J Prosthodont 1990;3(1):89–92.

11. Davis DM, Packer ME, Watson RM. Maintenance requirements of implant-supported fixed prostheses opposed by implant-supported fixed prostheses, natural teeth, or complete dentures: a 5-year retrospective study. Int J Prosthodont 2003;16(5):521–3.
12. Wittneben JG, Buser D, Salvi GE, et al. Complication and failure rates with implant-supported fixed dental prostheses and single crowns: a 10-year retrospective study. Clin Implant Dent Relat Res 2014;16(3):356–64.
13. Sailer I, Muhlemann S, Zwahlen M, et al. Cemented and screw-retained implant reconstructions: a systematic review of the survival and complication rates. Clin Oral Implants Res 2012;23(Suppl 6):163–201.
14. Goodacre CJ, Bernal G, Rungcharassaeng K, et al. Clinical complications with implants and implant prostheses. J Prosthet Dent 2003;90(2):121–32.
15. Priest G, Smith J, Wilson MG. Implant survival and prosthetic complications of mandibular metal-acrylic resin implant complete fixed dental prostheses. J Prosthet Dent 2014;111(6):466–75.
16. Salvi GE, Bragger U. Mechanical and technical risks in implant therapy. Int J Oral Maxillofac Implants 2009;24(Suppl):69–85.
17. Gealh WC, Mazzo V, Barbi F, et al. Osseointegrated implant fracture: causes and treatment. J Oral Implantol 2011;37(4):499–503.
18. Isidor F. Influence of forces on peri-implant bone. Clin Oral Implants Res 2006;17(Suppl 2):8–18.
19. Sheridan RA, Decker AM, Plonka AB, et al. The role of occlusion in implant therapy: a comprehensive updated review. Implant Dent 2016;25(6):829–38.
20. Benic GI, Thoma DS, Munoz F, et al. Guided bone regeneration of peri-implant defects with particulated and block xenogenic bone substitutes. Clin Oral Implants Res 2016;27(5):567–76.
21. Deeb GR, Deeb JG. Soft tissue grafting around teeth and implants. Oral Maxillofac Surg Clin North Am 2015;27(3):425–48.
22. Gjelvold B, Sohrabi MM, Chrcanovic BR. Angled screw channel: an alternative to cemented single-implant restorations–three clinical examples. Int J Prosthodont 2016;29(1):74–6.
23. Barwacz CA, Stanford CM, Diehl UA, et al. Electronic assessment of peri-implant mucosal esthetics around three implant-abutment configurations: a randomized clinical trial. Clin Oral Implants Res 2016;27(6):707–15.
24. Linkevicius T, Apse P. Influence of abutment material on stability of peri-implant tissues: a systematic review. Int J Oral Maxillofac Implants 2008;23(3):449–56.
25. Lemos CAA, Verri FR, Bonfante EA, et al. Comparison of external and internal implant-abutment connections for implant supported prostheses. A systematic review and meta-analysis. J Dent 2018;70:14–22.
26. Zembic A, Kim S, Zwahlen M, et al. Systematic review of the survival rate and incidence of biologic, technical, and esthetic complications of single implant abutments supporting fixed prostheses. Int J Oral Maxillofac Implants 2014;29(Suppl):99–116.
27. Balshi TJ, Hernandez RE, Pryszlak MC, et al. A comparative study of one implant versus two replacing a single molar. Int J Oral Maxillofac Implants 1996;11(3):372–8.
28. Sadid-Zadeh R, Kutkut A, Kim H. Prosthetic failure in implant dentistry. Dent Clin North Am 2015;59(1):195–214.
29. Jemt T. Single implants in the anterior maxilla after 15 years of follow-up: comparison with central implants in the edentulous maxilla. Int J Prosthodont 2008;21(5):400–8.

30. Ekfeldt A, Carlsson GE, Borjesson G. Clinical evaluation of single-tooth restorations supported by osseointegrated implants: a retrospective study. Int J Oral Maxillofac Implants 1994;9(2):179–83.
31. Glauser R, Sailer I, Wohlwend A, et al. Experimental zirconia abutments for implant-supported single-tooth restorations in esthetically demanding regions: 4-year results of a prospective clinical study. Int J Prosthodont 2004;17(3): 285–90.
32. Scheller H, Urgell JP, Kultje C, et al. A 5-year multicenter study on implant-supported single crown restorations. Int J Oral Maxillofac Implants 1998;13(2): 212–8.
33. Vigolo P, Mutinelli S, Givani A, et al. Cemented versus screw-retained implant-supported single-tooth crowns: a 10-year randomised controlled trial. Eur J Oral Implantol 2012;5(4):355–64.
34. Cooper LF, Ellner S, Moriarty J, et al. Three-year evaluation of single-tooth implants restored 3 weeks after 1-stage surgery. Int J Oral Maxillofac Implants 2007;22(5):791–800.
35. Duncan JP, Nazarova E, Vogiatzi T, et al. Prosthodontic complications in a prospective clinical trial of single-stage implants at 36 months. Int J Oral Maxillofac Implants 2003;18(4):561–5.
36. Lops D, Bressan E, Chiapasco M, et al. Zirconia and titanium implant abutments for single-tooth implant prostheses after 5 years of function in posterior regions. Int J Oral Maxillofac Implants 2013;28(1):281–7.
37. Spies BC, Stampf S, Kohal RJ. Evaluation of zirconia-based all-ceramic single crowns and fixed dental prosthesis on zirconia implants: 5-year results of a prospective cohort study. Clin Implant Dent Relat Res 2015;17(5):1014–28.
38. Chrcanovic BR, Kisch J, Albrektsson T, et al. Factors influencing the fracture of dental implants. Clin Implant Dent Relat Res 2018;20(1):58–67.
39. Chrcanovic BR, Kisch J, Albrektsson T, et al. Bruxism and dental implant treatment complications: a retrospective comparative study of 98 bruxer patients and a matched group. Clin Oral Implants Res 2017;28(7):e1–9.
40. Zurdo J, Romao C, Wennstrom JL. Survival and complication rates of implant-supported fixed partial dentures with cantilevers: a systematic review. Clin Oral Implants Res 2009;20(Suppl 4):59–66.
41. Henry PJ, Laney WR, Jemt T, et al. Osseointegrated implants for single-tooth replacement: a prospective 5-year multicenter study. Int J Oral Maxillofac Implants 1996;11(4):450–5.
42. Wahlstrom M, Sagulin GB, Jansson LE. Clinical follow-up of unilateral, fixed dental prosthesis on maxillary implants. Clin Oral Implants Res 2010;21(11): 1294–300.
43. Wennstrom JL, Ekestubbe A, Grondahl K, et al. Oral rehabilitation with implant-supported fixed partial dentures in periodontitis-susceptible subjects. A 5-year prospective study. J Clin Periodontol 2004;31(9):713–24.
44. Wady AF, Paleari AG, Queiroz TP, et al. Repair technique for fractured implant-supported metal-ceramic restorations. A clinical report. J Oral Implantol 2014; 40(5):589–92.
45. Kimmich M, Stappert CF. Intraoral treatment of veneering porcelain chipping of fixed dental restorations: a review and clinical application. J Am Dent Assoc 2013;144(1):31–44.
46. Kreissl ME, Gerds T, Muche R, et al. Technical complications of implant-supported fixed partial dentures in partially edentulous cases after an average observation period of 5 years. Clin Oral Implants Res 2007;18(6):720–6.

47. Bidra AS, Daubert DM, Garcia LT, et al. A systematic review of recall regimen and maintenance regimen of patients with dental restorations. Part 2: implant-borne restorations. J Prosthodont 2016;25(Suppl 1):S16–31.
48. Koyano K, Esaki D. Occlusion on oral implants: current clinical guidelines. J Oral Rehabil 2015;42(2):153–61.
49. Pjetursson BE, Thoma D, Jung R, et al. A systematic review of the survival and complication rates of implant-supported fixed dental prostheses (FDPs) after a mean observation period of at least 5 years. Clin Oral Implants Res 2012; 23(Suppl 6):22–38.
50. Cehreli MC, Karasoy D, Kokat AM, et al. Systematic review of prosthetic maintenance requirements for implant-supported overdentures. Int J Oral Maxillofac Implants 2010;25(1):163–80.
51. Chaffee NR, Felton DA, Cooper LF, et al. Prosthetic complications in an implant-retained mandibular overdenture population: initial analysis of a prospective study. J Prosthet Dent 2002;87(1):40–4.
52. Kreisler M, Behneke N, Behneke A, et al. Residual ridge resorption in the edentulous maxilla in patients with implant-supported mandibular overdentures: an 8-year retrospective study. Int J Prosthodont 2003;16(3):295–300.
53. Pjetursson BE, Bragger U, Lang NP, et al. Comparison of survival and complication rates of tooth-supported fixed dental prostheses (FDPs) and implant-supported FDPs and single crowns (SCs). Clin Oral Implants Res 2007; 18(Suppl 3):97–113.
54. Abdulmajeed AA, Lim KG, Narhi TO, et al. Complete-arch implant-supported monolithic zirconia fixed dental prostheses: a systematic review. J Prosthet Dent 2016;115(6):672–677 e1.
55. Bidra AS, Rungruanganunt P, Gauthier M. Clinical outcomes of full arch fixed implant-supported zirconia prostheses: a systematic review. Eur J Oral Implantol 2017;10(Suppl 1):35–45.
56. Stefanescu C, Ionita C, Nechita V, et al. Survival rates and complications for zirconia-based fixed dental prostheses in a period up to 10 years: a systematic review. Eur J Prosthodont Restor Dent 2018;26(2):54–61.
57. Romeo E, Storelli S. Systematic review of the survival rate and the biological, technical, and aesthetic complications of fixed dental prostheses with cantilevers on implants reported in longitudinal studies with a mean of 5 years follow-up. Clin Oral Implants Res 2012;23(Suppl 6):39–49.

Biomaterials

Ceramic and Adhesive Technologies

Robert R. Seghi, DDS, MS[a,*], Diana Leyva del Rio, DDS, MS[b]

KEYWORDS

• Y-TZP • Ceramics • Adhesive cements • Fracture

KEY POINTS

- Ceramic systems have varying degrees of research to support their use.
- Adhesive cements are changing based on knowledge gained from older materials. New cements are designed to accomplish durable bonding with fewer steps.
- The relationship between the cement used and crown survival is not well understood.

INTRODUCTION

Improvement in the optical and mechanical properties of dental ceramic materials coupled with improved production techniques have largely caused a shift in the type of fixed restorations dentists are prescribing. The complete crown procedure remains the most common fixed prosthodontic procedure prescribed by dentists. It has been estimated that in 2012 about 54.5 million indirect restorations were placed in the United States.[1] Most of those units were most likely single crowns. In a recent survey of 1777 dentists enrolled in the National Practice-Based Research Network, it was estimated that for single-unit crowns, the top 3 choices for anterior crowns were lithium disilicate (54%), layered zirconia (17%), and leucite-reinforced glass-ceramics (13%).[2] Less than 10% prescribed the more traditional metal-ceramic restorations. For posterior teeth, the top 3 choices for crowns were full contour zirconia (32%), porcelain fused to metal (31%), and lithium disilicate (21%).[2] The profession has made a dramatic shift toward the increased use of all-ceramic materials for crowns.

This review focuses on the ceramic materials most often prescribed and some newly developed glass-ceramic materials. There are many ceramic systems that will not be discussed, and more complete reviews on all-ceramic materials can be found elsewhere.[2–4] With respect to cements, this review focuses on the adhesive cements that are used in conjunction with dental ceramic crowns. Finally, this review discusses

Disclosure Statement: The Authors have nothing to disclose.

[a] Division of Restorative and Prosthetic Dentistry, The Ohio State University College of Dentistry, 305 West 12th Avenue, Room 3005H, Columbus, OH 43210-1267, USA; [b] Oral Biology, The Ohio State University College of Dentistry, 305 West 12th Avenue, Room 3037D, Columbus, OH 43210-1267, USA
* Corresponding author.
E-mail address: seghi.1@osu.edu

Dent Clin N Am 63 (2019) 233–248
https://doi.org/10.1016/j.cden.2018.11.005

crown fracture with respect to the ceramic/cement interface. For the purposes of discussion, the ceramics are characterized into 2 categories: silica-based ceramics and non–silica-based ceramics; this categorization method is related to the types of cementation techniques suggested.

ALL-CERAMIC MATERIALS

The silica-based ceramics are the oldest of the two categories, with the introduction of the feldspathic porcelain jacket crown in the early 1900s having evolved into the much stronger glass-ceramic materials in routine use today. The fluormica-based glass-ceramic (DICOR) introduced in 1984 was the first dental application of an all–glass-ceramic material for crown fabrication. The lithium disilicate (LDS) glass-ceramics have nearly a 20-year record in service with good clinical data to support their use. The new zirconia-containing lithium silicate (LS) glass-ceramics have been developed to compete with the very popular LDS glass-ceramics. InCeram (Vita), the first non–silica-based dental ceramic, was introduced into dentistry in 1990. The dense sintered zirconia polycrystalline ceramics have been the dominant ceramics in this category for some time and represent the product that is experiencing the most rapid developmental changes (**Table 1**).

Table 1
Ceramic categories with example products

	Silica-Based Ceramics	
Lithium disilicate glass-ceramics	Zirconia lithium silicate glass-ceramics	Other silica-based ceramics
IPS e.max Press (Ivoclar/Vivadent)	Obsidian (Glidewell Laboratory)	IPS Empress Esthetic (Ivoclar/Vivadent)
IPS e.max CAD (Ivoclar/Vivadent)	Celtra Press (Dentsply Sirona)	IPS Empress CAD (Ivoclar/Vivadent)
	Celtra Duo (Dentsply Sirona)	VitaBlocs Mark II (Vita Zahnfabrik)
	Suprinity (Vita Zahnfabrik)	
	Non–Silica-Based Ceramics (Y-TZP)	
Original zirconia formula	High-translucency zirconia	Ultrahigh-translucency zirconia
Lava Frame (3M ESPE)	Lava Plus (3M ESPE)	Lava Esthetic (3M ESPE)
Zenostar MO (Ivoclar/Vivadent)	Zenostar T (Ivoclar/Vivadent)	Zenostar MT (Ivoclar/Vivadent)
Cercon base (Dentsply Sirona)	Cercon ht (Dentsply Sirona)	Cercon xt (Dentsply Sirona)
	Prettau Zirconia (Zirconzahn)	Prettau Anterior (Zirconzahn)
	Bruxir (Glidwell Laboratory)	Bruxir Anterior (Glidwell Laboratory)
	Katana HT/ML (Kuraray/Noritake)	Katana UTML/STML (Kuraray/Noritake)

Silica-Based Dental Ceramics

Lithium disilicate glass-ceramics

LDS glass-ceramic, the first glass-ceramic developed,[5] provided knowledge from fundamental studies using this system, which formed the basis for further development of many different glass-ceramic materials. LDS glass-ceramic was introduced for crown application in 1998 by Ivoclar Vivadent. The material was marketed first as Empress 2 and later as eMax Press and eMax CAD. It is the most well documented and successful long-term all-ceramic crown material currently in use. Over time it has become a major restorative choice for single anterior crowns and to a lesser extent for posterior crowns.[2]

A more complex multicomponent LDS system with increased translucency, easy machinability, and decreased reactivity with the refractory investment were all modifications needed to accommodate esthetic crown fabrication.[6,7] LDS glass-ceramics required certain compositional and processing modifications to result in the strong (400 MPa), tough (2.5 MPa $m^{1/2}$), and translucent (55%) structure that is used today.[6]

Detailed analysis of the thermal process for this particular glass-ceramic formulation has shown that there are actually 2 major crystal phases that begin to form at about 500°C.[6,8,9] The lithium metasilicate (LMS) Li_2SiO_3 crystals dominate at the lower temperatures with only minor amounts of the LDS (Li_2Si2O_5) crystallites being present initially. At temperatures higher than 750°C, a secondary crystallization process occurs whereby the LMS crystals react with the surrounding glass to form additional LDS crystals with the aid of an intermediate lithium orthophosphate Li_3PO_4 (LOP) nucleating agent. Under very specific heating conditions, the LMS crystals can be fully dissolved and the final product is composed entirely of LDS crystals (70 vol%) and a small amount of residual glass. It is less well known that LDS glass-ceramics contain a small amount of ZrO_2 (3%–4%), which has been shown to help increase translucency.[6]

The LDS is supplied in 2 different crystalline states depending on the application. The CAD form (eMax CAD) is supplied in a precrystallized state that is more easily machined. The CAD form is primarily glassy with evidence of the presence of LMS and LOP crystals,[10] which gives the e.max CAD milling blanks their characteristic "blue block" appearance. The milled restoration is subsequently heat treated to allow the crystallization process to continue to completion. In the final form the glass-ceramic contains primarily LDS crystals. The pressable pellets (e.max Press) supplied by the manufacturer are in the fully crystallized state. The influence of these differences on clinical performance is unknown.

Several clinical trials and meta-analysis of its performance as single crowns (SCs) has been reported. The cumulative survival meta-analysis of LDS SCs reported a 5-year survival rate of 97.8%.[11] In another meta-analysis, which combined studies that included both LDS and leucite-reinforced glass-ceramics, the 5-year survival rate was 95.6% for SCs. The 8-year cumulative survival rates for Empress 2 were reported to be 94.8% for SCs.[11] Most recently the 10-year cumulative survival rates of Empress 2 restorations were reported to be 81% for SCs and 93.4% for implant-supported crowns.[12] A 10-year evaluation of molar crowns manufactured from e.max CAD materials was reported to be 83.5%.[13]

Lithium silicate glass-ceramics

LS glass-ceramics are the newest glass-ceramic materials designed for crown applications. They were introduced in 2013 as zirconia-reinforced lithium silicate (ZLS) glass-ceramics, a stronger alternative to the LDS material. Commercially this material is marketed as Celtra (Dentsply Sirona) and Suprinity PC (Vita). The materials are similar in composition, as they were developed in a collaborative effort between the 2 manufacturers and the Fraunhofer Institute for Silicate Research in Wurzburg, Germany. Glidwell Dental laboratories, has introduced its own version of this material that is marketed under the name of Obsidian.

The microstructure has been examined by several investigators.[10,14,15] In the fully crystallized form, these materials consist primarily of LMS crystals with minor amounts of LDS and LOP. The low concentration of tetragonal zirconia (10%) is not detectable by Raman spectroscopy and only slightly detectable by x-ray diffraction spectroscopy. Because the ZrO_2 crystals remain in the residual glass they are marketed as ZLS glass-ceramics. Whether they actually contribute to the overall strength of the final glass-ceramic product is unclear.

In the CAD form, the glass-ceramic is supplied in either a precrystallized or fully crystallized form. The precrystallized form is easier to machine because it is primarily a glassy structure with a small amount of very fine precipitated crystals of LMS and LOP.[10] The machined precrystallized crown is subsequently heat treated to produce the fully crystallized form of the glass-ceramic. In the fully crystallized form they have strengths comparable with or greater than e.max CAD.[16–18] These ceramics have demonstrated easier polishability[19] and slightly more translucency than e.max CAD.[17,20] There is little reported on the pressable form of this new glass-ceramic, but it would be expected to be similar. The manufacturer's information (Celtra Press FactFile) shows the pressing pellets to contain very small plate-like crystals initially and larger more needle-like crystals after pressing, indicating that some crystal growth occurs during the pressing cycle. The unique characteristic of Obsidian[21] is that this LS glass-ceramic composition containing 1% to 10% germanium, which claims to make the material more castable by lowering its viscosity and increasing the thermal expansion and the refractive index of the glass.[21] This allows the material to be pressed to metal. No independent laboratory or clinical data are available for this material, but it is expected to be similar to the other products in this category.

Only one clinical evaluation of Celtra Duo CAD/CAM LS restorations could be found in the literature. The success rate after 1 year was reported to be 96.7% with 2 failures out of 60 restorations being reported from bulk fractures.[22] Further long-term clinical results are needed to fully understand the clinical performance of these materials.

Non–Silica-Based Dental Ceramics

Polycrystalline zirconia

Of the non–silica-based ceramics in use today, dense sintered polycrystalline zirconia is the most commonly prescribed all-ceramic crown material.[2] Its rapid increasing rate of application is attributed to its high strength, high toughness, reasonable esthetics, and claims by manufacturers and laboratories to be strong enough for use on posterior teeth even with a relatively conservative preparation.

The first commercial application of a dense sintered polycrystalline core material was Procera (Nobel Biocare). The Procera process was significant because it was the first commercial application of CAD/CAM manufacturing used within the laboratory industry. In the initial introduction, 99.9% alumina was used as the core material. The initial alumina coping materials generated strengths in the area of 550 MPa. Later, yttria-stabilized tetragonal zirconia oxide (Y-TZP) copings became available with much higher strength (>1200 MPa) and toughness (4.4 MPa $m^{1/2}$).[23] The high cost of CAM equipment led to a business model, which had local laboratories scan the die with a digital scanner, design the coping, and send the design file via the Internet to one of two worldwide manufacturing sites. The coping was returned to the laboratory within 3 days. The local laboratory applied the porcelain veneer to the coping, completing the crown within the same timeframe as a metal-ceramic crown. The concept soon led other manufacturers to follow (ie, LAVA, 3M-ESPE, CERCON: Densply).

Unlike pure aluminum oxide (Al_2O_3) powders, pure zirconium oxide (ZrO_2) powders are not able to be formed into a dense solid structure directly.[24,25] The stresses generated on cooling from the smaller tetragonal crystals transforming to larger monoclinic crystals create stresses and cracking.[24,25] Strengthened zirconia was first developed in the 1970s[26,27] and details of the toughening mechanism have been described.[25] Since the initial introduction of this material to dentistry, it has undergone several formulation changes and these have been summarized in some detail.[28]

The zirconia products originally introduced in dentistry were 3 mol% yttria-stabilized tetragonal polycrystal (3Y-TZP). This material had the characteristics of high strength (>1100 MPa), high toughness (>4 GPa), high stiffness (>200 GPa), and high opacity. The high opacity limited their application to crown substructures. These original formulations are still applicable for layered crowns and very demanding structural applications such as implant-supported complete prostheses and long-span tooth-supported fixed dental prostheses. Much of the clinical longevity data that have been reported are from these layered crowns.[29,30] Layered zirconia was demonstrated to have higher chipping rates than metal-ceramics.[31,32] Several factors were thought to contribute to this clinical observation, and current chipping rates have been reduced.[33]

The opaque nature of zirconia arises because of the birefringence character of the tetragonal crystals, the size of the crystals, and issues related to light scattering at the grain boundaries, which contain pores and impurities.[34] Changes in formulations for the newer zirconia materials have been discussed.[28,35] The first improvements were designed to modify the grain size and the grain boundaries through improved heat treatments and minor dopant composition changes.[28,35] The translucency changes were modest and had little effect on the mechanical properties, making them suitable for monolithic posterior crowns.[35] Many clinicians were introduced to this application through an online video displaying a monolithic zirconia crown being hammered into a piece of wood with no damage to the crown. Although this test has no relationship to clinical performance, the visual did have an impact on encouraging dentists to try these ceramics for posterior crowns. In addition, it was purported that reduced preparation dimensions and survival rates were similar to those of cast metal, and laboratories were supporting the claims with a 5- to 7-year manufacturer material warranty. The clinical performances of conservative monolithic crowns are beginning to appear in the literature.[36–39] That there are few anecdotal or scientific reports of unusual problems with millions of units already in service is encouraging.

The ultrahigh-translucency zirconia is the latest generation of newly formulated compositions. These materials have increased their translucency by increasing the yttria dopant from 3 mol% to as high as 5 mol%. The higher yttria content stabilizes more cubic zirconia into the final polycrystalline structure. The cubic phase does not have the high scattering effect that the tetragonal stabilized crystals do, leading to higher translucencies. However, these materials do have a somewhat diminished fracture toughness (2.5 GPa) and strength (700 MPa).[28]

Much has been written concerning the potential susceptibility of Y-TZP to low-temperature degradation (LTD), and this process has been reviewed in detail.[40] The issue first arose from work done to understand a problem related to the premature failure of the Y-TZP ceramic heads on hip implants.[41] The basic mechanism that gives this ceramic its unusual toughness and strength characteristics also exposes a potential Achilles heel. The crystal transformation induced by stresses can slow crack propagation, but the same process also can occur spontaneously by reaction with water, potentially leading to microcracking and strength loss.[40] This reaction is autocatalytic, but the kinetics of the degradation process are greatly accelerated by temperature.[40,42] Researchers study the process at elevated temperatures of 137°C to accelerate the effect. It was estimated that 1 h under these conditions is equivalent to 4 years of service in vivo.[42] Numerous laboratory studies have reported on the effects of accelerated LTD on zirconia properties. The depth to which the LTD process penetrates the surface depends on the specific materials and amount of time held at 137°C, but is usually confined to the surface 5 to 10 μm.[43,44] Even under the most extreme aging conditions, strength and toughness are either unaffected or only modestly decreased.[44,45] Significant decreases in strength were noted only after more than 100 h of accelerated aging, comparable with 300 years.[44] Keuper and colleagues[46] have examined the LTD process at 37°C and have estimated the rate of progression to be 0.5 μm/y (1 grain/y). Although the process will progress over time, based on these findings the strength levels would not be affected for tens of years.[46] There is clearly a need to understand this process under more clinically relevant conditions.

ADHESIVE CEMENTS FOR ALL-CERAMIC RESTORATIONS

Adhesive cements are broadly categorized into 2 groups: water-based cements or resin-based cements (**Table 2**). The current range of cements actually exists as a spectrum of materials that share characteristics of each group. Cements that require the application of a dental adhesive before cementation are considered to be more "composite-like" while those requiring no adhesive before cementation are considered more "glass-ionomer–like." New developments in cements and adhesives have resulted from improved the understanding of the chemical and structural features of the interface that exists between dentin and adhesive materials. The use of visual and chemical analytical methods including transmission electron microscopy, field-emission scanning electron microscopy, x-ray photoelectron spectroscopy, infrared spectroscopy, and advanced sample preparation methods have advanced this knowledge, leading to the introduction of the newest class of cements and adhesives that are considered to be self-etching and self-adhesive.

Glass Ionomers and Resin-Modified Glass-Ionomer Cement

According to market research, the cement market was valued at US$784 million in 2016.[47] Overall this segment of the industry is dominated by glass-ionomer (GI) cements with the resin-modified glass ionomers (RMGI) being the most important. GI is still considered the one material that self-adheres to mineralized tissues.[48,49] Knowledge gained from understanding the nature of this interface has inspired the design of a new generation of self-etch adhesives and cements.

For GI restorative materials, the teeth are cleaned with polyacrylic acid to remove the smear layer and expose a clean surface of intact collagen fibrils allowing the cement mix to interdiffuse, establishing a micromechanical bond through a very thin (1 μm) hybrid layer.[50] Chemical bonding occurs through the interaction of the carboxylic acid groups on the polyacrylic acid chains with the calcium ions of the hydroxyapatite crystals that remain associated with the exposed collagen fibrils.[48,49] Because the polymer chains in the GI liquid are relatively large compared with the monomers found in dental adhesives, the hybrid layer formed is shallow. The high viscosity renders them unable to diffuse a phosphoric acid etched dentin surface, which is much deeper and more demineralized.

The RMGIs were developed to improve on the less desirable properties of conventional GIs while maintaining the desirable properties. Despite their relatively low reported

Table 2
Adhesive cement categories with example products

Water-Based Adhesive Cements		
Glass-Ionomer Cement	**Resin-Modified GI Cements**	**Other Water-Based Cements**
Ketac Cem (3M ESPE)	Rely X Luting (3M ESPE)	Zinc phosphate (Fleck's-Mizzy)
Fuji 1 Cement (GC America)	Fuji Cem 2 (GC)	Zinc polycarboxylate (Durelon-3M)
VivaGlas Cem PL (Ivoclar)	Rivia Luting Plus (SDI)	
Hy-Bond CX plus (Shofu)	Nexus RMGI (Kerr)	
Resin-Based Cements		
Self-Adhesive Resin Cements (DC)	**Adhesive-Assisted Resin Cements**	
[a]Rely X Unicem (3M ESPE)	DC Cements	SC-Only or LC-Only Cements[b]
[a]Panavia SA Cement Plus (Kuraray)	[a]Panavia F 2.0 with [a]SEA (Kuraray)	[a]Panavia 21 SC with [a]SEA (Kuraray)
[a]Maxcem Elite (Kerr)	Panavia V5 with [a]SEA (Kuraray)	
[a]SmartCem2 (Dentsply)	[a]Rely X Ultimate with [a]SEA or [a]ERA (3M)	[b]NX3 Nexus LC with [a]SEA or ERA (Kerr)
[a]SpeedCem (Ivoclar)	VariolinkEsthetics DC with [a]SEA or [a]ERA (Ivoclar)	[b]Variolink Esthetics LC with [a]ERA or [a]SEA (Ivolclar)
BisCem (Bisco)	Multilink with [a]SEA (Ivoclar)	[b]Rely X Veneer Cement LC with [a]ERA (3M)
	NX3 Nexus DC with SEA or ERA (Kerr)	
	NX3 XTR with [a]SEA (Kerr)	

Abbreviations: DC, dual cured; ERA, etch and rinse adhesive; SC, self-cured only; SEA, self-etch adhesive.

[a] Contains a phosphate ester modified resin in its formulation.

[b] LC = light cured: light cured-only cements are generally not recommended for complete crowns.

bond strengths, the interface between the RMGI and dentin has been shown to be very durable when used to restore class-5 noncarious lesions. Retention rates are comparable with or better than other adhesive strategies that report much higher bond strengths.[51,52] Their outstanding clinical retention rates caused researchers to examine more carefully the nature of this interface, revealing evidence that they undergo similar mechanical and ionic reactions demonstrated by conventional GI cements.[53–56] The formulations for these materials vary somewhat but are essentially high molecular weight polyacrylic acid chains that have a small proportion of functional methacrylate groups grafted along the polymer chains. The remaining carboxylic acid groups render the polymers hydrophilic enough to combine into a water/HEMA mixture.[57,58] When mixed with the typical acid-soluble glasses found in conventional GIs they have the capability of setting through both ionic and free radical polymerization reactions. The incorporation of a resin component gives them some improved physical properties and handling characteristics over conventional GIs. Morphologic examination of the RMGIs/dentin interface shows 2 distinct structures depending on the application technique. The RMGIs that use a conditioner before application form a submicron hybrid layer with a deposition of a submicron gel phase immediately adjacent.[55] Those that did not call for an application of a dentin conditioner made intimate contact with the unaffected dentin but showed no evidence of a similar submicron hybrid layer. Both interface types perform well clinically, suggesting that the primary bonding mechanisms for these materials is a chemical interaction with some micromechanical interlocking.[55] The manufacturers of RMGI cements do not generally require that the dentin be conditioned before cementation, perhaps because cement formulations are polyacrylic acid rich in their mixtures to assure lower viscosity than comparable restorative materials, allowing them to wet the surface more completely and leaving them more capable of self-etching. Until the introduction of high-strength zirconia, the RMGI cements had enjoyed more limited use for all-ceramic crown cementation.[59]

Adhesive-Assisted Resin Cements

Resin cements have been the most commonly used cements to support all-ceramic restorations.[59] Like resin composite restorations, they rely on the application of an adhesive before cementation to facilitate bonding. Changes to resin cement systems have essentially mirrored the developments of dental adhesives. The changes to adhesives have been a direct result of our improved knowledge of the interface chemistry and morphology. Although numerous products exist in this category, there are no clinical data that support the use of one resin cement system over another when used to support all-ceramic crowns.[59]

Adhesive-assisted resin cement systems can be categorized by either the curing modes—chemical or self-cured, light cured (LC), and dual cured (DC), or by the type of adhesive used—"total etch," etch and rinse, or self-etch.[60,61] The indication for each of these cements depends on the clinical situation. For thin, translucent ceramics, such as laminate veneers, LC resins provide infinite working time, and concerns about potential discolorations from the amine/BPO or unreacted bonds in self-cured and DC systems can be minimized.[62–64] For more opaque ceramics or areas where the cement is far from the surface of the ceramic, self-cured or DC cements are preferred because postcure discoloration does not affect the overall appearance of the restoration. The choice of resin cements is based on clinician preference rather than performance.

The etch and rinse techniques became popularized in the early 1990s.[65,66] Although these systems were available by 1978,[67] and the concept of the hybrid layer was first described in 1982,[68] it took more than a decade for most dentists in the United States to adopt the technique. Improved retention rates and bond strengths along with an improved understanding of the role of the smear layer helped popularize the etch and rinse techniques. The original 3-step systems utilize a low-viscosity hydrophilic monomer mixture in a solvent that is applied onto the etched dentin surface, allowing for good diffusion into the mineral-depleted collagen-rich dentin layer, forming a hybrid of cured resin and collagen fibrils. This layer seals the surface and allows a second layer of a more hydrophobic resin to be applied before cementation with a resin cement. The 3-step etch and rinse adhesive systems remain the gold standard by which clinical retention rates are judged.[59,60] The 2-step etch and rinse systems were followed by combining the components of the 2 bottles into one, simplifying the cementation and bonding procedure. As the interface of the etch and rinse systems were more carefully evaluated, it became clear that perfect hybridization between demineralized collagen was not possible and that by demineralizing the collagen we make it more susceptible to degradation. Details of the factors involved in the process have been recently reviewed.[69]

The clinicians' desire to simplify the adhesive process and improved scientific understanding of the interface of our current adhesives have helped researchers and manufacturers move away from etch and rinse systems in trying to establish a more durable interface akin to resin-modified GIs. The modern clinical application of self-etching adhesives is similar to the techniques used in the 1980s when the enamel was preferentially etched and the "smear layer modifier" adhesives were applied to the enamel and dentine surfaces. The phrase "selective etch" was not yet conceived, but was being applied. The formulations of these self-etch systems have changed; the components are often the components found in early adhesives. The clinical outcomes of these adhesives show the most variability in clinical trials because their formulations are different and have changed over time. In the class-5 restoration model used to evaluate clinical performance, the 2-step self-etch systems seem to outperform the 1-step self-etch systems lesion just as the 3-step etch and rinse systems seem to outperform the 2-step etch and rinse systems.[51,52,70]

Self-Adhesive Cements

The self-adhesive resin cements have captured the interest of clinicians because they are easy to use and offer the promise of adhesion to dentin without the prior application of bonding agent. The first cement marketed in this category was Rely X Unicem (3M/ESPE), and its popularity has driven other manufacturers to develop similar products in this category. A detailed review of this cement category has been reported by Ferracane and colleagues.[71] The components that make up these materials look similar to the polyacid modified resins referred to as compomers. They generally contain traditional hydrophobic dimethacrylates and silanated silica-based glass fillers traditionally found in resin composites. In addition, they contain acid-soluble fillers similar to those found in glass ionomers and carboxylated or phosphorylated methacrylates. The phosphorylated methacrylates are of most interest because they are highly acidic, hydrophilic, and often more reactive than the carboxylic acid derivatives, and are found in many self-etching adhesive formulations. The acid-functionalized monomers are used to achieve demineralization and attachment to the dentin. The ratio of hydrophilic acid functional groups to hydrophobic methacrylate groups can be controlled by the ratio of these monomers in the starting composition. The ratio of these components must be balanced to achieve an acceptable degree of self-etching character and dentin bonding without making the resin too hydrophilic to cause swelling. The initially hydrophilic nature of the material facilitates wetting and, thus, adaptation to the dentin. The surface acid groups can react with Ca^{+} ions in hydroxyapatite and with ions that are released from the acid-soluble glass fillers. As stable salts form, the material becomes more hydrophobic. Because these materials do not appear to contain water in their initial mix, the neutralization of the acid functional groups within the body of the cement cannot occur until water is absorbed or reaction products that generate water become available.

Morphologic examination of the interface shows that the cement is well adapted to the dentin, but there is little evidence of significant penetration through the smear layer to form a detectable hybrid zone.[72,73] In the case of one RMGI (Vitrebond), intimate contact without hybridization was observed and the clinical performance was comparable with that of the most effective dental adhesive systems.[51,52] Unicem has been shown an increase chemical interaction with Ca from HAp, which helps explain its reasonable bond strengths.[74,75] It is possible that these cement types could benefit from the prior application of a dentin conditioner to exposed the HAp associated with intact dentin.

Limited clinical studies have been reported for the use of self-etching cements with ceramic restorations. Three studies reported the survival of partial ceramic crowns cemented with Rely X Unicem on teeth that were unetched and teeth that were selectively etched.[76–78] The results after 2 to 3 years in all studies showed little difference between the 2 groups. However, one group reported the results after 6.5 years, revealing that the selective etch group had significantly higher survival rates (82%) compared with the unetched group (60%).[76] No studies could be found on the performance of this cement with monolithic Y-TZP crowns. Because of its reactive phosphate ester pendant groups the cement has some potential to attach to metal ions, making it suitable as a zirconia or metal cement. One study compared the use of Rely X Unicem with traditional zinc phosphate cement and found no difference at 6 years.[79]

THE CROWN TOOTH COMPLEX

Loads applied to the occlusal surfaces of crowns during mastication generate Hertzian contact stresses directly around the cusp contact area as well as tensile stresses on the intaglio or cement surface.[80] Fractographic analysis of failed clinical crowns suggest that the most common location for fracture initiation is from the intaglio surface of the crown and not from the contact surface.[81–86] Chipping results from stresses generated at the contact surface and is an important ceramic failure mode for layered ceramics. As the profession shifts from layered crowns toward monolithic crowns made from ceramics that are stronger and tougher, chipping is likely to be reduced. Fractographic analysis of failed crowns suggests that many cracks originate from areas close to the margins.[83,84,86,87] As the walls of ceramic crowns become thinner, the probability of failure is likely to increase. By providing patients with ceramic crowns on conservatively prepared teeth, there is a potential risk of earlier failures. Despite this potential risk, there are some data to suggest that these crown types are likely to have a reasonable lifespan.[88–90]

The role that the cement plays on the overall survival of a crown is unclear. Most reviews have concluded that adhesive cements are necessary to reinforce at least the moderate-strength glass-ceramics.[91,92] These conclusions are based on laboratory data demonstrating that ceramics cemented with resin can sustain greater loads to failure than ceramics with conventional cements. However, several clinical studies have found that the survival of ceramic crowns did not seem to be influenced by cement type (conventional versus resin).[93–97] To improve our understanding of the fracture process and the role that the cement plays on overall survival of a crown, there is a need for laboratory models that simulate clinical crown failure modes under clinical loading conditions.[98–100] More work is needed to understand this interaction.

The profession is shifting to the use of high-strength, thin-walled, monolithic ceramics to crown teeth. The claim that these ceramics are as strong as metal and can be utilized with conservative tooth preparations is an attractive one. Despite the lack of adequate scientific data, many dentists are choosing to believe the claims in the hope that the data will one day be supported. Failure from fracture is still the main concern for dentists. There is clearly a need to develop testing methods that can predict the clinical behavior of thin-walled ceramic crowns. For ceramics materials, the inherent flaws that are present at the time of restoration delivery are perhaps the most limiting factor with respect to fracture initiation and propagation. To optimize performance, we need to understand the failure process more completely.

REFERENCES

1. Christensen GJ. Is the rush to all-ceramic crowns justified? J Am Dent Assoc 2014;145(2):192–4.
2. Makhija SK, Lawson NC, Gilbert GH, et al. Dentist material selection for single-unit crowns: findings from the National Dental Practice-Based Research Network. J Dent 2016;55:40–7.
3. Denry I, Kelly J. Emerging ceramic-based materials for dentistry. J Dent Res 2014;93(12):1235–42.
4. Zhang Y, Kelly JR. Dental ceramics for restoration and metal veneering. Dent Clin North Am 2017;61(4):797–819.
5. Stookey S. Catalyzed crystallization of glass in theory and practice. Ind Eng Chem 1959;51(7):805–8.
6. Holand W, Beall GH. Glass ceramic technology. John Wiley & Sons; 2012.
7. Schweiger M, von Clausbruch SC, Höland W, et al. Process for the preparation of shaped translucent lithium disilicate glass ceramic products. Google Patents; 2002.
8. Lien W, Roberts HW, Platt JA, et al. Microstructural evolution and physical behavior of a lithium disilicate glass–ceramic. Dent Mater 2015;31(8):928–40.
9. Höland W, Apel E, van't Hoen C, et al. Studies of crystal phase formations in high-strength lithium disilicate glass-ceramics. J Non Cryst Solids 2006; 352(38–39):4041–50.
10. Belli R, Wendler M, de Ligny D, et al. Chairside CAD/CAM materials. Part 1: measurement of elastic constants and microstructural characterization. Dent Mater 2017;33(1):84–98.
11. Gehrt M, Wolfart S, Rafai N, et al. Clinical results of lithium-disilicate crowns after up to 9 years of service. Clin Oral Investig 2013;17(1):275–84.
12. Teichmann M, Göckler F, Weber V, et al. Ten-year survival and complication rates of lithium-disilicate (Empress 2) tooth-supported crowns, implant-supported crowns, and fixed dental prostheses. J Dent 2017;56:65–77.
13. Rauch A, Reich S, Dalchau L, et al. Clinical survival of chair-side generated monolithic lithium disilicate crowns: 10-year results. Clin Oral Investig 2018; 22(4):1763–9.
14. de Carvalho Ramos N, Campos TMB, de La Paz IS, et al. Microstructure characterization and SCG of newly engineered dental ceramics. Dent Mater 2016; 32(7):870–8.
15. Riquieri H, Monteiro JB, Viegas DC, et al. Impact of crystallization firing process on the microstructure and flexural strength of zirconia-reinforced lithium silicate glass-ceramics. Dent Mater 2018;34(10):1483–91.
16. Elsaka SE, Elnaghy AM. Mechanical properties of zirconia reinforced lithium silicate glass-ceramic. Dent Mater 2016;32(7):908–14.
17. Sen N, Us YO. Mechanical and optical properties of monolithic CAD-CAM restorative materials. J Prosthet Dent 2018;119(4):593–9.
18. Wendler M, Belli R, Petschelt A, et al. Chairside CAD/CAM materials. Part 2: flexural strength testing. Dent Mater 2017;33(1):99–109.
19. Vichi A, Fonzar RF, Goracci C, et al. Effect of finishing and polishing on roughness and gloss of lithium disilicate and lithium silicate zirconia reinforced glass ceramic for CAD/CAM systems. Oper Dent 2018;43(1):90–100.
20. Awad D, Stawarczyk B, Liebermann A, et al. Translucency of esthetic dental restorative CAD/CAM materials and composite resins with respect to thickness and surface roughness. J Prosthet Dent 2015;113(6):534–40.

21. Castillo R. Lithium silicate glass ceramic and method for fabrication of dental appliances. Google Patents; 2009.
22. Zimmermann M, Koller C, Mehl A, et al. Indirect zirconia-reinforced lithium silicate ceramic CAD/CAM restorations: preliminary clinical results after 12 months. Quintessence Int 2017;48(1):19–25.
23. Luthardt R, Holzhüter M, Sandkuhl O, et al. Reliability and properties of ground Y-TZP-zirconia ceramics. J Dent Res 2002;81(7):487–91.
24. Kelly JR, Denry I. Stabilized zirconia as a structural ceramic: an overview. Dent Mater 2008;24(3):289–98.
25. Denry I, Kelly JR. State of the art of zirconia for dental applications. Dent Mater 2008;24(3):299–307.
26. Garvie RC, Nicholson PS. Phase analysis in zirconia systems. J Am Ceram Soc 1972;55(6):303–5.
27. Garvie RCHR, Pascoe RT. Ceramic steel? Nature 1975;258(5537):703.
28. Zhang Y, Lawn BR. Novel zirconia materials in dentistry. J Dent Res 2018;97(2): 140–7.
29. Sailer I, Makarov NA, Thoma DS, et al. All-ceramic or metal-ceramic tooth-supported fixed dental prostheses (FDPs)? A systematic review of the survival and complication rates. Part I: single crowns (SCs). Dent Mater 2015;31(6):603–23.
30. Kassardjian V, Varma S, Andiappan M, et al. A systematic review and meta analysis of the longevity of anterior and posterior all-ceramic crowns. J Dent 2016; 55:1–6.
31. Christensen GJ. Porcelain-fused-to-metal versus zirconia-based ceramic restorations, 2009. J Am Dent Assoc 2009;140(8):1036–9.
32. Sax C, Hammerle CH, Sailer I. 10-year clinical outcomes of fixed dental prostheses with zirconia frameworks. Int J Comput Dent 2011;14(3):183–202.
33. Kimmich M, Stappert CF. Intraoral treatment of veneering porcelain chipping of fixed dental restorations: a review and clinical application. J Am Dent Assoc 2013;144(1):31–44.
34. Zhang Y. Making yttria-stabilized tetragonal zirconia translucent. Dent Mater 2014;30(10):1195–203.
35. Zhang F, Vanmeensel K, Batuk M, et al. Highly-translucent, strong and aging-resistant 3Y-TZP ceramics for dental restoration by grain boundary segregation. Acta Biomater 2015;16:215–22.
36. Bomicke W, Rammelsberg P, Stober T, et al. Short-term prospective clinical evaluation of monolithic and partially veneered zirconia single crowns. J Esthet Restor Dent 2017;29(1):22–30.
37. Moscovitch M. Consecutive case series of monolithic and minimally veneered zirconia restorations on teeth and implants: up to 68 months. Int J Periodontics Restorative Dent 2015;35(3):315–23.
38. Koenig V, Wulfman CP, Derbanne MA, et al. Aging of monolithic zirconia dental prostheses: protocol for a 5-year prospective clinical study using ex vivo analyses. Contemp Clin Trials Commun 2016;4:25–32.
39. Cheng CW, Chien CH, Chen CJ, et al. Randomized controlled clinical trial to compare posterior implant-supported modified monolithic zirconia and metal-ceramic single crowns: one-year results. J Prosthodont 2018. https://doi.org/10.1111/jopr.12767.
40. Lughi V, Sergo V. Low temperature degradation -aging- of zirconia: a critical review of the relevant aspects in dentistry. Dent Mater 2010;26(8):807–20.

41. Hummer CD 3rd, Rothman RH, Hozack WJ. Catastrophic failure of modular zirconia-ceramic femoral head components after total hip arthroplasty. J Arthroplasty 1995;10(6):848–50.
42. Chevalier J, Cales B, Drouin JMA. Low-temperature aging of Y-TZP ceramics. J Am Ceram Soc 1999;82(8):2150–4.
43. Flinn BD, Raigrodski AJ, Mancl LA, et al. Influence of aging on flexural strength of translucent zirconia for monolithic restorations. J Prosthet Dent 2017;117(2): 303–9.
44. Wille S, Zumstrull P, Kaidas V, et al. Low temperature degradation of single layers of multilayered zirconia in comparison to conventional unshaded zirconia: phase transformation and flexural strength. J Mech Behav Biomed Mater 2018; 77:171–5.
45. Guilardi LF, Pereira GKR, Gundel A, et al. Surface micro-morphology, phase transformation, and mechanical reliability of ground and aged monolithic zirconia ceramic. J Mech Behav Biomed Mater 2017;65:849–56.
46. Keuper M, Berthold C, Nickel KG. Long-time aging in 3 mol.% yttria-stabilized tetragonal zirconia polycrystals at human body temperature. Acta Biomater 2014;10(2):951–9.
47. Healthcare market research report: global dental cement market snapshot. Albany (NY): Transparency Market Research; 2018. Available at: https://www.transparencymarketresearch.com/dental-cement-market.html. Accessed September 18, 2018.
48. Yoshida Y, Van Meerbeek B, Nakayama Y, et al. Evidence of chemical bonding at biomaterial-hard tissue interfaces. J Dent Res 2000;79(2):709–14.
49. De Munck J, Van Landuyt K, Peumans M, et al. A critical review of the durability of adhesion to tooth tissue: methods and results. J Dent Res 2005;84(2):118–32.
50. Inoue S, Van Meerbeek B, Abe Y, et al. Effect of remaining dentin thickness and the use of conditioner on micro-tensile bond strength of a glass-ionomer adhesive. Dent Mater 2001;17(5):445–55.
51. Peumans M, Kanumilli P, De Munck J, et al. Clinical effectiveness of contemporary adhesives: a systematic review of current clinical trials. Dent Mater 2005; 21(9):864–81.
52. van Dijken JW, Pallesen U. Long-term dentin retention of etch-and-rinse and self-etch adhesives and a resin-modified glass ionomer cement in non-carious cervical lesions. Dent Mater 2008;24(7):915–22.
53. Sidhu SK, Watson TF. Interfacial characteristics of resin-modified glass-ionomer materials: a study on fluid permeability using confocal fluorescence microscopy. J Dent Res 1998;77(9):1749–59.
54. Sidhu SK, Sherriff M, Watson TF. Failure of resin-modified glass-ionomers subjected to shear loading. J Dent 1999;27(5):373–81.
55. Coutinho E, Yoshida Y, Inoue S, et al. Gel phase formation at resin-modified glass-ionomer/tooth interfaces. J Dent Res 2007;86(7):656–61.
56. Cardoso MV, Delme KI, Mine A, et al. Towards a better understanding of the adhesion mechanism of resin-modified glass-ionomers by bonding to differently prepared dentin. J Dent 2010;38(11):921–9.
57. Misra S. Photocurable ionomer cement systems. St Paul (MN): Minnesota Mining and Manufacturing Co; 1992. US patent #5,130,347.
58. Akahane S, Tosaki S, Kusayanagi S, et al. Dental glass ionomer cement compositions 1991.
59. van den Breemer CR, Gresnigt MM, Cune MS. Cementation of glass-ceramic posterior restorations: a systematic review. Biomed Res Int 2015;2015:148954.

60. Manso AP, Silva NR, Bonfante EA, et al. Cements and adhesives for all-ceramic restorations. Dent Clin North Am 2011;55(2):311–32.
61. Stamatacos C, Simon JF. Cementation of indirect restorations: an overview of resin cements. Compend Contin Educ Dent 2013;34(1):42–4.
62. Ferracane J, Moser J, Greener E. Ultraviolet light-induced yellowing of dental restorative resins. J Prosthet Dent 1985;54(4):483–7.
63. Smith DS, Vandewalle KS, Whisler G. Color stability of composite resin cements. Gen Dent 2011;59(5):390–4.
64. Asmussen E. Factors affecting the color stability of restorative resins. Acta Odontol Scand 1983;41(1):11–8.
65. Kanca J III. An alternative hypothesis to the cause of pulpal inflammation in teeth treated with phosphoric acid on the dentin. Quintessence Int 1990; 21(2):83–6.
66. Bertolotti RL. Total etch—the rational dentin bonding protocol. J Esthet Restor Dent 1991;3(1):1–6.
67. Nakamura M. A newly developed bonding restoration material—Clearfil Bond System F. Kokubyo Gakkai Zasshi 1978;45(1):234 [in Japanese].
68. Nakabayashi N, Kojima K, Masuhara E. The promotion of adhesion by the infiltration of monomers into tooth substrates. J Biomed Mater Res 1982;16(3): 265–73.
69. Breschi L, Maravic T, Cunha SR, et al. Dentin bonding systems: from dentin collagen structure to bond preservation and clinical applications. Dent Mater 2018;34(1):78–96.
70. Peumans M, De Munck J, Van Landuyt KL, et al. A 13-year clinical evaluation of two three-step etch-and-rinse adhesives in non-carious class-V lesions. Clin Oral Investig 2012;16(1):129–37.
71. Ferracane JL, Stansbury J, Burke FJT. Self-adhesive resin cements—chemistry, properties and clinical considerations. J Oral Rehabil 2011;38(4): 295–314.
72. De Munck J, Vargas M, Van Landuyt K, et al. Bonding of an auto-adhesive luting material to enamel and dentin. Dent Mater 2004;20(10):963–71.
73. Monticelli F, Osorio R, Mazzitelli C, et al. Limited decalcification/diffusion of self-adhesive cements into dentin. J Dent Res 2008;87(10):974–9.
74. Gerth HU, Dammaschke T, Züchner H, et al. Chemical analysis and bonding reaction of RelyX Unicem and Bifix composites—a comparative study. Dent Mater 2006;22(10):934–41.
75. Al-Assaf K, Chakmakchi M, Palaghias G, et al. Interfacial characteristics of adhesive luting resins and composites with dentine. Dent Mater 2007;23(7): 829–39.
76. Baader K, Hiller K-A, Buchalla W, et al. Self-adhesive luting of partial ceramic crowns: selective enamel etching leads to higher survival after 6.5 years in vivo. J Adhes Dent 2016;18(1):69–79.
77. Peumans M, Voet M, De Munck J, et al. Four-year clinical evaluation of a self-adhesive luting agent for ceramic inlays. Clin Oral Investig 2013;17(3): 739–50.
78. Schenke F, Federlin M, Hiller K-A, et al. Controlled, prospective, randomized, clinical evaluation of partial ceramic crowns inserted with RelyX Unicem with or without selective enamel etching. Results after 2 years. Clin Oral Investig 2012;16(2):451–61.

79. Behr M, Rosentritt M, Wimmer J, et al. Self-adhesive resin cement versus zinc phosphate luting material: a prospective clinical trial begun 2003. Dent Mater 2009;25(5):601–4.
80. Zhang Y, Sailer I, Lawn BR. Fatigue of dental ceramics. J Dent 2013;41(12): 1135–47.
81. Kelly JR, Giordano R, Pober R, et al. Fracture surface analysis of dental ceramics: clinically failed restorations. Int J Prosthodont 1990;3(5):430–40.
82. Øilo M, Gjerdet NR. Fractographic analyses of all-ceramic crowns: a study of 27 clinically fractured crowns. Dent Mater 2013;29(6):e78–84.
83. Øilo M, Hardang AD, Ulsund AH, et al. Fractographic features of glass-ceramic and zirconia-based dental restorations fractured during clinical function. Eur J Oral Sci 2014;122(3):238–44.
84. Thompson J, Anusavice K, Naman A, et al. Fracture surface characterization of clinically failed all-ceramic crowns. J Dent Res 1994;73(12):1824–32.
85. Øilo M, Quinn GD. Fracture origins in twenty-two dental alumina crowns. J Mech Behav Biomed Mater 2016;53:93–103.
86. Quinn JB, Quinn GD, Kelly JR, et al. Fractographic analyses of three ceramic whole crown restoration failures. Dent Mater 2005;21(10):920–9.
87. Scherrer SS, Quinn GD, Quinn JB. Fractographic failure analysis of a Procera® AllCeram crown using stereo and scanning electron microscopy. Dent Mater 2008;24(8):1107–13.
88. Schmitz JH, Cortellini D, Granata S, et al. Monolithic lithium disilicate complete single crowns with feather-edge preparation design in the posterior region: a multicentric retrospective study up to 12 years. Quintessence Int 2017;48(8): 601–8.
89. van den Breemer CR, Vinkenborg C, van Pelt H, et al. The clinical performance of monolithic lithium disilicate posterior restorations after 5, 10, and 15 years: a retrospective case series. Int J Prosthodont 2017;30(1):62–5.
90. Poggio CE, Dosoli R, Ercoli C. A retrospective analysis of 102 zirconia single crowns with knife-edge margins. J Prosthet Dent 2012;107(5):316–21.
91. Burke F, Fleming GJ, Nathanson D, et al. Are adhesive technologies needed to support ceramics? An assessment of the current evidence. J Adhes Dent 2002; 4(1):7–22.
92. Blatz M, Vonderheide M, Conejo J. The effect of resin bonding on long-term success of high-strength ceramics. J Dent Res 2018;97(2):132–9.
93. Malament KA, Socransky SS. Survival of Dicor glass-ceramic dental restorations over 16 years. Part III: effect of luting agent and tooth or tooth-substitute core structure. J Prosthet Dent 2001;86(5):511–9.
94. Sjögren G, Lantto R, Tillberg A. Clinical evaluation of all-ceramic crowns (Dicor) in general practice. J Prosthet Dent 1999;81(3):277–84.
95. Schmitz JH, Beani M. Effect of different cement types on monolithic lithium disilicate complete crowns with feather-edge preparation design in the posterior region. J Prosthet Dent 2016;115(6):678–83.
96. Selz CF, Strub JR, Vach K, et al. Long-term performance of posterior InCeram Alumina crowns cemented with different luting agents: a prospective, randomized clinical split-mouth study over 5 years. Clin Oral Investig 2014;18(6): 1695–703.
97. Zitzmann NU, Galindo ML, Hagmann E, et al. Clinical evaluation of Procera AllCeram crowns in the anterior and posterior regions. Int J Prosthodont 2007; 20(3):239–41.

98. Nasrin S, Katsube N, Seghi RR, et al. 3D statistical failure analysis of monolithic dental ceramic crowns. J Biomech 2016;49(10):2038–46.
99. Nasrin S, Katsube N, Seghi R, et al. Survival predictions of ceramic crowns using statistical fracture mechanics. J Dent Res 2017;96(5):509–15.
100. Nasrin S, Katsube N, Seghi RR, et al. Approximate relative fatigue life estimation methods for thin-walled monolithic ceramic crowns. Dent Mater 2018;34(5): 726–36.

Management of Edentulous Patients

Damian J. Lee, DDS, MS[a,*], Paola C. Saponaro, DDS, MS[b]

KEYWORDS

• Edentulism • Management • Complete dentures • Maintenance • Dental implants • Prosthesis • Digital

KEY POINTS

- Edentulism is a global phenomenon and it is projected to remain in high numbers for many countries.
- Complete dentures are widely used for edentulous patients and proper maintenance, timely recall, and patient education are essential for their success.
- With advanced technology in CAD/CAM, digital dentures may provide advantages in its material, method of fabrication, and favorable clinical outcomes.
- As dental implants have improved the treatment of edentulous patients the use of fewer numbers of implants has led to alternative treatment options.

INTRODUCTION

Prevalance of Edentulism

Edentulism, defined as the complete loss of all dentition,[1] is a worldwide phenomenon. According to the World Health Organization criteria, edentulous patients are considered physically impaired, disabled, and handicapped because of their inability to properly masticate and speak.[2]

Edentulism occurs because of biologic disease processes, such as dental caries, periodontal diseases, trauma, and oral cancer. Social and/or behavioral factors that have led to this disease state include poor access to care or third-party payer or insurance systems that may limit the types of care the patient receives.[3]

The estimated edentulous population in the United States is greater than 36 million.[4] For adults 18 and older, approximately 10% (9.7%) are edentulous, with the rate increasing with age.[5] About 26% of the population in the United States between the

Disclosure: The authors have nothing to disclose.
[a] Advanced Prosthodontics Program, Division of Restorative and Prosthetic Dentistry, The Ohio State University College of Dentistry, 305 West 12th Avenue, Room 2039L, Columbus, OH 43210, USA; [b] Division of Restorative and Prosthetic Dentistry, The Ohio State University College of Dentistry, 305 West 12th Avenue, Room 3005Q, Columbus, OH 43210, USA
* Corresponding author.
E-mail address: lee.6221@osu.edu

Dent Clin N Am 63 (2019) 249–261
https://doi.org/10.1016/j.cden.2018.11.006 dental.theclinics.com

ages of 65 years and 74 years, approximately 23 million people, are completely edentulous and another 12 million are edentulous in one arch.[4] Among the geriatric population that is greater than 65 years, the ratio of edentulous individuals to dentate individual is 2 to 1.[4] In Europe, prevalence of edentulism ranges from 15% to 72% for the elderly 65- to 74-year age group population in various countries.[6] Ren and colleagues[5] reported that in China adults aged 65 to 74 were 11 times more likely to become edentulous, and adults older than 75 were 24 times more likely to become edentulous compared with the 45 to 54 age group.

Although the trend of edentulism has been reported to have declined in prevalence in many countries, because of an increase overall in the elderly population, the number of edentulous individuals has not declined.[7] In the United States, the rate of edentulism has been declining and is projected to be reduced to a rate of 2.6% by 2050. It is projected that there will be less than 9 million edentulous people by 2050.[7] Other areas of the world are foreseeing an increase among their adult population. A study by Cardoso and colleagues[8] reported edentulous patients in Brazil were declining in the teenage and middle-aged adults, but will increase among the elderly population, reaching more than 64 million by 2040. Therefore, the need to restore edentulous patients to function will not only remain but will increase in the future globally.

The latest trends show that there are no gender biases for edentulism. Men and women are nearly equally likely to become edentulous.[4] However, socioeconomic status does seem to play a role. There are higher percentages of edentulism shown in those who are below the poverty level (14.3%).[4] By race, Wu and others[5,9] reported that Native Americans had the highest prevalence (23.98%) for edentulism, followed by African Americans (19.39%), white persons (16.90%), Asians (14.22%), and Hispanics (14.18%) for adults older than the age 50.

Edentulism is accompanied by several comorbidities that can significantly influence an individual. According to Felton,[3,10] edentulous patients were associated with poor dietary habits and nutritional intake, osteoporosis, and increased risk of having hypertension and coronary artery disease. The literature has reported edentulous patients are more likely to be smokers and have smoking-associated diseases, such as asthma, emphysema, and cancer. Health-related quality-of-life studies indicate that edentulism can affect the quality of life, where patients report to have unsatisfactory esthetics and lowered self-esteem.[3,10] Socially, denture wearers have revealed they keep their dentures a secret from friends, siblings, and spouses. Furthermore, some denture wearers may avoid certain social situations, such as eating at weddings and parties, and avoiding job interviews and networking with other professionals.[11]

COMPLETE DENTURE AS REPLACEMENT OF TEETH

Complete denture rehabilitation remains one of the most popular and traditional prosthodontic treatment options for edentulous patients who have systemic, anatomic, and/or financial limitations (**Fig. 1**).[12] Successful outcomes of complete denture patients may depend on prognostic factors, such as age of patient, patient demographic, psychological factors and personal traits, previous denture experience, expectation and attitudes, residual ridge form and anatomy, method of construction, quality of dentures and changes over time, and esthetics.[13] Although there has been much debate on the influence or significance of these factors on the outcome of denture therapy, one thing that is certain is the sequelae of prolonged denture use.

Residual ridge resorption is a phenomenon that describes the life-long remodeling of the alveolar ridge after dental extractions, where the size of the residual ridge is reduced most rapidly in the first 6 months and continues throughout life at a slower

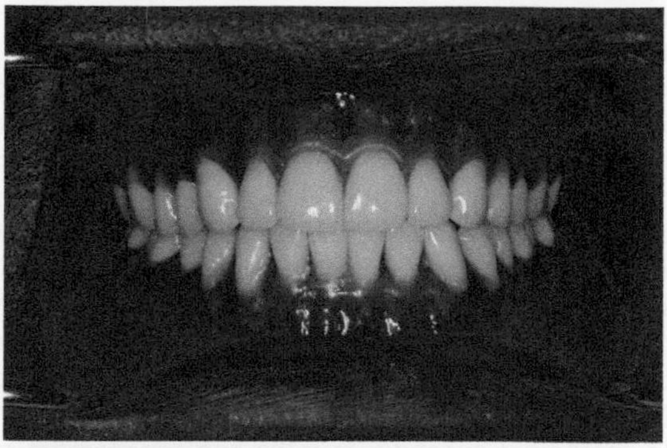

Fig. 1. Complete dentures as replacement of teeth.

rate.[14–17] Residual ridge resorption has been described as being chronic, progressive, irreversible, and catabolic. There are several studies that have examined this phenomenon in the past; describing the process by using standardized measurements in panoramic radiographs, lateral cephalographs, and diagnostic casts.[14–17] The rate of resorption can differ based on the individual and jaw location.[18] It is influenced by different anatomic, prosthetic, metabolic and systemic, and functional factors.[18] Additionally, studies have investigated the association of residual ridge resorption and systemic conditions, such as osteoporosis, menopause, age, and gender.[18–22] There was a higher tendency for narrower ridges with elderly women, estrogen deficiencies, and vitamin supplements helped with minimizing ridge resorption.[18–22] Different prosthetic and functional factors have been evaluated in their roles in residual ridge resorption, such as immediate dentures, zero degree teeth, and duration of denture wearing.[17,23–26] Previous studies have reported increased amount of ridge resorption associated with immediate dentures, zero degree or nonanatomic teeth, and prolonged denture use.

As the by-product of residual ridge resorption, adaptation of the denture base can change significantly. Ill-fitting dentures can cause the following mucosal changes: traumatic ulcers, denture stomatitis, candida infection, angular chelitis, and soft tissue hyperplasia.[27] Resilient lining material compensates for the resorbed tissue and allows tissue recovery to take place.[28] Reline is defined as "the procedure used to resurface the tissue side of a removable dental prosthesis with new base material, producing an accurate adaption to the denture foundation area."[1] Resilient lining materials are either an elastomeric silicone or plasticized acrylic resin. Over time, the plasticizers can leach out of the reline material and become much harder, whereas elastomeric silicone is more dimensionally stable.[29] However, the bonding of the silicone to the denture base is unreliable long-term.

Commercially available denture cleansers can roughen the surface of the lining materials, leading to biofilm formation and *Candida albicans* colonization.[30] Therefore, prolonged use of a resilient liner, compared with more stable laboratory rebasing, should be cautioned.

Denture relining materials are often used to accommodate hard and soft tissue changes during healing periods. When this is the case, the duration of need for the denture reline is unpredictable because of variability in healing times of individual patients. A recent study by Puri and colleagues[31] showed that bone turnover markers known as serum osteocalcin and C-terminal telopeptides, which are easily assessed in blood, were linked with increased number of relines among denture patients.

Therefore, in the future, certain biologic markers may potentially inform the clinician of the proper timing to perform the laboratory rebase.

Fit, retention, and stability of the prosthesis are hallmark to successful complete denture therapy. Therefore, establishing a recall regimen and consistent and periodic monitoring of soft and hard tissue health is essential for successful complete denture therapy. Felton and colleagues[32] published guidelines for proper care and maintenance for complete dentures. Properly educating patients regarding the significance of denture care and maintenance is recommended. Several key points, such as storage, biofilm formation, disinfection, and use of denture adhesives, were described in detail.[32] It was recommended that biofilm on dentures should be removed every day with an effective, nonabrasive cleaner; dentures should never be placed in boiling water or bleach solution for more than 10 minutes; and although use of denture adhesives is helpful, the period of usage should not exceed 6 months and assessment of oral health care provider for supporting tissue is recommended at that time.[31] Teaching patients to recognize the changes occurring in their own mouth and to return to their dental provider can prevent further problems and successfully prolong the use of their prostheses.

ADVANCEMENT IN COMPLETE DENTURES

The methods of conventional complete denture fabrication have remained unchanged for the past 70 years since the introduction of polymethylmethacrylate in 1936.[33] Over the decades, acrylic resin has demonstrated improvements in its physical properties and polymerization processes with the introduction of autopolymerizing, compression-molded, microwave-processed, and injection-molded techniques.[34] The conventional protocol for fabrication of complete dentures involves a complex sequence of clinical and laboratory steps. On average, this process requires at least five clinical appointments[35–37]; which can consist of recording the horizontal and vertical relationships of the jaws and transferring it accurately to the semiadjustable articulator, patient approval of the esthetics, and the unavoidable postinsertion adjustment visits.[38–40] This minimum number of appointments may discourage clinicians from offering rehabilitation of edentulism with complete dentures as part of their services.

Computer-aided design/computer-aided manufacturing (CAD-CAM) has made significant contributions in dentistry since its early introduction in the 1980s. With the advent of this technology and its successful application in the realm of maxillofacial, fixed, and implant prosthodontics,[41,42] CAD-CAM technology was recently applied to the fabrication of complete dentures to simplify the clinical and laboratory procedures,[43] and to establish cost- and time- efficient protocols that would provide favorable outcomes for edentulous patients.

These advancements in digital fabrication have had a significant impact on conventional complete denture fabrication processes. The methods for construction of complete denture using CAD-CAM technology have been previously reported (**Figs. 2** and **3**).[12,43–47] These methods simplify and shorten the number of patient visits. A recent review by Steinmassl and colleagues[48] described six different commercially available CAD-CAM denture systems and their methods of fabrication and the number of patient visits required.[48] Most of the companies described use subtractive technology to mill the dentures (ie, Wieland Digital Denture, Baltic Denture System Global Dental Sciences), whereas others use additive manufacturing with three-dimensional printing (ie, Dentca).[48] In both techniques, scanning of the clinical records obtained either through master casts or definitive impressions are digitized and allow for designing and milling of the monolithic prosthesis or the denture bases.[49,50]

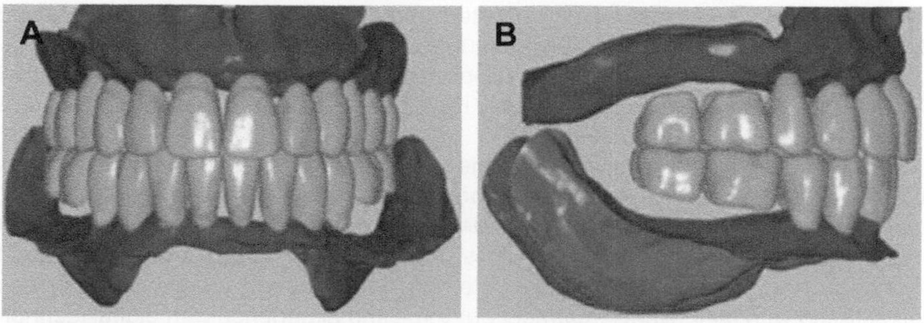

Fig. 2. Digital denture teeth arrangements. (*A*) Frontal view (*B*) Lateral view.

The subtractive manufacturing process uses prepolymerized resin pucks fabricated under high heat and pressure, which supposedly results in less monomer release, higher density, and less microporosity and polymerization volumetric shrinkage.[48] The decrease in monomer residual and porosity have been linked with having less microbial colonization on denture surfaces and increased biocompatibility with the oral environment compared with its conventional counterpart. This method of fabrication eliminates the errors of conventional denture processing, which include denture warpage, volumetric and linear shrinkage, porosity, and crazing.[34]

According to Goodacre and colleagues,[45] CAD-CAM monolithic complete dentures produced the most accuracy, reproducibility, and least overall denture tooth movement during fabrication when compared with other methods of complete denture fabrication. In regards to the accuracy of the available CAD-CAM systems, Steinmassl and colleagues[48] determined that AvaDent Digital Dentures system exhibited the highest precision in denture fit when compared with traditionally fabricated dentures. Further research in long-term prospective outcomes of the denture material, stability in the oral environment, and clinical outcome is still needed.[34]

Intraoral scanning of the edentulous tissues has been suggested and attempted with promising results.[45] However, difficulty lies in the digital program algorithm to recognize appropriately extended denture borders because of the functional movements and displaceability of the edentulous tissues.[49]

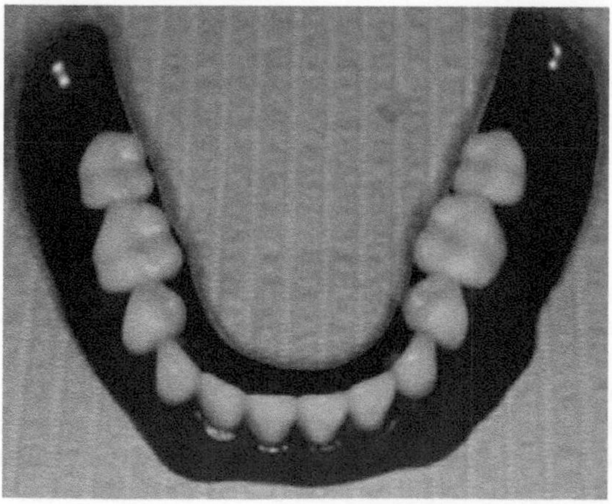

Fig. 3. Milled complete denture.

Kattadiyil and colleagues[12] have reported improved retention of the denture and reduced clinical chair time for milled dentures compared with the conventional dentures. Steinmassl and colleagues[48] supported these findings and reported that CAD-CAM systems were able to precisely reproduce the master cast surface in comparison with the traditional methods.

Bidra and colleagues[44] reported that one of the most important advantages of this technology is the decrease in clinical appointments whereby definitive impressions, maxillomandibular records, and tooth selection are completed in one appointment thus reducing the number of patient visits. Patient satisfaction has been measured through survey studies and it has been determined that patients are generally pleased and satisfied with their overall treatment outcome and experience with digital technologies suggesting that, regardless of the operator training and expertise, this method of denture fabrication may be predictable as long as prosthodontic fundamentals are applied.[37] "Electronically archiving" the patient and denture data for future fabrication has been another advantage of CAD-CAM dentures.[12,47]

Bidra and colleagues[44] also advocated that CAD-CAM fabricated complete dentures can positively influence patient care, dental curriculums, and research. A study surveying US dental schools showed 52% of program directors and 12% of restorative chairs that completed the questionnaire reported implementing this technology into their curriculum.[35] However, growing concerns exist because of the high cost of implementation compared with the low-cost traditional fabrication techniques.

Although most outcomes were favorable, a few minor complications of CAD-CAM dentures having poor esthetic outcomes or altered phonetics with the prostheses, and discrepancies with occlusal vertical dimension and tooth arrangements have been reported.[12,35] Some studies reported having additional appointments for small percentages of patients than what the manufacturers stated. Saponaro and colleagues[36] reported that 17 patients out of 48 (35.4%) needed an extra appointment for their two-visit protocol. A direct correlation exists between the number of postinsertion adjustments and patient satisfaction. The lower the number of recall visits, higher scores documented for patient satisfaction.[51]

In their systematic reviews, Kattadiyil and colleagues[12,47] published that careful patient selection seems critical for the success of computer-engineered dentures. The authors recommended that complex prosthodontic patients should be treated with caution to avoid the cost associated with prosthesis remakes.[12,47] Although the available literature on CAD-CAM dentures is scarce, this method using the latest technology has shown promising short-term results with improved material offering good fit, retention, and mechanical properties. Prospective clinical studies involving edentulous patients requiring CAD-CAM complete dentures are needed to improve patient-centered outcomes. Further research is needed, with substantial sample sizes and longer follow-up periods to validate the performance of this treatment alternative.

TOOTH-RETAINED OVERDENTURE

With the high expenses associated with dental implant treatment, saving a few teeth to fabricate a tooth-supported overdenture (**Fig. 4**) is a viable option for managing edentulous patients.[52] Carlsson in 2014[52] reiterated the continuous and unpredictable loss of residual bone after extraction and while using complete denture. It was suggested to not extract all remaining dentition but to preserve several teeth to fabricate overdentures to provide denture stability and retention.[52] This classical modality of simply using the reduced mandibular canines sealed with amalgam restorations has been shown to delay the ridge resorption process by eight times more than using a

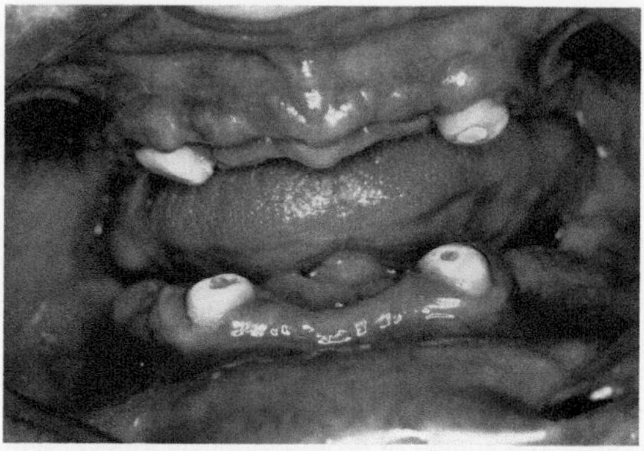

Fig. 4. Tooth-retained overdenture. (*Courtesy of* David M. Bohnenkamp, DDS, MS, FACP, Iowa City, IA.)

conventional complete denture in the mandible.[53] Sensory feedback from the periodontal receptors and enhancement of the masticatory system have been advocated as an advantage for the use overdentures for the edentulous patient compared with conventional complete dentures.[54,55] However, additional need for treatment before denture fabrication usually requires more time and cost on the patient's behalf, and third-party payment may have restrictions for tooth-supported overdentures.[54,55]

Several attachment systems are incorporated onto the canines to enhance the retention of the overdenture, such as ball attachments, locators, telescopic copings, and more. Various case reports have documented use of these retentive mechanisms to provide satisfactory treatment of edentulous patients.[56–58] Common causes for failure for tooth-retained overdentures have been caries, periodontal disease, endodontic failure, and trauma.[54,55] Although caries and recurrent caries of remaining roots have been a common reason for failure, daily use of fluoride to prevent demineralization has been advocated.[59] A recent study examining remineralization of root surfaces, suggested that combining dentrifices containing calcium phosphosilicate with fluoride may improve remineralization of root surfaces.[59] Ettinger and Qian[60] reported attachment loss of 116 abutment teeth of tooth-supported overdentures over a 42-month period. The authors attributed the loss to the rotation of the overdenture around the abutments in a buccolingual direction, especially for the mandibular overdenture. Strict protocols have been recommended for maintaining the overdenture patients: surgical elimination of periodontal pockets greater than 3 mm at the beginning of treatment, removal of dentures while sleeping, cleaning abutment teeth and dentures at least twice a day, and using a high concentration (500 ppm) neutral sodium fluoride gel once a day.[61] With a proper recall regimen, tooth-retained overdentures still are an effective treatment modality for edentulous patients.

IMPLANT CONSIDERATION

Dental implants have been effective in minimizing the rate of bone resorption. Carlsson[62] advocated for the use of implant-supported prosthesis, which have a bone preserving effect rather than the continuing bone resorption under a complete denture. He suggested the dental implants may even promote bone growth. A comparison between conventional dentures and implant overdentures on the effect on posterior mandibular residual ridge resorption showed that there was a mean reduction in alveolar height of 1.63 mm in the conventional denture group compared with 0.69 mm in the implant overdenture group over a 5-year period.[63]

It has been more than 15 years since the landmark McGill Consensus Statement that described "mandibular two-implant overdenture as first choice standard of care for edentulous patients."[64] Feine and colleagues[64] stated that although two-implant overdenture has a greater cost than conventional dentures, the difference is "not as large as one might expect and should be made affordable to edentulous patients." Similarly, the York Consensus in 2009 advocated that two-implant-supported mandibular overdenture should be the "minimum offered to edentulous patients as a first choice of treatment."[65] Cost is stated as a "real perceived barrier" for the delivery of implant-supported prostheses. Advocates of this treatment modality justify the cost over the life span of the patient.[64]

Although dental implant treatment options for edentulous patients are plenty, the use of dental implants for this group of patients globally may be different. Kronstrom and Carlsson[66] reported in a survey of prosthodontists in 33 countries that less than 20% of their patients received implant treatment of edentulous mandibles. Financial costs related to implant-supported prostheses were estimated to be 5 to 12 times more expensive than conventional dentures.[67] Regardless, the initial cost for implant therapy remains high for edentulous patients and uptake of dental implants as standard of care remains slow.[65]

There has been a growing body of evidence that suggest a single-implant-supported overdenture is a viable alternative to the traditional two-implant modality.[68–72] The use of one endosseus implant at the midline of the mandible has shown to have good clinical outcome and high level of patient satisfaction compared with two-implant overdenture.[71,72] A systematic review by Nogueira and colleagues[71] reported that within the available publications, single-implant mandibular overdenture reported a significant improvement in comfort, function, and stability in the mandibular denture after receiving one implant in the mandible for 158 patients. A randomized clinical trial published by Kern and colleagues[70] showed that most single-implant-supported overdentures had high success in delayed loading protocol and immediate loading should be considered only in exceptional cases. Although better controlled clinical trials of longer duration with larger sample size are advocated,[71] this modality seems to have a realistic potential to become the "new" minimum standard of care for edentulous patients and replacement of dentition.

With the long-term success of full arch implant-supported fixed complete denture supported by four to six implants[73] patients with failing dentitions are able to be rehabilitated using prostheses that look, feel, and perform similar to the natural dentition. A review by Goodacre and Goodacre[73] discussed various outcomes comparing fixed versus removable complete arch implant prostheses. The variables analyzed were implant and prosthesis survival, prosthesis maintenance/complications, bone changes, patient satisfaction/quality of life, cost-effectiveness, and masticatory performance. Although one modality provided advantage compared with the other in some of the factors investigated, implant survival, patient satisfaction, and masticatory performance were comparable.[73]

The cost of fixed complete implant-supported prostheses as a treatment modality is significantly high. Clinicians have investigated the use of fewer numbers of implants per arch with great success.[74–78] Maló and colleagues[74] reported cumulative implant survival rate of 95.4%, and prosthetic survival of 99.7% after 7 years of service of fixed implant-supported prostheses using the All-on-4® treatment concept. The success of this technique is based on implant length and distribution, which provides a broad dispersal of functional force acting on the implants and bone. The concept of using only three implants was introduced as the Branemark Novum protocol in early 2000.[76–78] This method used a preformed titanium substructure that guided the

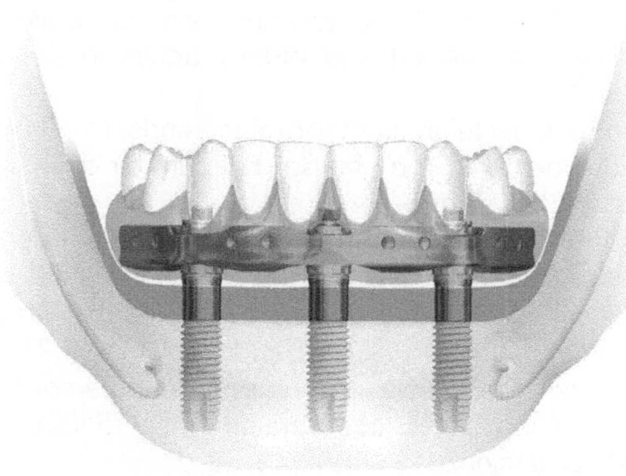

Fig. 5. Using three implants for full-arch fixed complete denture. (*Courtesy of* Nobel Biocare USA, Yorba Linda, CA; with permission.)

implant placement in an edentulous mandible and served as a primary bar. Then, a secondary prefabricated titanium substructure was used to create the definitive prosthesis using acrylic teeth and polymethylmethacrylate, which allowed for prosthesis placement on the same day.[78] Clinically, this method showed 93% to 95% implant survival and 99% prosthesis survival over 5 years.[77]

This concept was recently reintroduced as Trefoil™ from Nobel Biocare (**Fig. 5**)[79] and it has gained prominence for being able to offer full arch implant-supported prosthesis with lower cost with fewer implants. According to the manufacturer, through CAD-CAM technology the prefabricated bar is anatomically designed to fit the mandibular arch and has improved passive fit through an adaptive joint that accounts for horizontal, vertical, and angular deviations.[79] With the use of cone beam computed tomography and digital planning, the outcome may be more favorable than its previous generation.

Regardless of the type of prostheses, dental implants are capable of enhancing the outcomes of prosthodontic rehabilitation for edentulous patients and truly change their lives. Ways to use this technology must be explored so that more edentulous individuals are treated more globally.

SUMMARY

Because of the growing population across the world, the need for managing edentulous patients will continue to remain globally. The dental profession will continue to face the challenge of how best to treat these patients in the future. Although there is not one modality that is considered most effective, the minimum standard for the treatment of this population is to restore them to health, function, comfort, and esthetics.

REFERENCES

1. The glossary of prosthodontic terms. J Prosthet Dent 2017;117(5S):e1–105.
2. Bouma J, Uitenbroek D, Westert G, et al. Pathways to full mouth extraction. Community Dent Oral Epidemiol 1987;15(6):301–5.
3. Felton DA. Edentulism and comorbid factors. J Prosthodont 2009;18(2):88–96.
4. Dye B, Thornton-Evans G, Li X, et al. Dental caries and tooth loss in adults in the United States, 2011-2012. NCHS Data Brief 2015;(197):197.

5. Ren C, McGrath C, Yang Y. Edentulism and associated factors among community-dwelling middle-aged and elderly adults in China. Gerodontology 2017;34(2):195–207.
6. Mojon P. The world without teeth: demographic trends. In: Feine JS, Carlsson GE, editors. Implant overdentures: the Standard of care for edentulous patients. Chicago: Quentessence; 2003. p. 3–14.
7. Slade GD, Akinkugbe AA, Sanders AE. Projections of U.S. edentulism prevalence following 5 decades of decline. J Dent Res 2014;93(10):959–65.
8. Cardoso M, Balducci I, Telles Dde M, et al. Edentulism in Brazil: trends, projections and expectations until 2040. Cien Saude Colet 2016;21(4):1239–46.
9. Wu B, Liang J, Plassman BL, et al. Edentulism trends among middle-aged and older adults in the United States: comparison of five racial/ethnic groups. Community Dent Oral Epidemiol 2012;40(2):145–53.
10. Felton DA. Complete edentulism and comorbid diseases: an update. J Prosthodont 2016;25(1):5–20.
11. Healthcare GC. The biting into denture care. Cisionn PR Newswire; 2015. Available at: https://www.prnewswire.com/news-releases/new-us-oral-care-survey-reveals-over-half-56-of-denture-wearers-avoid-eating-certain-foods1-also-feel-limitations-in-work-social-and-romantic-lives-300104859.html. Accessed July 26, 2018.
12. Kattadiyil MT, AlHelal A, Goodacre BJ. Clinical complications and quality assessments with computer-engineered complete dentures: a systematic review. J Prosthet Dent 2017;117(6):721–8.
13. Critchlow SB, Ellis JS. Prognostic indicators for conventional complete denture therapy: a review of the literature. J Dent 2010;38(1):2–9.
14. Atwood DA. Some clinical factors related to rate of resorption of residual ridges. J Prosthet Dent 1962;12:441–50.
15. Atwood DA, Coy WA. Clinical, cephalometric, and densitometric study of reduction of residual ridges. J Prosthet Dent 1971;26(3):280–95.
16. Tallgren A. Alveolar bone loss in denture wearers as related to facial morphology. Acta Odontol Scand 1970;28(2):251–70.
17. Tallgren A. The continuing reduction of the residual alveolar ridges in complete denture wearers: a mixed-longitudinal study covering 25 years. J Prosthet Dent 1972;27(2):120–32.
18. Jahangiri L, Devlin H, Ting K, et al. Current perspectives in residual ridge remodeling and its clinical implications: a review. J Prosthet Dent 1998;80(2):224–37.
19. Prevention: calcium and vitamin D. Arlington (VA): National Osteoporosis Foundation; 2004.
20. Ortman LF, Hausmann E, Dunford RG. Skeletal osteopenia and residual ridge resorption. J Prosthet Dent 1989;61(3):321–5.
21. Wical KE, Brussee P. Effects of a calcium and vitamin D supplement on alveolar ridge resorption in immediate denture patients. J Prosthet Dent 1979;41(1):4–11.
22. Yang J, Farnell D, Devlin H, et al. The effect of ovariectomy on mandibular cortical thickness in the rat. J Dent 2005;33(2):123–9.
23. Bergman B, Carlsson GE. Clinical long-term study of complete denture wearers. J Prosthet Dent 1985;53(1):56–61.
24. Campbell RL. A comparative study of the resorption of the alveolar ridges in denture-wearers and non-denture-wearers. J Am Dent Assoc 1960;60:143–53.
25. Carlsson GE. Measurements on casts of the edentulous maxilla. Odontol Revy 1966;17(4):386–402.

26. Nicol BR, Somes GW, Ellinger CW, et al. Patient response to variations in denture technique. Part II: five-year cephalometric evaluation. J Prosthet Dent 1979;41(4):368–72.
27. Carlsson GE. Clinical morbidity and sequelae of treatment with complete dentures. J Prosthet Dent 1998;79(1):17–23.
28. Garcia RM, Leon BT, Oliveira VB, et al. Effect of a denture cleanser on weight, surface roughness, and tensile bond strength of two resilient denture liners. J Prosthet Dent 2003;89(5):489–94.
29. Sakaguchi RL, Powers JM. Craig's restorative dental materials: e-book. St Louis (MO): Elsevier Health Sciences; 2012.
30. Mohammed HS, Singh S, Hari PA, et al. Evaluate the effect of commercially available denture cleansers on surface hardness and roughness of denture liners at various time intervals. Int J Biomed Sci 2016;12(4):130–42.
31. Puri S, Kattadiyil MT, Puri N, et al. Evaluation of correlations between frequencies of complete denture relines and serum levels of 3 bone metabolic markers: a cross-sectional pilot study. J Prosthet Dent 2016;116(6):867–73.
32. Felton D, Cooper L, Duqum I, et al. Evidence-based guidelines for the care and maintenance of complete dentures: a publication of the American College of Prosthodontists. J Am Dent Assoc 2011;142(Suppl 1):1s–20s.
33. Murray MD, Darvell BW. The evolution of the complete denture base. Theories of complete denture retention–a review. Part 1. Aust Dent J 1993;38(3):216–9.
34. Srinivasan M, Gjengedal H, Cattani-Lorente M, et al. CAD/CAM milled complete removable dental prostheses: an in vitro evaluation of biocompatibility, mechanical properties, and surface roughness. Dent Mater J 2018;37(4):526–33.
35. Fernandez MA, Nimmo A, Behar-Horenstein LS. Digital denture fabrication in pre- and postdoctoral education: a survey of U.S. dental schools. J Prosthodont 2016;25(1):83–90.
36. Saponaro PC, Yilmaz B, Heshmati RH, et al. Clinical performance of CAD-CAM-fabricated complete dentures: a cross-sectional study. J Prosthet Dent 2016;116(3):431–5.
37. Saponaro PC, Yilmaz B, Johnston W, et al. Evaluation of patient experience and satisfaction with CAD-CAM-fabricated complete dentures: a retrospective survey study. J Prosthet Dent 2016;116(4):524–8.
38. Drago CJ. A retrospective comparison of two definitive impression techniques and their associated postinsertion adjustments in complete denture prosthodontics. J Prosthodont 2003;12(3):192–7.
39. Kivovics P, Jahn M, Borbely J, et al. Frequency and location of traumatic ulcerations following placement of complete dentures. Int J Prosthodont 2007;20(4):397–401.
40. Sadr K, Mahboob F, Rikhtegar E. Frequency of traumatic ulcerations and post-insertion adjustment recall visits in complete denture patients in an Iranian faculty of dentistry. J Dent Res Dent Clin Dent Prospects 2011;5(2):46–50.
41. McLaughlin JB, Ramos V Jr, Dickinson DP. Comparison of fit of dentures fabricated by traditional techniques versus CAD/CAM technology. J Prosthodont 2017. [Epub ahead of print].
42. Miyazaki T, Hotta Y, Kunii J, et al. A review of dental CAD/CAM: current status and future perspectives from 20 years of experience. Dent Mater J 2009;28(1):44–56.
43. Yilmaz B, Azak AN, Alp G, et al. Use of CAD-CAM technology for the fabrication of complete dentures: an alternative technique. J Prosthet Dent 2017;118(2):140–3.

44. Bidra AS, Farrell K, Burnham D, et al. Prospective cohort pilot study of 2-visit CAD/CAM monolithic complete dentures and implant-retained overdentures: clinical and patient-centered outcomes. J Prosthet Dent 2016;115(5):578–86.e1.
45. Goodacre BJ, Goodacre CJ, Baba NZ, et al. Comparison of denture tooth movement between CAD-CAM and conventional fabrication techniques. J Prosthet Dent 2018;119(1):108–15.
46. Infante L, Yilmaz B, McGlumphy E, et al. Fabricating complete dentures with CAD/CAM technology. J Prosthet Dent 2014;111(5):351–5.
47. Kattadiyil MT, AlHelal A. An update on computer-engineered complete dentures: a systematic review on clinical outcomes. J Prosthet Dent 2017;117(4):478–85.
48. Steinmassl O, Dumfahrt H, Grunert I, et al. CAD/CAM produces dentures with improved fit. Clin Oral Investig 2018;22(8):2829–35.
49. Kanazawa M, Iwaki M, Arakida T, et al. Digital impression and jaw relation record for the fabrication of CAD/CAM custom tray. J Prosthodont Res 2018;62(4): 509–13.
50. Wimmer T, Eichberger M, Lumkemann N, et al. Accuracy of digitally fabricated trial dentures. J Prosthet Dent 2018;119(6):942–7.
51. Regis RR, Cunha TR, Della Vecchia MP, et al. A randomised trial of a simplified method for complete denture fabrication: patient perception and quality. J Oral Rehabil 2013;40(7):535–45.
52. Carlsson GE. Implant and root supported overdentures: a literature review and some data on bone loss in edentulous jaws. J Adv Prosthodont 2014;6(4):245–52.
53. Crum RJ, Rooney GE Jr. Alveolar bone loss in overdentures: a 5-year study. J Prosthet Dent 1978;40(6):610–3.
54. Morrow RM, Feldmann EE, Rudd KD, et al. Tooth-supported complete dentures: an approach to preventive prosthodontics. J Prosthet Dent 1969;21(5):513–22.
55. Schwartz IS, Morrow RM. Overdentures. Principles and procedures. Dent Clin North Am 1996;40(1):169–94.
56. Bansal S, Aras MA, Chitre V. Tooth supported overdenture retained with custom attachments: a case report. J Indian Prosthodont Soc 2014;14(Suppl 1):283–6.
57. Mensor MC Jr. Attachment fixation of the overdenture: part II. J Prosthet Dent 1978;39(1):16–20.
58. Tancu AM, Melescanu Imre M, Preoteasa CT, et al. Therapeutical attitudes in tooth supported overdentures with ball attachments. Case report. J Med Life 2014;7(Spec No. 4):95–8.
59. Goettsche ZS, Ettinger RL, Wefel JS, et al. In vitro assessment of 3 dentifrices containing fluoride in preventing demineralization of overdenture abutments and root surfaces. J Prosthet Dent 2014;112(5):1257–64.
60. Ettinger RL, Qian F. Incidence of attachment loss of canines in an overdenture population. J Prosthet Dent 2014;112(6):1356–63.
61. Ettinger RL, Qian F. Longitudinal assessment of denture maintenance needs in an overdenture population. J Prosthodont 2018. [Epub ahead of print].
62. Carlsson GE. Responses of jawbone to pressure. Gerodontology 2004;21(2): 65–70.
63. Kordatzis K, Wright PS, Meijer HJ. Posterior mandibular residual ridge resorption in patients with conventional dentures and implant overdentures. Int J Oral Maxillofac Implants 2003;18(3):447–52.
64. Feine JS, Carlsson GE, Awad MA, et al. The McGill consensus statement on overdentures. Mandibular two-implant overdentures as first choice standard of care for edentulous patients. Gerodontology 2002;19(1):3–4.

65. Thomason JM, Feine J, Exley C, et al. Mandibular two implant-supported overdentures as the first choice standard of care for edentulous patients–the York Consensus Statement. Br Dent J 2009;207(4):185–6.
66. Kronstrom M, Carlsson GE. An international survey among prosthodontists of the use of mandibular implant-supported dental prostheses. J Prosthodont 2017. [Epub ahead of print].
67. MacEntee MI, Walton JN. The economics of complete dentures and implant-related services: a framework for analysis and preliminary outcomes. J Prosthet Dent 1998;79(1):24–30.
68. Alqutaibi AY, Esposito M, Algabri R, et al. Single vs two implant-retained overdentures for edentulous mandibles: a systematic review. Eur J Oral Implantol 2017; 10(3):243–61.
69. Alqutaibi AY, Kaddah AF, Farouk M. Randomized study on the effect of single-implant versus two-implant retained overdentures on implant loss and muscle activity: a 12-month follow-up report. Int J Oral Maxillofac Surg 2017;46(6):789–97.
70. Kern M, Att W, Fritzer E, et al. Survival and complications of single dental implants in the edentulous mandible following immediate or delayed loading: a randomized controlled clinical trial. J Dent Res 2018;97(2):163–70.
71. Nogueira TE, Dias DR, Leles CR. Mandibular complete denture versus single-implant overdenture: a systematic review of patient-reported outcomes. J Oral Rehabil 2017;44(12):1004–16.
72. Passia N, Att W, Freitag-Wolf S, et al. Single mandibular implant study: denture satisfaction in the elderly. J Oral Rehabil 2017;44(3):213–9.
73. Goodacre C, Goodacre B. Fixed vs removable complete arch implant prostheses: a literature review of prosthodontic outcomes. Eur J Oral Implantol 2017; 10(Suppl 1):13–34.
74. Maló P, de Araujo Nobre MA, Lopes AV, et al. Immediate loading short implants inserted on low bone quantity for the rehabilitation of the edentulous maxilla using an all-on-4 design. J Oral Rehabil 2015;42(8):615–23.
75. Malo PS, de Araujo Nobre MA, Ferro AS, et al. Five-year outcome of a retrospective cohort study comparing smokers vs. nonsmokers with full-arch mandibular implant-supported rehabilitation using the all-on-4 concept. J Oral Sci 2018; 60(2):177–86.
76. Branemark PI, Engstrand P, Ohrnell LO, et al. Branemark Novum: a new treatment concept for rehabilitation of the edentulous mandible. Preliminary results from a prospective clinical follow-up study. Clin Implant Dent Relat Res 1999;1(1):2–16.
77. Engstrand P, Grondahl K, Ohrnell LO, et al. Prospective follow-up study of 95 patients with edentulous mandibles treated according to the Branemark Novum concept. Clin Implant Dent Relat Res 2003;5(1):3–10.
78. Engstrand P, Nannmark U, Martensson L, et al. Branemark Novum: prosthodontic and dental laboratory procedures for fabrication of a fixed prosthesis on the day of surgery. Int J Prosthodont 2001;14(4):303–9.
79. Trefoil™ the next full-arch revolution. Nobelbiocare.com. Available at: https://www.nobelbiocare.com/content/microsite/us/en/trefoil.html. Accessed July 29, 2018.

Revisiting the Removable Partial Denture

Jiyeon J. Kim, DMD, MS

KEYWORDS

- Removable partial denture • Partial edentulism • Classification systems
- Treatment considerations • Framework design
- Distal extension RPD considerations • Implant-assisted RPD • CAD/CAM

KEY POINTS

- Removable partial denture therapy will remain a cost- and time-effective treatment for partially edentulous patients.
- Most basic concepts, framework design, and treatment considerations for metal-framework RPD remain unchanged.
- Implant-assisted RPD significantly improves the quality of life and satisfaction of patients.
- Computer-assisted design and manufacturing for RPD framework provides high-quality treatment with its accuracy and precision.
- More research is necessary to examine changing design principles to better serve the new polymer framework materials.

INTRODUCTION

The percentage of complete edentulism has decreased in the aging population because of better understanding and reduction of dental diseases, establishment of effective maintenance and preventive programs, and improvement of dental materials. However, the proportion of the partially edentulous population is increasing because of increased life expectancy, an increasing aging population, and more teeth being retained within this population.[1,2] The American College of Prosthodontists predicted the number of individuals with partial edentulism could increase to more than 200 million in the United States in the next 15 years, and currently almost 50% of all adults are missing one or more teeth.[1] Therefore, the need for fixed and removable partial prostheses remains high and will continue to grow in the future.[2]

Fixed dental prostheses (FDPs) have traditionally been the gold standard to treat partial edentulism. However, when there is no abutment tooth distal to the edentulous

Disclosure: The author has nothing to disclose.

Department of Restorative Dentistry, University of Illinois at Chicago, 801 South Paulina Street Room 359., Chicago, IL 60612, USA
E-mail address: Jkim439@uic.edu

Dent Clin N Am 63 (2019) 263–278
https://doi.org/10.1016/j.cden.2018.11.007 dental.theclinics.com
0011-8532/19/

space or in a long-spanning edentulous space, FDP therapy is contraindicated. When these patients would have had no other treatment choice in the past but to receive a removable partial denture (RPD), now they may have a fixed option in the form of dental implants. Frequently, dental implants today provide the best practice alternative. However, financial considerations often contribute to the decision-making process for many of these patients, leading to RPDs being the treatment option selected.

Dental implants come at a cost, both financial and time-related. The financial expense of dental implants is high, especially when additional therapies are required to prepare the implant site. Because the treatment period is generally longer than for nonsurgical interventions, there is an additional expense of time. When compared with an implant placed without site development, bone augmentation procedures can easily double the treatment time. For patients who have a significant medical history or dental anxiety, the surgical therapy may be considered more aggressive and may be contraindicated.

In contrast to implant therapy, RPD treatment is minimally invasive, and allows cost-effective and timely care for partially edentulous patients. When replacing lost hard and soft tissues to provide esthetic support, for long-term transitional prosthesis for a terminal dentition, and when restoring long edentulous spans,[1] it is the best practice therapy for many clinical scenarios (**Figs. 1** and **2**). Therefore, RPDs will remain an important treatment alternative and viable option for a large proportion of the partially edentulous population.

The purpose of this article is to review RPD classification systems, treatment concerns, and framework design, and to discuss advances in implant-assisted RPD (IARPD), computer-assisted design (CAD)/computer-assisted manufacturing (CAM) in RPD framework design and fabrication, and the use of new materials such as milled polymer frameworks that allow metal-free options.

REMOVABLE PARTIAL DENTURE CLASSIFICATION SYSTEMS

The most widely used classification system for partial edentulism is the Kennedy method of classification and Applegate's rule for applying the Kennedy classification. This classification system divides RPD scenarios according to the location of the edentulous region and its popularity. Kennedy classification class I designates bilateral edentulous areas located posterior to the natural teeth, and Kennedy class II describes a unilateral edentulous area located posterior to the remaining natural teeth.[3] Kennedy defined a unilateral edentulous area bound by natural teeth to be class III, and for a single edentulous area crossing the midline located anterior to the remaining natural teeth, class IV was the designation.[3] Applegate provided 8 rules that help with the application of the Kennedy classification in more complex situations. Although the

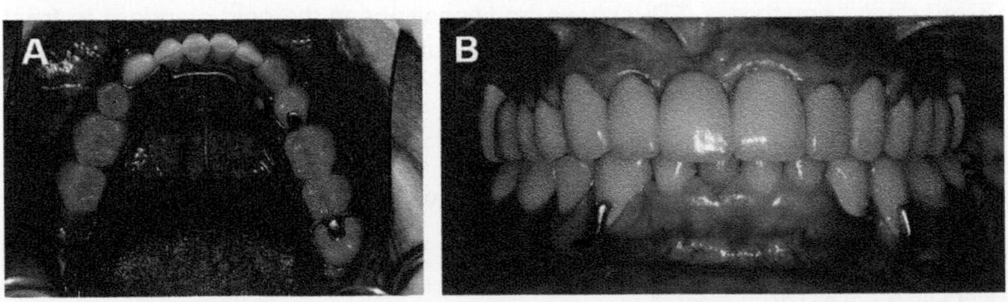

Fig. 1. (*A, B*) Because of the severely resorbed edentulous ridge, mandibular RPD was the only option to restore function.

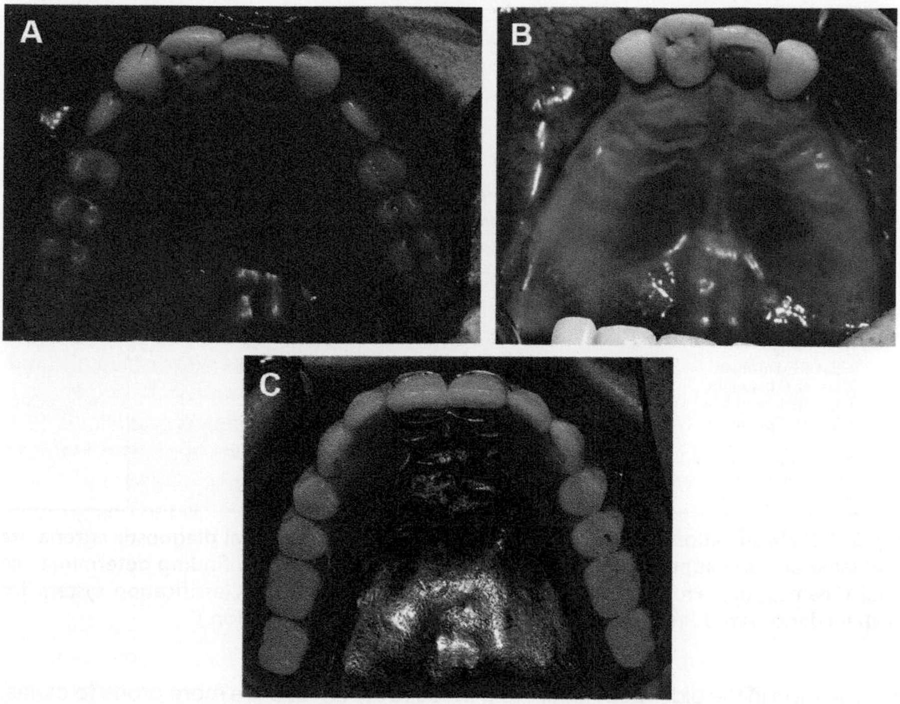

Fig. 2. (*A–C*) Prolonged use of a nonmetal clasp denture resulted in severe resorption of edentulous ridges, lacking retention and resistance form for a complete denture. Remaining teeth were used for a long-term transitional RPD prosthesis for terminal dentition.

Kennedy and Applegate classifications are useful in visualizing the partially edentulous arch and communicating, they do not address the detailed complexity that is necessary for billing issues and distinguishing complex situations that need referral. The Prosthodontic Diagnostic Index (PDI) classification system for partially edentulous patients was developed to address this issue. This classification distinguishes partially edentulous scenarios according to complexity determined by 5 criteria, namely location and extent of edentulous areas, abutment tooth condition, occlusal scheme, residual ridge morphology, and other conditions, to facilitate consistent and predictable treatment-planning decisions.[4] The descriptive nature of this classification system (**Fig. 3**) provides a more detailed communication with dental providers, laboratory technicians, and others. The adoption of this system has the potential to benefit dentistry greatly through emphasis of the PDI classification system in dental education and its usage for billing, compensation/reimbursements, and establishing referrals. Unfortunately, this classification system currently has limited use in dentistry because of its complexity, resistance to change, and diagnostic basis in a profession that is largely therapy driven.

REMOVABLE PARTIAL DENTURE TREATMENT CONSIDERATIONS

Partially edentulous patients must be cautious of the development of caries, periodontal diseases, and resorption of the residual ridge. These disease states may be detrimental to the long-term survival of tissues supporting the RPD. Exposed root surfaces caused by periodontal disease or gingival recession from mechanical brushing

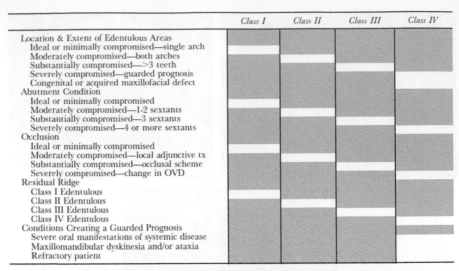

	Class I	Class II	Class III	Class IV
Location & Extent of Edentulous Areas				
Ideal or minimally compromised—single arch				
Moderately compromised—both arches				
Substantially compromised—>3 teeth				
Severely compromised—guarded prognosis				
Congenital or acquired maxillofacial defect				
Abutment Condition				
Ideal or minimally compromised				
Moderately compromised—1-2 sextants				
Substantially compromised—3 sextants				
Severely compromised—4 or more sextants				
Occlusion				
Ideal or minimally compromised				
Moderately compromised—local adjunctive tx				
Substantially compromised—occlusal scheme				
Severely compromised—change in OVD				
Residual Ridge				
Class I Edentulous				
Class II Edentulous				
Class III Edentulous				
Class IV Edentulous				
Conditions Creating a Guarded Prognosis				
Severe oral manifestations of systemic disease				
Maxillomandibular dyskinesia and/or ataxia				
Refractory patient				

Fig. 3. PDI classification for partial edentulism worksheet. Individual diagnostic criteria are evaluated and the appropriate box is checked. The most advanced finding determines the final classification. (*From* McGarry TJ, Nimmo A, Skiba JF, et al. Classification system for partial edentulism. J Prosthodont. 2002;11(3):181–93; with permission.)

are common in the older population, and these root surfaces are more prone to caries. Increased plaque accumulation with the use of RPD prostheses has been well documented,[5] and directly contribute to the high incidences of caries for patients wearing RPDs. When appropriate etiologic factors are present, RPDs may accelerate bone loss and tooth mobility.[6] Therefore, an attentive framework design that minimizes accumulation of plaque and has favorable biomechanical forces is necessary. Continuous maintenance and excellent oral hygiene are necessary for long-term survival of the prosthesis, the abutment teeth, and the periodontium.[6]

A retrospective study found that 39% of RPDs were no longer in use within 5 years of delivery.[7] To be successful, RPDs must be worn by the patient with minimal complications. Therefore, framework design should take the patient's comfort and esthetic expectations into consideration to ensure patient compliance. Because ill-fitting RPDs transferring detrimental forces to the ridge may accelerate the progression of residual ridge resorption, the fit and occlusion of the RPD must be verified during fabrication of the prosthesis and subsequent maintenance appointments to delay the progression of residual ridge resorption. Partially dentate patients most likely lost their teeth as a result of caries or periodontal disease from poor oral hygiene. Therefore, it is essential that dental care providers help patients improve their oral hygiene habits through proper home-care instructions while enforcing an appropriate maintenance schedule for their removable prosthesis.

The challenge of RPD therapy is to restore function, esthetics, and comfort while minimizing potentially damaging forces to the abutment teeth and supporting tissues. Although the design of the RPD framework is important to minimize detrimental forces to abutment teeth and supporting tissue, most classic RPD concepts are based on empirical observations and philosophic biases of the clinician presenting the concepts.[8] Several concepts are based on attempts to integrate scientific research into the philosophic and biological biases that were acquired during professional practice.[8] The basic concepts of RPD design that are widely accepted are reviewed in the following sections, and are in part based on the properties of conventionally used metal framework.

REVIEW OF BASIC CONCEPTS AND FRAMEWORK DESIGN

Rests

The main function of a rest is to serve as a vertical support for the RPD to resist movement toward the tissue[3]; it also provides the positional placement and reproducibility for all of the other components of the RPD. All rest preparations should have a positive seat that transmits the occlusal forces to the center long axis of the tooth without slippage of the prosthesis away from the abutment. Any preparation must be free of sharp angles with smooth finishing.

Occlusal rest seats on posterior teeth should be one-third the buccolingual width and one-third the mesiodistal length of premolars or one-fourth the mesiodistal length of molars. These rest preparations should be triangular in shape with dovetails on the marginal ridge to meet the proximal plate of the correct width. A longer rest preparation that extends beyond half of the occlusal surface, mesiodistal width, may be used in special clinical scenarios to transfer forces along the vertical axis, to the center of the tooth, especially in mesially inclined molars.

Cingulum rests can be prepared on anterior teeth with distinct anatomic cingula, which are typically limited to maxillary canines. A cingulum rest seats is prepared into the incisal most extent of the cingulum where there is a bulk of enamel, not above the cingulum (**Fig. 4**). These rests should have adequate thickness—at least 1 mm at the center and tapered as it moves away from the center. Any undercuts created above the rest preparation should be conservatively removed. When an anterior tooth does not have a prominent cingulum, a lingual ball rest may be used. Because a lingual ball rest is placed on either the mesial or distal part of the marginal ridge, it may transmit tipping forces to the teeth. Careful framework design and a well-fitting framework will help minimize these tipping forces. Although incisal rests have been used in the past, their use has declined in recent years because of unfavorable lever forces and esthetic concerns.

A common cause of framework failure is rest fracture at the junction between the rest seat and the proximal surface. A 1.5-mm minimal thickness of metal is advocated to prevent this type of a complication. At times it is difficult to prepare a posterior

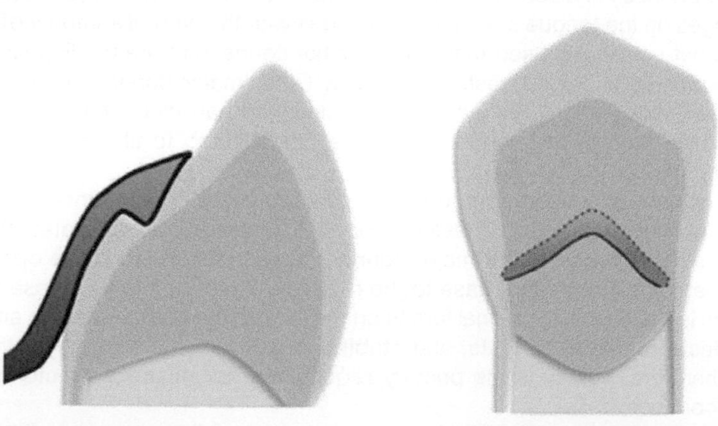

Fig. 4. Ideal location and preparation of a cingulum rest. (*Courtesy of* Jay Jayanetti, DDS, Los Angeles, CA.)

occlusal rest seat on sound enamel structure without penetrating into dentin when a minimal preparation of 1.5 mm is required. Therefore, it is critical that the patient's occlusion be evaluated before initiating any treatment, either through clinical evaluation or by articulating opposing diagnostic casts. If the opposing tooth does not directly contact the marginal ridge area or if the patient is edentulous on the opposing arch, a more conservative rest seat preparation may be allowed without compromising the integrity of the metal framework as long as it does not interfere with patient's static and dynamic occlusion. In this clinical situation, the metal can be designed to meet the minimum thickness and not interfere with opposing occlusion.

Major Connectors and Minor Connectors

The major connector joins components of the prosthesis on one side to those on the opposite side of the same arch.[3] The marginal gingiva of teeth is highly vascular and susceptible to injury from pressure.[9] Therefore, the major connector must maintain a safe distance of 6 mm away from the gingival margin of maxillary teeth and 3 mm away from that of mandibular teeth.

The most important requirement of a major connector is rigidity for cross-arch stability, resulting in effective distribution of occlusal forces to supporting teeth, bone, and soft tissue. A flexible major connector is detrimental because it will concentrate forces on individual teeth and areas of edentulous residual ridges, and not allow other components of the prosthesis to fulfill their purposes. Ben-Ur and colleagues[10] characterized major connectors based on their rigidity. For maxillary RPDs, anteroposterior palatal straps on different planes were deemed most rigid, followed by a palatal strap and U-shape.[10] Campbell[11] investigated patient preferences for the various major connector designs, rank ordering them by ability to speak, chew, swallow, overall comfort, and satisfaction. Based on patient perceptions, the preferred rank order was broad strap, anteroposterior palatal straps (no anterior plating), anteroposterior strap (with plating), and full palatal coverage.[11] It is no surprise that both studies rated lingual bar higher than lingual plating in the mandible.[10,11] The most commonly used maxillary major connectors are the single palatal strap for short-span tooth-supported scenarios and the anterior-posterior strap for most partially edentulous scenarios. Complete palatal coverage may be used in compromised anatomic situations and a U-shaped palatal major connector may be used when a palatal torus or a sensitive gag reflex is present. The use of the bar type of maxillary major connector is decreasing because of discomfort created in patients from the bulk required for rigidity as it impinges on the tongue space and coincides with the natural anatomy of the palate. The most commonly used mandibular major connectors are the lingual bar and plate, when there is limited vestibular space. Other major connectors with limited use include sublingual bar, lingual bar with cingulum bar, cingulum bar, and labial bar.[3] The best type of major connector must be selected to fit individual patients and their needs.

Minor connectors are the components that unite other components of the prosthesis to the major connector. These components include proximal plates, the rests, indirect retainers, clasps to the major connector, tissue stops, and the open lattice or mesh that joins the denture base to the major connector.[3,9] The purpose of minor connectors is to transfer functional forces on the RPD to the abutment teeth and transfer the effects of retainers, rests, and stabilizing components throughout the prosthesis.[3] Therefore, rigidity is the primary requirement for minor connectors, as it is for major connectors.

Although the concepts proposed by Kratochvil and Krol are relevant to distal extension clasp assemblies, it is important to mention their differences and discuss the length of the proximal plate. Kratochvil[12] advocated the use of long proximal plates to maximize contact with the abutment tooth to improve stabilization, prevent food impaction, and prevent hypertrophy of soft tissue in the area. Krol[13] advocated the use of a short proximal plate to provide physiologic relief, and disengagement of the proximal plate from the abutment tooth during function, thereby avoiding torquing of the abutment tooth. It is widely accepted to use a proximal plate somewhere in between, that is, one-half to one-third of the clinical crown height. The width of the proximal plate should be one-third of the buccal lingual width of the tooth and follow the natural curvature of the tooth.

Retainers

Direct retainers are used to provide retention for the RPD; resisting the movement of the prosthesis away from the tissue surface. The terminal tip of a direct retainer (retentive clasp) passes below the height of contour (HOC) to engage a 0.01-inch or 0.02-inch undercut. Extracoronal retainers are the most widely used and taught in dental curriculums. There are 2 types of clasps, suprabulge and infrabulge. Because the suprabulge clasp approaches the undercut from above the HOC, it is crucial to have a low HOC to allow sufficient room for the approach arm of the clasp to originate from the rest or the proximal plate (**Fig. 5**), thereby providing improved flexibility and esthetics. An infrabulge clasp approaches the undercut from below the HOC. Its use is not recommended when there is a significant amount of soft tissue undercut or a shallow vestibular depth.

The retentive clasp arm must be designed with a reciprocal component on the opposite tooth surface to provide bracing of the abutment tooth during placement and removal of the prosthesis.[3] If the reciprocation is provided by a bracing arm, it must stay above the HOC and directly contact the abutment tooth before or as the retentive tip passes over the HOC on the opposite side. The HOC may need to be lowered to allow proper placement of a reciprocal clasp arm at the junction of middle to lower third of the clinical crown height (**Fig. 6**).

Once seated, the RPD should passively be seated on the abutment teeth and tissues. The retentive clasp of the RPD should only engage the tooth when resisting movement away from the tissue. The proximal plates may provide additional retention in certain situations.

The clasp assembly, which includes the rest, retentive clasp, reciprocal component, and minor connectors, provides encirclement of the abutment tooth and reinforces

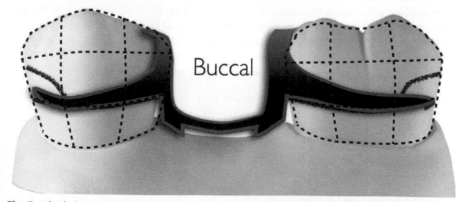

Fig. 5. Ideal placement of suprabulge clasp. *Dotted lines* represent the thirds and *solid line* represents the ideal height of contour. (*Courtesy of* Jay Jayanetti, DDS, Los Angeles, CA.)

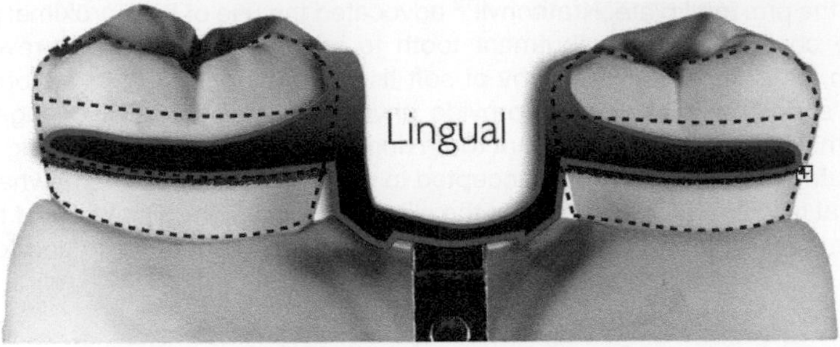

Fig. 6. Ideal placement of reciprocal clasp. *Dotted lines* represent the thirds and *solid line* represents the ideal height of contour. (*Courtesy of* Jay Jayanetti, DDS, Los Angeles, CA.)

stabilization of the RPD. Encirclement is important to prevent tooth movement away from the partial denture. The purpose of stabilization is to distribute the stress equally to all supporting teeth and efficiently resist horizontal movement of the prosthesis.

FRAMEWORK DESIGN CONSIDERATIONS

The selection of a clasp assembly for a tooth-supported RPD (Kennedy class III) is relatively simple because the occlusal forces are directly transferred to the adjacent abutment teeth, similar to an FDP. Akers clasp assemblies, also known as circumferential, are universally used for these scenarios. If the anterior abutment tooth is in the esthetic zone, an I-bar may be used to improve esthetics. On the other hand, careful selection of a stress-breaking clasp assembly is advocated for tooth- and tissue-supported RPDs such as in distal extension scenarios. Because tissue is more compressible than a tooth, potentially destructive class I lever forces may be applied onto the distal abutment tooth. Mesial positioning of the rest alters the fulcrum position and resulting clasp movement to minimize the class I lever forces and prevent harmful engagement of the abutment tooth.[3,12,13] Commonly used stress-breaking clasp assemblies for distal extension scenarios are the RPI, RPA(C), and combination clasp assemblies. The I-bar of the RPI clasp assembly must be placed at the greatest mesial distal curvature of the buccal surface[12,13] or slightly mesial to it, as long as it is not more mesial than the center of the mesial rest (**Fig. 7**). Combination clasp assemblies may be used when an RPI is contraindicated, but the wrought wire retentive clasp requires a 0.02-inch undercut because of its flexibility (**Fig. 8**). RPA(C) is more technique sensitive because the Akers (Circumferential) clasp must lie below the HOC with only the superior border of the clasp having a point contact at the HOC (**Fig. 9**).

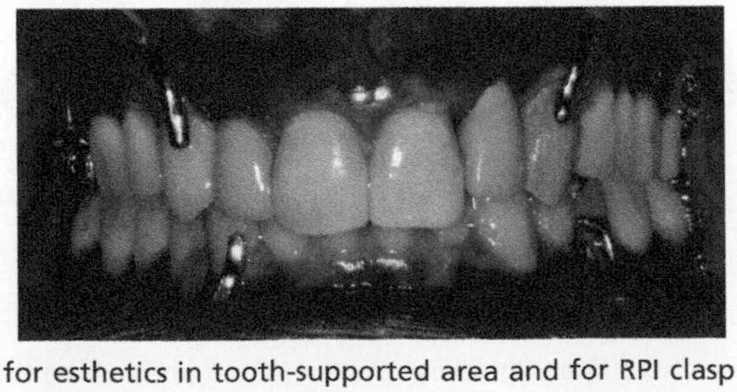

Fig. 7. I-bar used for esthetics in tooth-supported area and for RPI clasp assembly in distal extension area.

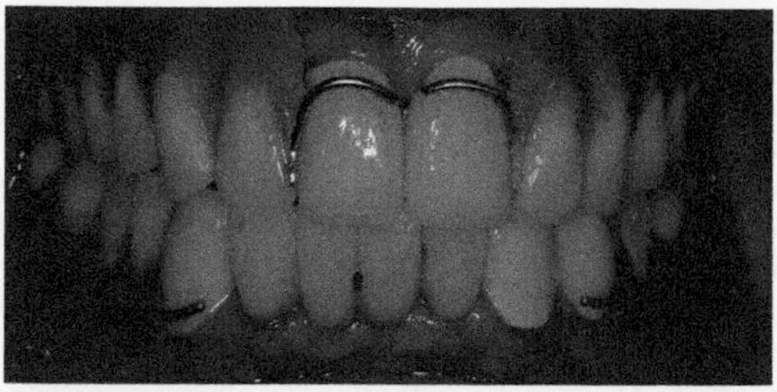

Fig. 8. Wrought wire/combination clasp assemblies used for distal extension area.

The board stress distribution philosophy is based on elements of RPD design to maximize support across multiple abutments and supporting anatomic structures to minimize destructive forces.[9] A key tenet of this design philosophy is based on the clasp assembly selected, to include locating rest seats immediately adjacent to an edentulous area, placing direct retention on the most distal abutment tooth or teeth adjacent to the edentulous space, and identifying the clasp preference based on location of retention on the abutment tooth. In addition, denture bases provide broad coverage of anatomic supporting structures and distribute occlusal forces, increasing resistance to lateral forces while minimizing forces on a single tooth or onto a limited area of the residual alveolar ridge.[9] Regardless of the desired design philosophy, all components of an RPD are prescribed to minimize potentially destructive biomechanical forces and address individual patient needs and expectations to achieve a successful treatment outcome.

ADVANCEMENTS IN REMOVABLE PARTIAL DENTURE

Implant-Assisted Removable Partial Denture

Implants may be used in RPD therapy to improve support, retention, and stability of the prosthesis while maintaining alveolar height in the region where the implant is placed. Successful treatment of implant-supported RPDs (ISRPDs) has shown to improve the oral health quality of life for patients.[14,15] The benefit of an implant is significant in distal extension scenarios (Kennedy class I and II), as it efficiently serves to improve support, creating a tooth-supported situation (Kennedy class III). This minimizes the potentially damaging class I lever force that is placed on the distal abutment tooth during function. Many studies, including a systematic review in 2012, report

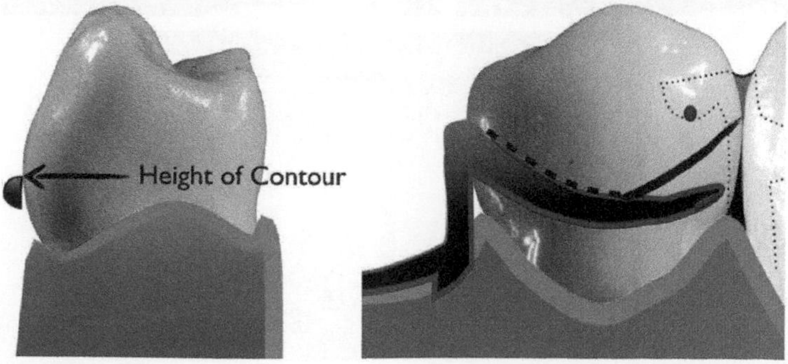

Fig. 9. Correct application of RPA(C) clasp assembly. *Dotted lines* represents the height of contour in point contact with the Akers clasp and the *red circle* represents rest seat. (*Courtesy of* Jay Jayanetti, DDS, Los Angeles, CA.)

a significant increase in patient satisfaction and high survival rates of implants associated with mandibular RPDs with distal extensions.[16] ISRPD is commonly recommended as an economical and beneficial rehabilitation that significantly improves patient satisfaction.[15–17] In addition to support, an implant can be used to improve retention. Therefore, it may be more suitable to use the term implant-assisted RPD (IARPD) than the term implant-supported RPD (ISRPD) (**Fig. 10**A, B).

The preferred location of the implants may be different depending on the purpose they will serve and bone availability. If extensive augmentation procedures were required to allow implant placement, it is questionable as to the advantage the patient would receive.[3] When used to improve retention, implants can provide the advantage of eliminating a visible clasp when placed in the anterior region of the edentulous span[3] (**Fig. 10**C). To increase support, many clinicians advocate placing an implant in the distal region to replace the missing distal abutment and essentially convert the situation to a Kennedy class III scenario. An implant that is placed parallel to the path of insertion of the RPD will have a more favorable outcome with fewer prosthetic complications.[3] Although many finite-element analysis (FEA) studies have been used to evaluate the biomechanical stress on implants to determine preferred implant position, these studies are limited because they are in vitro studies and fail to simulate the natural anatomy, oral environment, and function. A recent FEA by a group in Barcelona[18] attempted to simulate the partially edentulous mandible of a patient by printing a 3D stereolithographic model from an existing cone-beam CT of a patient and including soft-tissue and periodontal ligament (PDL) elements of the distal abutment tooth. Within the limitations of the study, they found more favorable stress distribution and dissipation along the peri-implant bone with implants placed in the first molar position compared with that of second molar and premolar area.[18] Closer proximity to distal abutment tooth helped with decreasing the stress placed on the PDL fibers of

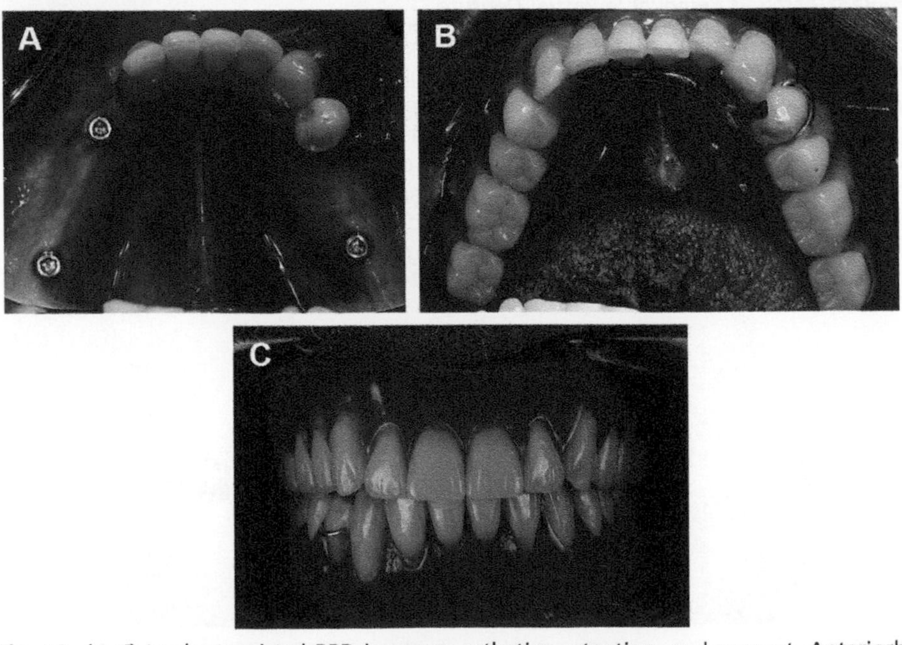

Fig. 10. (*A–C*) Implant-assisted RPD improves esthetics, retention, and support. Anteriorly placed implant may improve esthetics by eliminating a visible retainer clasp. (*Courtesy of* Laura Koo Min Chee, DMD, Chicago, IL.)

the distal abutment tooth.[18] These results were consistent with those observed in other FEA studies.[19,20] In a patient-based outcomes study, Jensen and colleagues[15] found that implants significantly improved patient satisfaction and quality of life, and more patients preferred the implant in the molar region over the premolar region.

Another debate regarding IARPD prosthodontic practices is the preferred retention system. One study compared Stern ERA (Sterngold, Attleboro, MA, USA) and O-ring attachments in a 2D finite-element model by inducing axial and oblique forces. The authors demonstrate that the ERA attachment system had more favorable stress distribution and was therefore the preferred system in IARPD cases.[21] Locator and housing systems seem to be the most widely used attachment system in IARPD. This system, though similar to the ERA, is often used in place of the ERA because of its shorter vertical height requirement and because many dentists are more familiar with its use for mandibular overdentures. A recent in vitro study evaluating and comparing the strain around abutment teeth found ball attachments to have the lowest strain, followed by the locator housing and the magnetic system.[22] The highest strain was observed in the control group with a distal RPD without any implants.[22] Although the axial loading of this study is a limitation and does not reflect the complexity of the masticatory forces, it provides evidence that implants improve the strain of the RPD abutment teeth with any attachment system.[22]

Computer-Aided Design/Computer-Aided Manufacturing and Removable Partial Dentures

CAD/CAM systems have been developed and widely used in dentistry in fixed and implant therapy to provide efficient and precise treatment.[1] The use of CAD/CAM systems in removable dental therapy, including complete dentures and RPDs, has been evolving to improve the accuracy and fit while reducing costs, time, and labor. An advantage of this technology is that digital files of the prosthesis can be saved and easily reproduced without additional clinical appointments for an impression if another prosthesis is necessary.

Many dental laboratory technicians are using laboratory scanners to image the master dental cast and then using design software to digitally design the RPD frameworks (**Fig. 11**). This process replaces the conventional technique. Instead of fabricating an

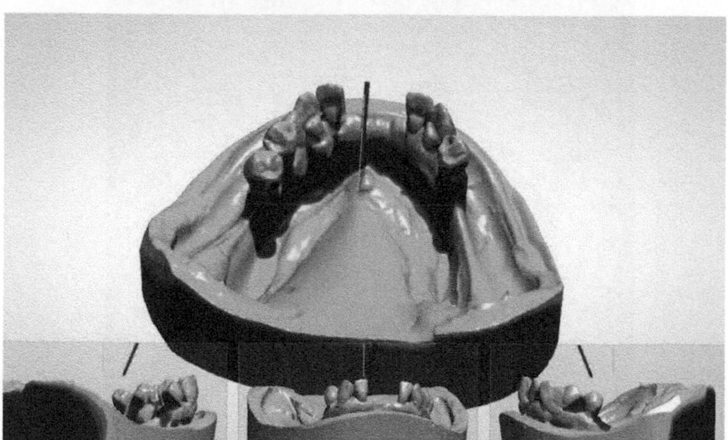

Fig. 11. Digital survey. *White arrow* is the purposed path of insertion and the *red arrow* is manipulating the path of insertion. (*Courtesy of* Timothy J. Shary, MS, Alpharetta, GA; and Solvay Dental 360, Alpharetta, GA.)

investment cast with wax patterns, a wax pattern of the framework is printed (**Fig. 12**). The printed wax pattern of the framework is used to traditionally cast a metal framework. These digitally designed frameworks prove to have similar, if not better, accuracy and fit compared with those fabricated by traditional methods.[1,23] With the increasing use of digital technology for RPDs, it is crucial that the dental curriculum follows this change and includes digital learning opportunities in the RPD dental curriculum. This potentially provides better 3D visualization for designing framework for students.

RPD metal frameworks may be directly fabricated from other digital fabrication methods such as selective laser sintering and milling[23] (**Figs. 13** and **14**). However, the use of direct printing of the frameworks rather than casting printed patterns has been used only limitedly to date. Although manufacturing capabilities are rapidly changing and offer engineering levels of precision and accuracy, the use of CAM in RPD framework fabrication is restricted by its high cost and accessibility.[1] CAD also has the advantage of improved communications by allowing the clinician to view and approve the design before manufacturing. In addition, CAD/CAM provides improved alternatives to RPD materials that may lead to significant improvements in the future.

New Removable Partial Denture Framework Materials

Traditionally RPDs have had metal frameworks, usually cobalt-chromium (vitallium) or nickel-chromium (ticonium). The use of metal frameworks has been advocated for reasons of their high strength and stiffness, heat conductivity, resilience, and biocompatibility.[1] Although the metal framework is inexpensive and predictable, its unesthetic display of metal clasps (**Fig. 15**), increased weight, incidences of metallic taste, and allergic reactions has made it unpopular to patients.[24] Despite decades of using metal frameworks, an increasing number of patients are hesitant to have metal in their mouth. Patients' preference for nonmetallic materials led to the development of

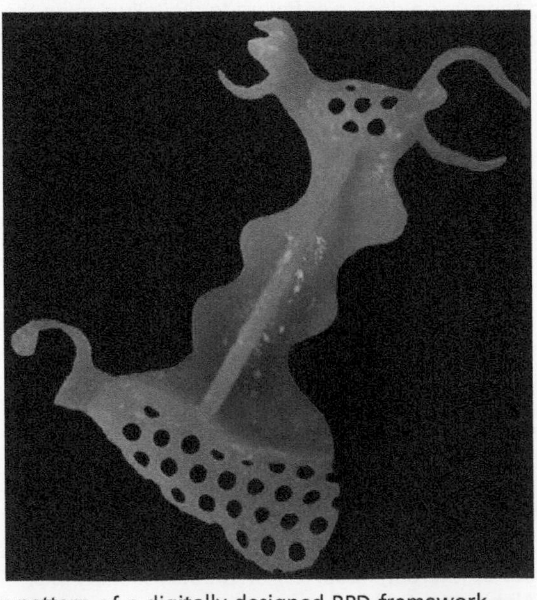

Fig. 12. Milled wax pattern of a digitally designed RPD framework.

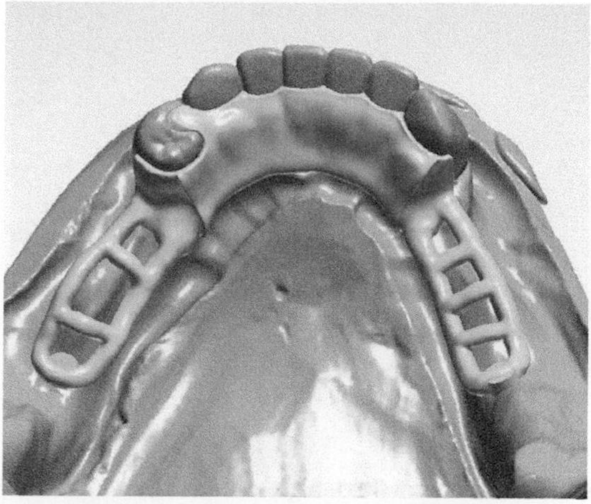

Fig. 13. RPD framework. (*Courtesy of* Cory Fibbs, CDT, Ottawa, IL.)

alternative materials such as thermoplastic resins including polyamide (nylon), polyester, polycarbonate, acrylic resins, and polypropylenes.[25] Most of these materials have yet to undergo the complete physical evaluation needed to advocate their clinical use as a permanent prosthesis.[25] Some of the problems encountered with these materials include color stability, difficulty for repair, high risk for fracture, and surface changes, but most importantly, they lack rigidity and support.[25] In addition, the lack of rests and other basic RPD components of fundamental design philosophy can lead to complications (see **Fig. 2**A, B).

Because these materials have different properties, it is important to understand them and recommend the correct maintenance protocol for these nonmetal clasp dentures (NMCDs). With increased use of digital technology, these NMCDs are more widely available because they can be directly milled or printed without the high cost associated with metal frameworks. Although the clinical use of NMCDs is increasing, they have never been advocated to replace metal frameworks as a definite treatment RPD because of their properties and lack of scientific evidence. This may in part be due to their variance from accepted RPD design components such as rests. Therefore, their use must be limited to temporary treatment or patients who cannot tolerate alloys.[25]

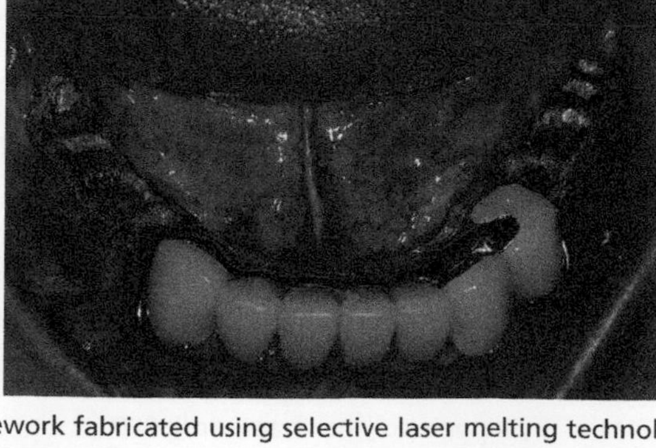

Fig. 14. RPD framework fabricated using selective laser melting technology.

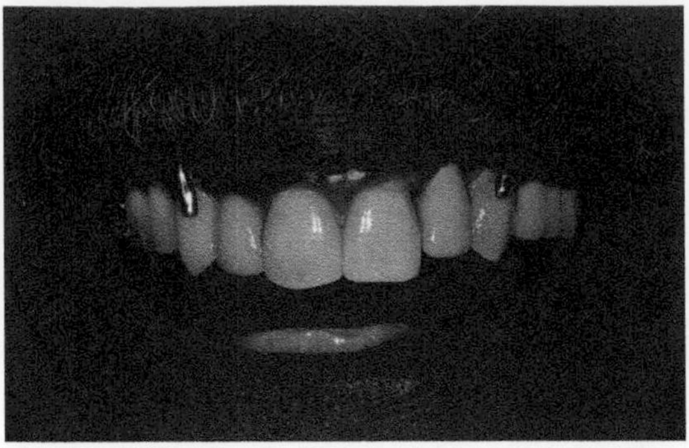

Fig. 15. Unesthetic display of metal clasps.

Successfully used in the medical field, high-performance medical-grade arylketone polymer (AKP) presents a promising alternative to RPD metal frameworks.[24] This material has overcome many of the disadvantages of thermoplastic resins. AKP includes supportive elements and has high biocompatibility, good mechanical properties, high temperature resistance, chemical stability, and more rigidity than thermoplastic resins.[24] Although this polymer framework material uses the traditional design concepts of RPD metal framework with minor modifications, its clasps require more thickness and bulk to increase their functional rigidity when compared with metal suprabulge retentive clasp arms. It offers potential improvements in esthetics because the clasps may be characterized to match abutment tooth shade. It is lighter in weight, and significantly decreases manufacturing costs while improving precision and accuracy (**Fig. 16**). Studies are needed to examine the impact of the increased flexibility of these prostheses on the hard and soft tissues as well as patient satisfaction. New approaches to design concepts such as the possible elimination of reciprocal/bracing arms with the use of dual flexible retentive clasps also need to be considered.

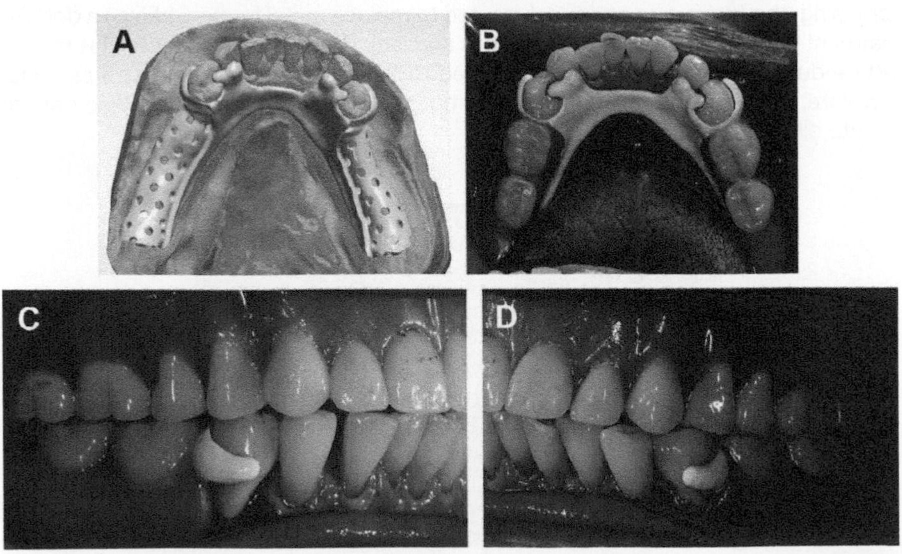

Fig. 16. (*A–D*) CAD/CAM of arylketone polymer framework RPD.

Research should examine changing design principles based on the properties of the new materials compared with the traditional design concepts of metal RPD frameworks.

Future Needs in Removable Partial Denture

RPDs are underappreciated compared with FDPs or dental implant therapy for the replacement of missing teeth. This negative attitude may be due to problems associated with wearing an RPD and concerns with comfort, esthetics, function, and maintenance of oral hygiene.[26] It is the clinician's responsibility to fabricate a well-fitting RPD that maximizes support and framework design while satisfying the patient's realistic expectations for function and esthetics. Maintenance and oral hygiene habits must also be emphasized.

Even with the advent of new materials and RPD design concepts, techniques and materials used in their fabrication process have seen minimal change. Therefore, RPD research more than ever needs to investigate new design principles to follow the development of new materials such as polymer frameworks and advanced technologies including digital design and production.

REFERENCES

1. Campbell SD, Cooper L, Craddock H, et al. Removable partial dentures: the clinical need for innovation. J Prosthet Dent 2017;118(3):273–80.
2. Douglass CW, Watson AJ. Future needs for fixed and removable partial dentures in the United States. J Prosthet Dent 2002;87(1):9–14.
3. Carr AB, Brown DT. McCracken's removable partial prosthodontics-e-book. 13th edition. Philadelphia: Elsevier Health Sciences; 2016.
4. McGarry TJ, Nimmo A, Skiba JF, et al. Classification system for partial edentulism. J Prosthodont 2002;11(3):181–93.
5. Addy M, Bates JF. The effect of partial dentures and chlorhexidine gluconate gel on plaque accumulation in the absence of oral hygiene. J Clin Periodontol 1977;4(1):41–7.
6. Rissin L, House JE, Conway C, et al. Effect of age and removable partial dentures on gingivitis and periodontal disease. J Prosthet Dent 1979;42(2):217–23.
7. Koyama S, Sasaki K, Yokoyama M, et al. Evaluation of factors affecting the continuing use and patient satisfaction with Removable Partial Dentures over 5 years. J Prosthodont Res 2010;54(2):97–101.
8. Becker CM, Kaiser DA, Goldfogel MH. Evolution of removable partial denture design. J Prosthodont 1994;3(3):158–66.
9. Stewart KL, Rudd KD, Kuebker WA. Clinical removable partial prosthodontics. St Louis (MO): Ishiyaku EuroAmerica Publishing Co.; 1992.
10. Ben-Ur Z, Matalon S, Aviv I, et al. Rigidity of major connectors when subjected to bending and torsion forces. J Prosthet Dent 1989;62(5):557–62.
11. Campbell LD. Subjective reactions to major connector designs for removable partial dentures. J Prosthet Dent 1977;37(5):507–16.
12. Kratochvil FJ. Influence of occlusal rest position and clasp design on movement of abutment teeth. J Prosthet Dent 1963;13(1):114–24.
13. Krol AJ. Clasp design for extension-base removable partial dentures. J Prosthet Dent 1973;29(4):408–15.
14. Gates WD 3rd, Cooper LF, Sanders AE, et al. The effect of implant-supported removable partial dentures on oral health quality of life. Clin Oral Implants Res 2014;25(2):207–13.

15. Jensen C, Raghoebar GM, Kerdijk W, et al. Implant-supported mandibular removable partial dentures; patient-based outcome measures in relation to implant position. J Dent 2016;55:92–8.
16. de Freitas RF, de Carvalho Dias K, da Fonte Porto Carreiro A, et al. Mandibular implant-supported removable partial denture with distal extension: a systematic review. J Oral Rehabil 2012;39(10):791–8.
17. Goncalves TM, Campos CH, Garcia RC. Implant retention and support for distal extension partial removable dental prostheses: satisfaction outcomes. J Prosthet Dent 2014;112(2):334–9.
18. Ortiz-Puigpelat O, Lazaro-Abdulkarim A, de Medrano-Rene JM, et al. Influence of implant position in implant-assisted removable partial denture: a three-dimensional finite element analysis. J Prosthodont 2017. https://doi.org/10.1111/jopr.12722.
19. Memari Y, Geramy A, Fayaz A, et al. Influence of implant position on stress distribution in implant-assisted distal extension removable partial dentures: a 3D finite element analysis. J Dent (Tehran) 2014;11(5):523–30.
20. Cunha LD, Pellizzer EP, Verri FR, et al. Evaluation of the influence of location of osseointegrated implants associated with mandibular removable partial dentures. Implant Dent 2008;17(3):278–87.
21. Pellizzer EP, Verri FR, Falcon-Antenucci RM, et al. Evaluation of different retention systems on a distal extension removable partial denture associated with an osseointegrated implant. J Craniofac Surg 2010;21(3):727–34.
22. MA EL, Omran AO, Fouad MM. Strains around abutment teeth with different attachments used for implant-assisted distal extension partial overdentures: an in vitro study. J Prosthodont 2017;26(1):42–7.
23. Williams RJ, Bibb R, Eggbeer D, et al. Use of CAD/CAM technology to fabricate a removable partial denture framework. J Prosthet Dent 2006;96(2):96–9.
24. Zoidis P, Papathanasiou I, Polyzois G. The use of a modified poly-ether-ether-ketone (PEEK) as an alternative framework material for removable dental prostheses. A clinical report. J Prosthodont 2016;25(7):580–4.
25. Fueki K, Ohkubo C, Yatabe M, et al. Clinical application of removable partial dentures using thermoplastic resin. Part II: material properties and clinical features of non-metal clasp dentures. J Prosthodont Res 2014;58(2):71–84.
26. Budtz-Jorgensen E, Bochet G. Alternate framework designs for removable partial dentures. J Prosthet Dent 1998;80(1):58–66.

Making the Best Clinical Decisions for Patients

The Pros-CAT Protocol™

Kent L. Knoernschild, DMD, MS[a,*], Stephen D. Campbell, DDS, MMSc[b]

KEYWORDS

• Evidence-based • PICO • Prognosis • Therapy • Harm • Systematic review • Pros-CAT • Critical appraisal

KEY POINTS

- A thorough patient assessment identifies clinical questions about prognostic factors that affect patient care outcomes.
- Clinical questions in the population, intervention, comparison, outcome format organize terms and assist the development of focused publication database searches.
- The Pros-CAT worksheets guide meaningful assessment of identified publications that are prognosis, therapy, harm, or systematic review formats.
- The Pros-CAT index compares identified articles validity and patient applicability in the context of the evidence hierarchy to determine the most relevant, highest quality information that answers the clinical question.
- Using the Pros-CAT protocol and index, clinicians are able to identify current, relevant, best evidence to answer patient care decisions.

INTRODUCTION

Patient-centered decision making is the principle on which successful treatment plans are developed. Patients seek predictable, state-of-the-art solutions for their concerns with goals of health promotion, disease prevention, disability recognition, and rehabilitation with a decreased incidence of maintenance and complications. Clinicians must have full awareness of patient expectations regardless of the therapeutic intervention. Clinicians must integrate patient expectations with clinical experience and the available published knowledge regarding a multitude of prognostic factors. These fundamentals are essential for patient-centered decision making and care.

Disclosure Statement: The authors have nothing to disclose.
[a] Advanced Education Program in Prosthodontics, Department of Restorative Dentistry, University of Illinois at Chicago College of Dentistry, 801 South Paulina Street, MC555, Chicago, IL 60612, USA; [b] Department of Restorative Dentistry, University of Illinois at Chicago College of Dentistry, 801 South Paulina Street, MC555, Chicago, IL 60612, USA
* Corresponding author.
E-mail address: kentk@uic.edu

Dent Clin N Am 63 (2019) 279–296
https://doi.org/10.1016/j.cden.2018.11.008
dental.theclinics.com

A clinician's knowledge must continuously grow as the dental profession's knowledge expands. Evidence-based decision making is described as the conscientious, explicit, and judicious use of the current best evidence in making decisions about the care of individual patients.[1] Contemporary dental practice is therefore founded on treatment decisions supported by a meaningful synthesis of the current clinical research. Health care professionals risk antiquated practice when their knowledge growth is less than that of the profession as a whole.

A straightforward, patient focused, critically appraised topic (CAT) method for literature appraisal was named Pros-CAT because it evolved within the accredited University of Illinois at Chicago Advanced Education Program in Prosthodontics, and for recognition that the method originated from the prosthodontic community. The format was developed following the *Journal of Prosthetic Dentistry* Evidence-Based Dentistry article series.[2–9] The series was written by 10 prosthodontists who visited McMaster University Medical School in the early 1990s to learn the decision-making process developed by Dr David Sackett, who is known as the father of evidence-based medicine. As a nephrologist and epidemiologist, Dr Sackett applied his skills in epidemiology and biostatistics in appraising the quality and validity of evidence for patient application, thereby setting the stage for structured appraisal in prosthodontics[10,11] and dentistry as a whole.

The Pros-CAT approach has meaningful application for clinical decision making. Considering patient presentation and care goals, specific prognostic factors that relate to clinical concerns are recognized, and concise clinical questions for treatment decisions are developed. Clinicians can have confidence when applying current best information identified with skills in literature analysis and synthesis. After the pertinent clinical literature is identified and appraised, the publications of greatest merit are synthesized into meaningful and brief topic summaries for immediate clinical application. The goal is to improve care outcomes when clinicians are empowered by an organized approach that guides patient-centered decisions.

Beginning with the development of the clinical question, 2 straightforward dental implant patient scenarios will be presented to provide examples for using the Pros-CAT protocol:

Scenario 1: Immediate Implant Placement, Immediate Restoration, and Esthetics; and

Scenario 2: Implant Fixed Complete Denture Prostheses and Veneer Fracture Incidence.

ASSESSING THE PATIENT

The goal of patient assessment is to maximize success and minimize the risk of complications by first identifying relevant prognostic factors. Patient medical and dental history, signs, symptoms, and diagnoses are examples of prognostic factors that must be recorded accurately to identify care outcomes. For example, prosthodontists consider the implications of many factors in the decision of prosthesis design, support, and esthetics. Depending on patient need and care considerations, the medical history, patient ability to tolerate surgical procedures, dental condition, caries risk, history of periodontitis, and bruxism are only a few of the many factors that could affect care outcome. Incomplete information can compromise care results.

The effects of prognostic factors individually and in combination on short- and long-term dental implant prognosis are difficult to determine. Indicated prosthodontic care options, which meet patient esthetic and functional expectations, determine predictable prosthesis design, prosthesis support, and decisions for adjunctive care. Melding of objective clinical findings with patient concerns leads to the initial care goal, for example, fixed or removable prosthesis designs. Patient presentation, patient expectations, and determined prosthesis design guide required prosthetic support, for example, tooth, implant or oral mucosa. Each support type leads to different prognostic factor considerations, for example, periodontal history, bone quantity and quality, and the presence of keratinized tissue. The influence of these factors is complex, because each patient has unique medical and dental status, treatment expectations, prosthesis design considerations, and long-term maintenance needs.

For patient-centered decision making, the careful assessment and identification of prognostic factors leads the clinician into a concise, answerable clinical question that directly applies to a specific patient's needs and expectations. Favorable or less favorable outcomes may be identified when such goals and factors are investigated in depth in the literature. Well-defined questions developed from correctly identified prognostic factors lead to the identification of patient-relevant literature and confidence in clinical decisions.

DEVELOPING THE CLINICAL QUESTION

Clinical questions can be developed in the straightforward population, intervention, comparison, outcome (PICO) format described by Sackett and colleagues.[12] The PICO format describes the patient population in question. The intervention is the considered patient or prosthesis factor that could influence therapy. The comparison is the factor that may lead to a different therapy result, and the outcome is the specific therapy result of interest. Patient-specific prognostic factors are carefully related to these areas to define publication database search terms leading to a meaningful literature search. Concise PICO components lead to a well-defined database search and the best evidence for decision making.

Population

The population is the group of patients found in published clinical research that best describes an individual patient who will receive care. A clear description of the patient is the first critical step in developing an effective literature search, because the population later identified in the researched literature directly arises from the patient's need. The conclusion from the investigation and critical appraisal then directly applies. Literature application for patient-centered relevant decision making brings greatest clinical meaning to the process.

A description of the patient population is infinitely broad and limited only by the clinician's imagination and the clinical question's applicability to the patient. Descriptions could include but are not limited to the surgical therapy they received, the specific prosthesis type, or the complications they developed. For example, the population might be described as (1) patients desiring dental implant therapy, (2) patients with mandibular dental implant overdentures, or (3) patients with periimplantitis. A clear definition of this population with carefully designed descriptors limits the literature search and identifies the articles most applicable to the patient about whom the question is generated.

Intervention and Comparison

The intervention is the potential prognostic factor or therapy approach that could directly affect the treatment results. Interventions could include but are not limited to medical history factors, clinical observations about the patient, prosthesis design factors, or proposed adjunctive therapy. As an example, for any patient receiving dental implants, interventions could include a (1) history of diabetes, (2) severe maxillary residual ridge resorption, (3) number of implants used in prosthesis design, or (4) the use of maxillary sinus augmentation. For any patient, each factor could predict care results.

The comparison describes the alternative patient descriptor or therapy approach that represents a potential pathway to a different therapeutic result. For example, with implant prognosis in the posterior maxilla, an intervention of long implants could be compared with short implants. If one is concerned with patient satisfaction based on therapy, a second intervention and comparison example could be single implant therapy compared with 3-unit, tooth-supported fixed partial denture therapy. Regarding periimplant bone loss, an intervention and comparison might be presence of periimplant keratinized tissue compared with a lack of keratinized tissue.

In the PICO question, the intervention and comparison concisely describe factors the clinician finds particularly important for treatment decisions. These suspected factors may influence the therapeutic outcomes.

Outcome

The outcome identifies a potential treatment result. Outcomes were described in 4 major categories, including (1) longevity, (2) physiologic, (3) psychological, and (4) economic outcomes.[13] An additional update from Carr and colleagues 2011[14] provided further category clarity. Each outcome group can be further divided into subcategories (**Table 1**). Within each category and subcategory, many prognostic factors with influence on outcome can be imagined. **Table 2** presents a small sample of the outcomes and possible prognostic factors associated with dental implant survival. Each prognostic factor suggests possible interventions or comparisons that affect outcomes.

The outcome describes one discreet aspect of patient therapy and does not represent the overall treatment result. For patients a mandibular implant supported fixed-complete prosthesis, the implant survival, prosthesis survival, occlusal force, nutritional intake, and patient satisfaction with esthetics or function each contribute to care success. Weighing the importance of these outcomes for an individual patient following literature appraisal is the defining action of the Pros-CAT analysis strategy. With these definitive clinical questions, a well-guided literature search focused on applicable prognostic factors can follow.

Table 1
Dental implant patient outcomes by category

Longevity	Functional	Psychological	Economic
Maintenance/follow-up	Speech	Treatment satisfaction	Direct costs
Implant survival	Swallowing	Self-image/confidence	Indirect costs
Implant success	Mastication	Esthetics	Disparities in health care
Prosthesis complications	Nutrition	Perception of function	Third-party policies
Prosthesis success	Motor/sensory function	Treatment preference	
Time to retreat		Health-related QoL Overall QoL Food preferences	

Abbreviation: QoL, quality of life.

Data from Guckes AD, Scurria MS, Shugars DA. A conceptual framework for understanding outcomes of oral implant therapy. J Prosthet Dent 1996;75:633–9; and Carr A, Wolfaardt J, Garrett N. Capturing patient benefits of treatment. Int J Oral Maxillofac Implants 2011;26(suppl):85–92.

Table 2
Longevity and survival outcome categories, example prognostic factor categories and example potential prognostic factors

Longevity/Survival	Outcome Categories	Prognostic Factor Categories	Example Prognostic Factors
Implant level	Implant success	Systemic health	Chemotherapy
	Implant survival	Oral health	Periodontitis
		Implant site	Bone quantity
		Implant design	Bone quality
		Timing for prosthetic restoration	Bone graft
			Implant length
			Implant diameter
		Oral habits	Implant surface
			Implant angulation
			Occlusion
			Bruxism

Assembling the Population, Intervention, Comparison, Outcome Question

Clear decision making results from a concise identification of the applicable prognostic factors and outcomes. The PICO question is assembled from the defined population, intervention, comparison, and outcome. The following clinical scenarios provide relevant examples for developing meaningful questions.

Scenario 1: Immediate implant placement, immediate restoration, and esthetics
A 35-year-old, partially edentulous patient desires a single implant to replace a maxillary central incisor. She requests immediate implant placement after extraction to expedite therapy, and she is focused on favorable esthetics throughout the care process. A thorough clinical evaluation suggests adequate alveolar bone and soft tissue quality exist to achieve favorable initial esthetics with immediate placement and immediate restoration. Decisions for the use of an immediate restoration compared with a more conventional, delayed approach are of interest. Stability of the periimplant soft tissue height is in question as it directly relates to prosthesis emergence, single implant crown dimensions, and the short- and long-term esthetic results.

For scenario 1, the PICO components are: P = patients with single maxillary incisor implants who desire immediate implant placement; I = immediate provisionalization; C = delayed provisionalization; and O = esthetics as determined by periimplant soft tissue dimensional change. The assembled PICO question is, "For patients who desire single maxillary incisor implant immediate placement, does immediate restoration compared with delayed restoration affect the esthetics as measured by soft tissue stability?" Implant survival is assumed with this question. Additional prognostic factors must be considered, such as bone volume and quality, soft tissue phenotype, immediate implant stability, immediate implant survival, and occlusal considerations. The risk of immediate implant failure or complications may be greater. Each of these relevant factors would be given full consideration during decision making when exploring immediate implant placement and restoration by constructing specific PICO questions.

Scenario 2: Implant fixed complete denture prostheses and complications incidence
A 50-year-old, edentulous patient is dissatisfied with the esthetics and function of her maxillary complete denture and mandibular implant-supported fixed complete denture she has worn for 5 years. Occlusal wear occurred with both prostheses, and her mandibular prosthesis has had frequent lost teeth and veneer fractures.

Mandibular implants have no bone loss or periimplant inflammation. Consideration for care includes replacement of the existing prostheses. Further consideration includes additional implants in the maxilla for an opposing fixed complete prosthesis. Zirconia prostheses are an option, but further investigation is necessary to determine the incidence of complications with zirconia and veneered zirconia compared with other designs.

Based on this scenario, the PICO components could be: P = edentulous patients with implant-supported fixed complete denture prostheses; I = zirconia prostheses; C = resin-metal prostheses; and O = complications. The assembled PICO question would be: "For edentulous patients who desire implant supported fixed complete denture prostheses, do zirconia prostheses compared with resin-metal prostheses have different incidence of complications?" Many relevant patient factors can be considered. For example, this question does not define the potential incidence of complications as influenced by opposing prosthesis designs and material. When comparing opposing complete denture, a resin-metal fixed complete denture, or a zirconia fixed complete denture option, bite force and supporting structure compliance (soft tissue vs implant) may influence the rate of occlusal wear and prosthesis fracture. Additional concise questions are necessary to identify trends such as these in greater detail.

CONDUCTING THE LITERATURE SEARCH

Only clinical research literature specifically applicable to the PICO question is of value in answering a clinical question. Consider the patient in scenario 1 with immediate implant placement after maxillary incisor extraction. One must search for only those articles that report esthetics as determined by measurable soft tissue height and discount those that report survival for other sites. Other prosthesis designs are not considered, because prosthesis design, loading conditions, maintenance, and complications could be quite different in those studies. Only when no relevant information evidence is identified can parallel literature with disparate patient characteristics or prosthesis designs be related to the question with understanding that the results do not directly apply.

A literature search is conducted through electronic and hand searching methods. Well-recognized and reliable databases exist including the Cochrane Library, TRIP, PubMed, EMBASE, and Web of Science. Each has their individual strengths based on purpose. PubMed and EMBASE are a broad access starting point for literature, whereas the Cochrane Library and TRIP focuses on high-quality evidence in different ways. Not all evidence is indexed in all databases. Access to more than 1 database may be necessarily followed by hand searching for thorough literature search identification.

Specific terms are used to categorize articles in the National Library of Medicine MEDLINE database. Search engines such as PubMed are helpful in finding the primary references of interest. Population, intervention, comparison, and outcome search terms can be identified using Medical Subject Headings (MeSH) directly related to PICO by entering a relevant term in the search field. For example, if one searches dental implant, the search engine will identify MeSH headings of (1) dental implants, (2) dental implantation, (3) dental implants, single-tooth, (4) dental implant-abutment design, (5) immediate dental implant loading, and (6) dental prosthesis, implant supported. These are patient population descriptors. Similar searches can be completed for the intervention, comparison, and outcome groups. When all terms are identified through the MeSH heading search, Boolean operators (AND, OR, or NOT) can be used to best develop the search strategy. During the search, limits are imposed for clinical trial, randomized controlled trial, metaanalysis, and systematic review references to find the reference of greatest strength and applicability. After this search, additional electronic and hand searching methods can be used.

Clinicians must have access to published literature. Online periodic subscriptions are available, and these accounts can be used to maintain the clinician's current practice standard. Single pay-per-view articles can provide access to the most relevant information in decision making in a broad range of periodicals most feasible. The cost for access to this information could be considered a necessary expense for contemporary practice and care.

The search focus is to identify systematic review and metaanalyses, followed by randomized controlled trials, clinical trials, and clinical studies. Straightforward searches arising from MeSH headings are likely to identify critical publications. Searches described in systematic reviews may help to develop additional search terms and searches that relate to the clinical question. Many searches may be required to identify the highest quality available evidence.

The following searches are examples that arise from a PICO question. Search strategy format must be consistent with search engine principles. For example, search field descriptors and tags can be added with PubMed to further focus the search. Scenario 2 applies as a mechanism to identify search terms within a publication's title or abstract. The search focus is to preferably identify systematic reviews and higher order evidence, followed by evidence lower in the hierarchy.

Scenario 1: Immediate Implant Placement, Immediate Restoration, and Esthetics

Search terms for immediate implant placement and loading are assembled for the PubMed search limited for systematic reviews are ("Immediate Dental Implant Loading"[Mesh]) AND ("Esthetics, Dental"[Mesh]).

Scenario 2: Implant Fixed Complete Denture Prostheses and Veneer Fracture Incidence

Terms for the PubMed search limited for systematic reviews are ("zirconia"[tiab] OR "methacrylate"[All Fields] OR "polymethyl methacrylate"[All Fields] OR metal-resin [All Fields] OR metal-acrylic[All Fields]) AND ("dental implant"[tiab] OR "Dental Implants"[Mesh] OR "Dental Prosthesis, Implant-Supported"[Mesh] OR "Dental Prosthesis"[Mesh] OR "implant-supported"[tiab] OR "full arch restorations"[tiab] OR "full arch restoration"[tiab] OR "complete-arch"[tiab]). A modified search not limited to systematic reviews includes zirconia AND ("methacrylate"[All Fields] OR "polymethyl methacrylate"[All Fields] OR metal-resin[All Fields] OR metal-acrylic[All Fields]) AND ("dental implant"[tiab] OR "Dental Implants"[Mesh] OR "Dental Prosthesis, Implant-Supported"[Mesh] OR "Dental Prosthesis"[Mesh] OR "implant-supported"[tiab] OR "full arch restorations"[tiab] OR "full arch restoration"[tiab] OR "complete-arch"[tiab]). A portion of this search strategy was previously described.[15]

CRITICALLY APPRAISING THE LITERATURE

The highest form of available evidence must be applied to the PICO question. Evidence is evaluated for validity and patient applicability, and the best evidence supports focused clinical decision making for each patient.

Identifying the Best Evidence

Literature is assessed based on its strength in research design (**Table 3**).[12] Expert opinion and personal clinical experience are the lowest forms of evidence. Stronger

Table 3
Hierarchy of study design and evidence strength from highest to lowest

Strength	Study Design
High	Systems (computerized decision support systems)
	Summaries (evidence-based clinical practice guidelines)
	Synopses (evidence-based abstraction journals)
	Systematic reviews (eg, Cochrane Library)
	Metaanalyses
	Randomized, controlled, double-blind studies
	Randomized, controlled studies
	Cohort designs
	Case-control designs
	Cross-sectional studies
↓	Descriptive designs (case series, case reports)
Low	Expert opinion

Data from Sackett DL, Richardson S, Rosenberg W, et al. Evidence-based medicine: how to teach and practice EBM. Edinburgh (United Kingdom): Churchill Livingston; 1999. p. 16; and DiCenso A, Bayley L, Haynes B. Accessing preappraised evidence: fine-tuning the 5S model into a 6S model. Evid Based Nurs 2001;12:99–101.

evidence includes clinical research of various designs, with the randomized controlled trials having greater strength. The true systematic review in which several randomized, controlled trials are selected based on specific, well-planned inclusion factors is higher on the clinical evidence pyramid. Cochrane Collaboration Study Groups have generated in-depth systematic reviews on a variety of topics in many areas of medicine and dentistry. The Cochrane reviews are considered higher order evidence because they strictly apply prospective randomized controlled trials for reviews.

A 6S hierarchy of evidence was introduced in 2009[16] as the publication of critical appraisal articles grew. The 6S model includes single studies, syntheses (structured systematic reviews), synopses (short critical analyses of studies or systematic reviews), summaries (assimilation of best evidence from lower evidence to form clinical practice guidelines), and systems (computer-automated focused analyses of prognostic factors and outcomes for a specific patient). These are included in **Table 3**.

Clinicians regularly apply recently published prospective or retrospective designs that are not included in advanced metaanalyses or higher level reviews, although according to the 6S hierarchy individual original articles are low on the hierarchy. Traditional recognition of the publication hierarchy prefers as example, prospective randomized controlled trials with well-defined patient populations, well-controlled prognostic factors, and adequate patient follow-up. Such studies are difficult to control, require possibly years of long-term follow-up, and are expensive. For these reasons, cohort, case control, and case series designs may be suitable to answer patient-centered questions.

Prognosis, therapy, harm, and overview article analyses are frequently used to predict if a patient prognostic factor or care intervention might influence the care outcome. Incorrect article designation leads to an irrelevant critical analysis. Recognition of the correct article design is necessary for analysis of research validity and applicability. Sackett's primer[12] and the *Journal of Prosthetic Dentistry* series[2–9] are sample references.

Study design and outcome type designate the format for critical appraisal. Prognosis articles are generally associated with prospective or retrospective cohort or case control studies. Therapy articles present comparative care within 1 study using

2 similar, well-identified patient populations, and these studies are ideally represented with prospective, randomized, controlled trials. Harm articles present comparative outcomes and may be presented in randomized, controlled trials, cohort studies, case control studies, and case series. Overview articles, or metaanalysis and systematic review articles, seek to provide a well-controlled assimilation of lower level studies that present similar data and outcomes. The study design and outcome type determine the assessment criteria for research validity and patient applicability. Incorrect article designation leads to an irrelevant critical analysis.

Research Validity

Tables 4–7 present focused question matrices that arise from the *Journal of Prosthetic Dentistry* series to assesses validity for prognosis, therapy, harm or overview articles. More favorable answers imply potentially greater perceived evidence strength. For example, with prognosis or therapy articles, a greater number of favorable answers in all categories are consistent with a well-designed randomized, controlled trial, high-level evidence among individual studies. Information from lower level studies (case series, cohort studies, case control studies) may also be useful when 10% to 50% of the answers to the worksheet questions are affirmative. Fewer affirmative answers are a commentary on the difficulty in completing a well-controlled, long-term trial, but studies lower in the hierarchy may still be relevant and valuable for the patient under consideration.

Patient Applicability

Patients described in the appraised literature are ideally similar to the patient for whom the PICO question is developed. Patient applicability questions in **Tables 4–7** outline these concepts. When answers are affirmative, the usefulness of the reference in addressing a patient's PICO question can increase further.

Table 4
Prognosis article critical appraisal worksheet

Were the results valid?	Was a well-defined sample population used?	Yes No
	Were inclusion and exclusion criteria clearly defined?	Yes No
	Was patient selection unbiased?	Yes No
	Were all patients at a similar stage of the disease?	Yes No
	Were all groups treated equally?	Yes No
	Were the patients followed for a sufficient period of time with all patients accounted for?	Yes No
	Were objective, unbiased outcome measures used?	Yes No
	Were the investigators blinded?	Yes No
	Was there adjustment for important prognostic factors?	Yes No
What were the results?	Were survival results presented (Kaplan-Meier survival curve)?	Yes No
	Was the likelihood of outcomes presented (relative risk, confidence intervals)?	Yes No
Do the results apply to my patient?	Was the sample similar in demographics, comorbidity, disease stage, and potentially contributing prognostic factors?	Yes No
	Is there a compelling reason to apply results to the patient in question based on study inclusion/exclusion criteria, etc?	Yes No
	Do the results lead one to select a therapy?	Yes No
	Are the results useful for patient reassurance?	Yes No

Table 5
Therapy article appraisal worksheet

Were the results valid?	Was the assignment of patients to treatment randomized?	Yes	No
	Were all patients who entered the trial properly accounted for and attributed at its conclusion?	Yes	No
	Were patients, clinicians, and study personnel blinded to the treatment?	Yes	No
	Were all groups similar at the start of the trial?	Yes	No
	Aside from the intervention were the groups treated equally?	Yes	No
What were the results?	Was a treatment effect reported?	Yes	No
	Can absolute risk reduction or relative risk reduction be calculated?	Yes	No
Do the results apply to the patient?	Was the sample similar in demographic, comorbidity, disease stage, and potentially contributing prognostic factors?		
	Is there a compelling reason to apply results to the patient in question based on study inclusion/exclusion criteria?	Yes	No
	Were all clinically important outcomes considered?	Yes	No
	Are the treatment benefits worth the potential harm and cost?	Yes	No

When applicable research specific to a patient's situation is difficult to identify, a study population modified to include individuals similar to the patient in question is used for inference of results. This process introduces a selection bias and compromises patient applicability, but the results may be valuable for patient reassurance.

SYNTHESIZING THE LITERATURE

Literature appraisal and synthesis requires objective and subjective examination. Objective, accurate, in-depth analysis of the research methods and results for each study is mandatory and involves recognition of study validity arising from its strengths,

Table 6
Harm article appraisal worksheet

Were the results valid?	Are there clearly identified comparison groups similar with respect to important determinants of outcome other than the one of interest?	Yes	No
	Are the outcomes and exposures for both groups measured in the same way?	Yes	No
	Is follow-up sufficiently long and complete?	Yes	No
	Is the temporal relationship of cause and effect correct, consistent, and reasonable?	Yes	No
	Is there a dose–response gradient?	Yes	No
What were the results?	Is the association between exposure and outcome strong?	Yes	No
	Is the estimate of the risk precise?	Yes	No
Will the results help in caring for the patient?	Are the results applicable to my practice?		
	Is the magnitude of the risk clinically relevant?	Yes	No
	Should the exposure be stopped or therapy discontinued?	Yes	No

Table 7
Systematic review article appraisal worksheet

Were the results valid?	Was a clearly defined question identified? (Who? What? Outcome?)	Yes	No
	Were specific article search strategies used?	Yes	No
	Were specific article inclusion and exclusion criteria used?	Yes	No
	Was the quality of the article methods assessed?	Yes	No
	Was justification made to combine articles of different evidence levels?	Yes	No
	Were results from the primary study reported in sufficient detail?	Yes	No
What were the results?	Was the preparation of results detailed? (eg, metaanalysis, confidence intervals)	Yes	No
	Were the overall results appropriate?	Yes	No
Do the results apply to the patient?	Was the sample similar in demographic, comorbidity, disease stage, and potentially contributing prognostic factors?	Yes	No
	Is there a compelling reason to apply results to the patient in question based on the study inclusion/exclusion criteria?	Yes	No
	Do results lead to selecting therapy?	Yes	No
	Are the results useful for patient reassurance?	Yes	No

weaknesses, and patient applicability. Subjective analysis of methods, results, and outcomes is based on one's knowledge, personal experiences, and beliefs. Patient desires, patient values, and perceived cost-benefit of the proposed therapy are considered.

Although prospective, randomized, controlled trials are desired, the consideration of all relevant evidence is necessary for qualitative literature synthesis. The proportion of prospective, randomized, controlled trials is small compared with other designs such as cohort and case series studies. When relevant higher order evidence is not available, relevant studies lower in the hierarchy are used to better understand reported outcomes.

The following are 2 sample objective synthesis of identified literature for the previously presented patient scenarios. From the PubMed identified articles, publications are selected for thorough analysis and synthesis using the Pros-CAT worksheets. Within the summary, a Pros-CAT index identifies the proportion of affirmative answers in the analysis worksheets. With this information, qualitative syntheses are made.

Scenario 1: Immediate Implant Placement, Immediate Restoration, and Esthetics

The previously described search focused on measurable soft tissue volume after immediate implant placement with or without the use of immediate restoration. The 3 identified articles were systematic reviews, and the systematic review appraisal worksheet was applied to all publications (**Table 8**).

For Chen and Buser (2014),[17] quantitative estimates were determined addressing the esthetic outcomes of immediately placed implants. Specific search strategies were used and specific article inclusion and exclusion criteria were presented. Quality evaluation occurred using the Cochrane Collaboration assessment method. Applicable randomized, controlled trials and cohort studies were assessed for bias. The authors recognized that most studies identified were cases series. One reported randomized, controlled trial (De Rouck and colleagues[18] 2009) was identified that described baseline to 1-year follow-up with significantly greater midfacial soft tissue

Table 8
Systematic review article appraisal worksheet for scenario 1 (immediate implant placement, immediate restoration, and esthetics)

		Chen and Buser[17] 2014	Yan et al,[19] 2016	Kinaia et al,[20] 2017
Were the results valid?	Was a clearly defined question identified? (Who? What? Outcome?)	Yes	Yes	Yes
	Were specific article search strategies used?	Yes	Yes	Yes
	Were specific article inclusion and exclusion criteria used?	Yes	Yes	Yes
	Was the quality of the article methods assessed?	Yes	Yes	Yes
	Was justification made to combine articles of different evidence levels?	Yes	Yes	No
	Were results from the primary study reported in sufficient detail?	Yes	Yes	No
What were the results?	Was the preparation of results detailed? (eg, metaanalysis, confidence intervals)	Yes	Yes	Yes
	Were the overall results appropriate?	Yes	Yes	No
Do the results apply to the patient?	Was the sample similar in demographic, comorbidity, disease stage, and potentially contributing prognostic factors?	Unknown	Yes	Unknown
	Is there a compelling reason to apply results to the patient in question based on the study inclusion/exclusion criteria?	No	Yes	No
	Do results lead to selecting therapy?	No	Yes	No
	Are the results useful for patient reassurance?	Yes	Yes	Yes
Analysis summary	Number of affirmative responses	9/12	12/12	6/12
	Pros-CAT index	0.75	1.00	0.60
	Results (mean difference [95% confidence interval]) of applicable results	Midfacial −0.75 [-1.16 to -0.34]	Midfacial −0.22 [-1.29 to 0.85]	Midfacial −0.25 (−0.31 to 0.82)
	Sample size	24	35	55
	Study design	Systematic review, but results are taken from a single paper with 1 y of follow-up	Systematic review, but results are from incisors, canines, premolars	Systematic review Articles with high design heterogeneity

recession with delayed restoration (-1.16 [0.66]) compared with the immediate restoration group (-0.41 [0.75]; $P = .005$). Studies regardless of design generally demonstrated a trend of mean height loss in midfacial and proximal periimplant soft tissue areas for immediate or delayed restoration.

In Yan and colleagues[19] (2016), the effects of all immediate protocols on soft and hard tissue changes were presented. Specific search strategies were used and specific article inclusion and exclusion criteria were presented with 6 months or greater of follow-up. Quality evaluation including GRADE analysis occurred. Mean values and standard deviations were used to calculate the standardized mean differences and 95% confidence intervals for continuous outcomes (marginal bone and soft tissue levels). Confidence intervals were used when similar data were combined to describe osseous and soft tissue positions. Results from the assimilation of studies for each of mesiofacial, midfacial, and distofacial positions suggest similarity in outcomes regarding periimplant soft tissue height with immediate restoration compared with a conventional, delayed protocol.

In Kinaia and colleagues[20] (2017), a portion of the systematic review described immediate implant placement with considerations of immediate provisionalization versus delayed loading. Cochrane assessment methods were used for validity and randomization evaluation. This article also identified De Rouck and colleagues[18] 2009. Additional reported randomized, controlled trial references focused on esthetic areas and included mandibular anterior and premolar teeth, or on canines and premolars. These do not relate to the presented maxillary anterior scenario and were not considered further. Nevertheless, the presented trends of periimplant soft tissue height loss across all reported studies with immediate placement were consistent and demonstrated mean change often between −0.2 to −1.0 mm with variability in confidence intervals among studies.

Scenario 2: Implant Fixed Complete Denture Prostheses and Veneer Fracture Incidence

Articles were identified using the previously described search strategy that focused on implant fixed prosthesis design and reported incidence of complications. None of the identified articles compared prosthesis material and design within a randomized, controlled trial. Two articles were systematic reviews, but they primarily described the incidence of complications associated with retrospective case series. One publication retrospectively compared metal-resin, zirconia, porcelain veneered zirconia, and replaceable crown prostheses. This study was considered a case series. **Tables 9** and **10** present appropriate systematic review or prognosis worksheet appraisals for the 3 publications.

Bidra and colleagues[15] (2017) described the incidence of complications associated with zirconia full arch fixed complete prostheses associated with edentulous patients. Twelve observational articles were identified that were prospective (n = 3) and retrospective (n = 9). Ten studies reported that at least a few patients in their study had fixed complete dentures made of various materials (zirconia, metal-resin, metal-ceramic). Follow-up was 2 months to 8 years. Pooled data from 285 zirconia fixed complete dentures with 223 patients showed prosthesis fracture (1.4%), and chipping of veneered porcelain (14.7%). Data could not be combined for further statistical analysis owing to the small sample size and limited number of complications.

Hogsett Box and colleagues[21] (2018) described the incidence of complications associated with metal-resin, retrievable crown, monolithic zirconia, and porcelain veneered zirconia prostheses after a retrospective record review. Although different types of

Table 9
Implant fixed complete denture prostheses and veneer fracture incidence systematic review appraisal worksheet for scenario 2 (implant fixed complete denture prostheses and veneer fracture incidence)

		Bidra et al,[15] 2017	Wong et al,[22] 2018
Were the results valid?	Was a clearly defined question identified? (Who? What? Outcome?)	Yes	Yes
	Were specific article search strategies used?	Yes	Yes
	Were specific article inclusion and exclusion criteria used?	Yes	Yes
	Was the quality of article the methods assessed?	Yes	Yes
	Was justification was made to combine articles of different evidence levels?	No	No
	Were results from the primary study reported in sufficient detail?	No	No
What were the results?	Was the preparation of results detailed? (eg, metaanalysis, confidence intervals)	No	No
	Were the overall results appropriate?	Yes	Yes
Do the results apply to the patient?	Was the sample similar in demographic, comorbidity, disease stage, and potentially contributing prognostic factors?	Unknown	Unknown
	Is there a compelling reason to apply results to the patient in question based on the study inclusion/exclusion criteria?	No	No
	Do results lead to selecting therapy?	No	No
	Are results useful for patient reassurance?	Yes	Yes
Analysis summary	Number of affirmative responses	6/12	6/12
	Pros-CAT index	0.50	0.50
	Results (mean difference, 95% confidence interval) of applicable results	14.7% PVZ veneer fracture incidence at 2 mo to 8 y	Metal–ceramic veneer fracture 22.1% at 5 y
	Sample size	285 prostheses	169 Metal-ceramic 70 All ceramic
	Study design	Systematic review, primarily retrospective, complications incidence data were combined	Systematic review, primarily retrospective, complications incidence data were combined

prostheses were compared in this study, the therapy appraisal worksheet could not be applied, because all clinical factors with the exception of material were not controlled. Although bias was introduced by patient and clinician in deciding the best path for care, a comparison of the incidence of complications associated with different prosthesis

Table 10
Implant fixed complete denture prostheses and veneer fracture incidence prognosis appraisal worksheet for scenario 2 (implant fixed complete denture prostheses and veneer fracture incidence)

		Hogsett Box et al,[21] 2018
Were the results valid?	Was a well-defined sample population used?	No
	Were patient inclusion and exclusion criteria clearly defined?	No
	Was patient selection unbiased?	No
	Were all patients at a similar stage of the disease?	No
	Were all groups treated equally?	No
	Were the patients followed for a sufficient period of time with all patients accounted for?	Yes
	Were objective, unbiased outcome measures used?	Yes
	Were the investigators blinded?	No
	Was there adjustment for important prognostic factors?	No
What were the results?	Were survival results presented (Kaplan-Meier survival curve)?	No
	Was the likelihood of outcomes presented (relative risk, confidence intervals)?	No
Do the results apply to my patient?	Was sample similar in demographics, comorbidity, disease stage, and potentially contributing prognostic factors?	Unknown
	Is there a compelling reason to apply results to the patient in question based on study inclusion/exclusion criteria, etc?	No
	Do results lead one to select a therapy?	Yes
	Are the results useful for patient reassurance?	Yes
Analysis summary	Number of affirmative responses	4/15
	Pros-CAT index	0.27
	Results (mean difference, 95% confidence interval) of applicable results	For incidence of all complications at 12-70 mo, MZ < MR < RC < PVZ
	Sample size	37 total patients, 49 prostheses, but low number of MZ (7) or PVZ (6)
	Study design	Retrospective cohort

Abbreviations: MR, metal-resin; MZ, monolithic zirconia; PVZ, porcelain veneered zirconia; RC, retrievable crown.

designs is valuable. A total of 37 patients with 49 prostheses were followed from 12 to 70 months in this cohort of edentulous patients. Chipping was associated with 2 of 6 porcelain veneered zirconia prosthesis compared with 0 of 7 monolithic zirconia prostheses. The incidence of all complications across materials was monolithic zirconia < metal-resin < retrievable crown < porcelain veneered zirconia.

Wong and colleagues[22] (2018) completed a systematic review and metaanalysis to determine veneer fracture incidence associated with metal-ceramic and all-ceramic prostheses. Clinical studies were included with a follow-up of more than 1 year. The Cochrane Collaboration protocol was used to identify bias. With combined data from comparable studies, metal-ceramic veneer fracture incidence within 8 studies at 5, 10, and 15 years was 22.1%, 29.3%, and 52.8%, respectively. For all-ceramic prostheses, 2 studies with a total of 70 prostheses were reported. One of the 2 studies reported veneer fracture events with 19 of 48 prostheses. With nonincluded studies, the least fractures were observed with facial porcelain veneered zirconia.

The previous brief syntheses recognize research validity and applicability arising from study design and patient inclusion criteria. Although more affirmative answers on the worksheets may relate to well-designed studies, controlling all prognostic factors is not possible. Lower Pros-CAT indices may be the only possible resource for decision making. Many clinical studies have lower Pros-CAT indices (case series, cohort studies) because the designs higher in the hierarchy (prospective, randomized, controlled trials with adequate follow-up) are expensive and difficult to complete. Lower order studies continue to provide valuable evidence to support decisions, and the data are often combined for systematic reviews.

The syntheses further emphasize that patient care decisions must be made with available evidence that often does not provide a clear, definitive answer. In fact, many PICO questions may not be directly answered with the limited number of published dental implant articles. Clinical experience is, therefore, crucial and must be included in sound patient care decision making.

APPLYING THE SYNTHESIS TO THE PATIENT

Evidence-based decisions are tempered by patient values. Patient desires, as well as patient perceived therapy cost and convenience, are driving forces in literature search, appraisal, synthesis, and therapy selection. The vision of the Pros-CAT decision-making approach is in applying the highest form of available contemporary evidence to the personal concerns of the patient. Effective communication skills with the patient with an emphasis on listening to patient concerns are crucial in making the best decisions. With informed consent, the clinician fully understands goals and expectations toward providing patient-centered care.

Scenario 1: Immediate Implant Placement, Immediate Restoration, and Esthetics

The identified systematic reviews recognized 2 randomized, controlled trials that included maxillary anterior teeth with data addressing midfacial tissue height. Results suggested that, with thoughtful patient selection, the loss of midfacial height may be less with immediate implant placement followed by immediate restoration compared with delayed restoration. All sites tend to lose soft tissue height over 1 year of healing. Additional studies identified in these systematic reviews, with different sites than described in the scenario, also reported trends in mean loss of soft tissue height of 0.2 to 1.0 mm.

Results from limited evidence suggest that immediate restoration after immediate implant placement can support a favorable esthetic outcome. A loss of midfacial soft tissue height is expected over time. Although the patient believes care could be completed more quickly, other prognostic factors must be reviewed carefully to determine if the proposed care is appropriate. The patient must be informed of the implant, prosthetic, and esthetic risks associated with immediate placement and immediate restoration as she considers care options.

Scenario 2: Implant Fixed Complete Denture Prostheses and Veneer Fracture Incidence

Synthesis of these studies indicates that the level of complications associated with monolithic zirconia prostheses is lowest compared with other designs, including metal-resin, replaceable crown, or PVZ. This conclusion is made with only a limited number of full-arch zirconia papers and few prostheses. Furthermore, the level of evidence is low, and advanced statistical analyses are not possible. Future studies are indicated.

Results from limited evidence suggest the use of monolithic zirconia may lead to the lowest incidence of veneer fracture. Although some patients had metal-resin, metal-ceramic, or porcelain veneered zirconia prostheses, which have a reportedly greater risk of complications, patients were nevertheless pleased with their prostheses regardless of material design, and the oral health quality of life was improved.[21] Prognostic factors must be considered carefully, and the patient should be informed of her risk for veneer fracture depending upon material and prosthesis design.

SUMMARY

The Pros-CAT protocol provides a straightforward framework for evidence identification and comparison, thereby leading to recognition of highest quality available evidence. The Pros-CAT index is unique in that it includes patient applicability in study comparisons. Appraisal using the protocol leads to identification, synthesis, and application of best evidence that is, focused on a specific patient's situation. Collaborative communication among patients and oral health care professionals is enhanced. Patients receive care based on decisions supported with best available evidence.

REFERENCES

1. Sackett DL, Rosenberg WM, Gray JA, et al. Evidence based medicine: what it is and what it isn't. Br Med J 1996;312:71–2.
2. Carr AB, McGivney GP. User's guides to the dental literature: how to get started. J Prosthet Dent 2000;83:13–20.
3. Jacob RF, Carr AB. Hierarchy of research design used to categorize the "strength of evidence" in answering clinical dental questions. J Prosthet Dent 2000;83:137–52.
4. Carr AB, McGivney GP. Measurement in dentistry. J Prosthet Dent 2000;83:266–71.
5. Eckert SE, Goldstein GR, Koka S. How to evaluate a diagnostic test. J Prosthet Dent 2000;83:386–91.
6. Anderson JD, Zarb GA. Evidence-based dentistry: prognosis. J Prosthet Dent 2000;83:495–500.
7. Goldstein GR, Preston JD. How to evaluate an article about therapy. J Prosthet Dent 2000;83:266–71.
8. Jacob RF, Lloyd PM. How to evaluate a dental article about harm. J Prosthet Dent 2000;84:8–16.
9. Felton DA, Lang BR. The overview: an article that interrogates the literature. J Prosthet Dent 2000;84:17–21.
10. Goldstein GR, Preston JD. Therapy: anecdote, experience, or evidence. Dent Clin North Am 2002;46:21–8.
11. Jacob RF, Goldstein GR, Layton DM. Evidence-based prosthodontics: 25 years later. J Prosthet Dent 2018;119:1–3.
12. Sackett DL, Richardson S, Rosenberg W, et al. Evidence-based medicine: how to teach and practice EBM. Edinburgh (United Kingdom): Churchill Livingston; 1999. p. 16.
13. Guckes AD, Scurria MS, Shugars DA. A conceptual framework for understanding outcomes of oral implant therapy. J Prosthet Dent 1996;75:633–9.

14. Carr A, Wolfaardt J, Garrett N. Capturing patient benefits of treatment. Int J Oral Maxillofac Implants 2011;26(suppl):85–92.
15. Bidra A, Rungruanganunt P, Gauthier M. Clinical outcomes of full arch fixed implant-supported zirconia prostheses: a systematic review. Eur J Oral Implantol 2017;10(Suppl1):35–45.
16. DiCenso A, Bayley L, Haynes B. Accessing preappraised evidence: fine-tuning the 5S model into a 6 S model. Evid Based Nurs 2001;12:99–101.
17. Chen ST, Buser D. Esthetic outcomes following immediate and early implant placement in the anterior maxilla – a systematic review. Int J Oral Maxillofac Implants 2014;29:186–215.
18. De Rouck T, Collys K, Wyn I, et al. Instant provisionalization of immediate single-tooth implants is essential to optimize esthetic treatment outcome. Clin Oral Implants Res 2009;20:566–70.
19. Yan Q, Xiao L, Su M, et al. Soft and hard tissue changes following immediate placement or immediate restoration of single-tooth implants in the esthetic zone: a systematic review and meta-analysis. Int J Oral Maxillofac Implants 2016;31:1327–40.
20. Kinaia BM, Ambrosio F, Lamble M, et al. Soft tissue changes around immediately placed implants: a systematic review and meta-analyses with at least 12 months of follow-up after functional loading. J Periodontol 2017;88:876–86.
21. Hogsett Box V, Sukotjo C, Knoernschild KL, et al. Patient-reported and clinical outcomes of implant-supported fixed complete dental prostheses: a comparison of metal-acrylic, milled zirconia, and retrievable crown prostheses. J Oral Implantol 2018;44:51–61.
22. Wong CKK, Narvekar U, Petridis H. Prosthodontic complications of metal-ceramic and all-ceramic, complete-arch fixed implant prostheses with minimum 5 years mean follow-up period. A systematic review and meta-analysis. J Prosthodont 2018. [Epub ahead of print].

Obstructive Sleep Apnea

The Role of Gender in Prevalence, Symptoms, and Treatment Success

Reva Malhotra Barewal, DDS, MS

KEYWORDS

• Sleep apnea • Mandibular advancement • Oral appliances • Gender differences • Symptoms • Prevalence • Practice guidelines • Review

KEY POINTS

- Women with sleep apnea are often unrecognized owing to differing symptomology.
- The prevalence of women with obstructive sleep apnea increases with age but more specifically with the menopausal transition.
- There is a lack of gender difference in bruxism and risk of obstructive sleep apnea with bruxism.
- Oral appliances seem to have more successful outcomes with women than men.
- There is a tremendous need for more research in the area of gender-specific indications and outcomes with oral appliance therapy.

INTRODUCTION

Obstructive sleep apnea (OSA) is characterized by repetitive upper airway collapse during sleep. This condition can lead to a complete cessation of breathing for 10 seconds or more (apnea) or partial collapse of the airway, resulting in either an arousal or oxyhemoglobin desaturation exceeding 3% (hypopnea). The resultant effect of this decreased airflow is episodic oxygen desaturation, sleep fragmentation, and marked negative intrathoracic pressures. In the past, sleep-disordered breathing (SDB) with symptoms of snoring and sleepiness were viewed as comical by others, an embarrassment for the individual, and an annoyance for the sleep partner. However, a multitude of studies have proven that OSA over time can negatively impact cardiovascular and metabolic health and is associated with hypertension, type II diabetes,[1] myocardial infarction, coronary artery disease, stroke, heart failure, pulmonary hypertension, and arrhythmias.[2] It can also lead to a lack of concentration and insomnia and

---

Disclosure: The author has nothing to disclose.

Department of Pulmonology and Critical Care, Oregon Health and Science University, 3181 Southwest Sam Jackson Park Road, Portland, OR 97239-3098, USA
E-mail address: barewalr@gmail.com

Dent Clin N Am 63 (2019) 297–308
https://doi.org/10.1016/j.cden.2018.11.009

contribute to psychiatric disorders such as depression.[3] At present, OSA is recognized as a major public health issue on a global scale, the prevalence of which is increasing owing to the obesity pandemic, the aging of our society, and improvements in screening and testing methods.[4] In the United States alone, the number of people affected with untreated SDB is approximately 12 to 18 million adults and this number is increasing.[5]

SDB has traditionally been assumed to be a condition occurring in men. The stereotypical overweight, snoring, middle-aged, sleepy man was an easy identifier to clinicians and led to easy identification of cases for further screening or evaluation. Epidemiologic studies using population samples free of clinical selection bias have raised our awareness of the magnitude of this condition and the presence of many subgroups of individuals with remarkably disparate presentations.

Relevant to this review, it has been suggested that the prevalence of symptoms and conditions associated with OSA can vary according to gender. Women who do not present with the classical clinical picture of the syndrome (loud snoring, witnessed apneic events, daytime sleepiness, obesity) might not get referred for screening for OSA and suffer the consequences of this condition unnecessarily. Ultimately, the recognition of gender differences in symptoms and associated comorbidities could improve screening and early diagnosis. Before 1993, women with SDB were not reported in the literature simply owing to a lack of awareness that this condition could exist in the female population. This lack led to many women suffering from this condition owing to the lack of a diagnosis. Young and associates[6] were the first to include women in a large study of prevalence of OSA syndrome (OSAS) in a general population sample. Over the past 2 decades, this knowledge deficit is slowly being filled with research found in sleep medicine publications, yet this area of study remains underrepresented.[7] Furthermore, information is relatively absent in the dental sleep medicine literature and is the basis for the presentation of this review.

GENDER DIFFERENCES IN THE PREVALENCE OF OBSTRUCTIVE SLEEP APNEA

Sleep apnea is measured with a home study or overnight sleep study (polysomnogram) by a qualified sleep physician and is a requirement for proper diagnosis and treatment. The total number of apnea, hypopnea events divided by total sleep time in hours observed in the study yields the apnea–hypopnea index (AHI). A diagnosis based on AHI is shown in **Table 1**.

In the landmark 2009 Wisconsin Sleep Cohort Study,[5] of the 352 men and 250 women, 30 to 60 years of age, 24% of the men and 9% of the women were found to OSA measure at an AHI 5 or greater. OSAS is defined as OSA plus excessive daytime sleepiness occurred in 4% of men and 2% of women. Since then, a review on the epidemiology of sleep apnea[8] revealed that an AHI of 5 or greater occurred in population-based studies at a mean frequency of 22% in men and 17% in women. Wide variation in the prevalence was noted in the various studies, which could be

Table 1
Grading of obstructive sleep apnea

Severity	Grading
Mild OSA	AHI $\geq$5 and <15 per hour of sleep + symptoms or comorbidity factors
Moderate OSA	AHI $\geq$15 and <30 events per hour of sleep
Severe OSA	AHI $\geq$30 events per hour of sleep

Abbreviations: AHI, apnea–hypoxia index; OSA, obstructive sleep apnea.

due to the heterogeneity in the diagnostic criteria used for AHI and the age and sex of the study population.[4]

What is intriguing is that, although this higher risk in men stays consistent in the elderly population, the prevalence in both genders increases markedly. For example, comparing the prevalence of OSA in a general population ages 40 or older to less than 60 versus 60 years or older, it was found that the younger age group was positive for OSA in 11.7% of men and 4.3% of women, and this finding increased to 21.1% of men and 10.8% of women in the older age groups.[9] This study was conducted in Switzerland on an exclusively white European population with a low prevalence of obesity and could possibly portend a higher prevalence in an American population. However, this study highlights not only the surprisingly high prevalence of this condition in the population, but also the remarkably close ratio of prevalence of SDB in men and women, which ranges between 2.7:1.0 in the middle-aged population to 2:1 in the older aged groups. Both these ratios show much greater risk in women than ratios found in earlier studies of 9:1.[5]

PREVALENCE ACCORDING TO MENOPAUSAL TRANSITION

The increase in sleep disturbances with age in women has been studied according to stages of menopause. In the perimenopausal period, there is an increase in sleep fragmentation, increased awakenings, and poorer sleep quality.[10] Chronic insomnia may develop in as many as 31% to 42% of perimenopausal women with increasing prevalence in the later stages of perimenopause.[11] In addition, the rates of occurrence of mood disorders, such as depression, can double during the menopausal transition, independent of other known factors.[12] With transition from premenopause to postmenopause, the severity of SDB as measured by AHI, increases independent of chronologic age and body size.[13] It is suggested that there is an exposure–response model between time in menopause and degree of severity of AHI. Interestingly, the prevalence of OSA is decreased in menopausal women on hormone replacement therapy, suggesting a hormonal effect on risk for sleep apnea independent of age and body mass index (BMI).[14]

The time period of pregnancy has a widespread association with poor sleep quality, frequent awakenings, and nocturia. However, what is less commonly known is that distinct changes in sleep characteristics occur between the first and third trimesters. Not only are there shorter sleep durations, more awakenings, poorer sleep efficiency, and less REM sleep in the late stages of pregnancy, but there is an increase in the severity of sleep apnea and periodic limb movements.[15] Risk factors for SDB during pregnancy are high BMI and more advanced age.[16] It has been demonstrated that SDB during pregnancy increases a woman's vulnerability to pregnancy-induced hypertension and gestational diabetes.[17]

Because the consequences can be serious for untreated SDB in the pregnant woman, our awareness should be heightened. However, the current screening tools for SDB are not targeted to the pregnant population and can have poor predictive ability.[18] Improvement in screening tools and awareness among all providers treating this population needs to occur to better identify and manage maternal and fetal well-being.

GENDER DIFFERENCES IN THE CLINICAL PRESENTATION AND SEVERITY OF THE CONDITION

Clinical Presentation

People initially seek treatment because of the symptoms associated with OSA. Although we are familiar with the presenting complaint of snoring and witnessed apneic events, there are many other night time symptoms that can disrupt sleep and contribute to overall sleep quality. Additionally, there are many daytime symptoms associated with SDB. People with symptoms of sleep problems are at a higher risk of motor vehicle accidents, reduced work productivity, reduced socialization, and reduced overall quality of life as compared with the general population.[19,20] It is believed that the diagnosis of SDB in women is often missed because the clinical presentation is different than the traditional presentation first identified predominantly in men, and women underreport their symptoms.[21]

These female-specific symptoms and medical comorbidities associated with SDB could lead to reduced recognition of risk for SDB and lack of referral to a sleep specialist for sleep testing. Thus, it is important to understand the gender-related differences in symptoms and increase our recognition of risk of OSA in women and potentially develop better screening tools in our history and examination.

Demographic

Obesity is more prevalent in female patients with OSA, especially those in perimenopause.[13,22,23] An average BMI of 36 for women compared with an average of 32 for men was found in 2 studies.[5,22] A statistically significant difference in age was found with female OSA patients being older.[22–24]

Comorbid Conditions

Hypertension, diabetes mellitus, thyroid disease, and asthma are reported to be more common in women as are insomnia and depression.[22,25] Gastroesophageal reflux disease has a higher prevalence in those diagnosed with primary snoring and OSAS, regardless of severity, as compared with the general population.[26,27] Although in 1 study by Basoglu and colleagues study[26] there was no gender preference found, in another study Hesselbacher and colleagues[27] found a significant increase in female patients with OSAS patients gastroesophageal reflux disease, necessitating further investigation.

Sleep Bruxism

The prevalence of bruxism among middle-aged patients is estimated to be 6.0% to 8.6%.[28,29] However, the method of diagnosis ranged from self-report to practitioner opinion, which lack sensitivity. The gold standard in the diagnosis of bruxism is polysomnography. The association between sleep bruxism and OSA has been studied by several authors.[30,31] In 1 study,[30] 30 patients diagnosed with a worn dentition received a polysomnogram. Of these patients, 93% tested positive for sleep apnea suggesting a relationship between sleep bruxism and OSA. This positive association has been shown in other studies as well.[31] Although an association does exist between bruxism and OSA, there is no evidence showing a higher prevalence of bruxism in women. It is interesting to note that sleep bruxism peaks in the premenopausal years of 45 to 54,[32] and yet the mean age of diagnosis of OSAS in women is 56, further distancing a potential relationship between sleep bruxism, OSA, and gender. More extensive studies need to be done in this area to validate this association as well as to determine the pathophysiology of OSAS and sleep bruxism.

Temporomandibular Disorder

A positive correlation has been found between temporomandibular disorder and OSA.[33–35] There is no evidence to show an increased correlation of temporomandibular disorder and OSA in the female population. However, the current evidence raises the question of improvement in screening for OSA risk in our current population with temporomandibular disorder.

Severity of Obstructive Sleep Apnea

In studying the severity of sleep apnea by gender, it is apparent that women tend toward milder forms of sleep apnea than men. It was also found that their apneic episodes were shorter than those in men, and that they had a higher occurrence of partial airway collapse.[36] Mohsenin[37] found that women were almost twice as likely to have primary snoring as OSAS. Conversely, men were almost 3 times more likely to have OSAS as primary snoring. Epidemiologic studies have reported on the higher prevalence of women with mild OSA with AHI of 5 or greater as compared with moderate OSA with AHI of 15 or greater.[22,38] The risk of presence of OSA increases dramatically to 68% when combining factors of a BMI of 40 or greater and age greater than 50 in women.[38]

Symptoms

There is a growing awareness of symptom differences by gender and degree of severity of these symptoms. Without knowledge of these differences, underrecognition of OSAS can occur, leading to a lack of referral to a sleep clinic for laboratory or home study evaluation. The classical symptom presentation of a patient with a partner complaint of witnessed apneas is specific to men.[22,39] Women present more commonly with excessive daytime sleepiness and daytime fatigue, insomnia, and sleep fragmentation.[22] However, daytime sleepiness as a standalone symptom does not seem to be a good differentiator between males and females positive for SDB.[22]

Females referred for a sleep study present more often than males with headaches. The odds ratio male to female is 1.0:2.7 for headaches.[40] Shepertycky and colleagues[25] found that the main presenting symptom for women was insomnia, not witnessed apnea. Unfortunately, the risk is that these presenting symptoms are believed to be associated with depression and do not lead to an evaluation for OSA.

In the literature, an opinion has been formed that there are female distinctive symptoms of OSA as well as some that are not gender specific.[22] An overview of the literature revealed similarities in findings on female distinctive symptoms compared with those that were not gender specific.[12,39–43] These symptoms and their gender association are presented in **Table 2**.

The clinical underrecognition of the disorder in women is due to the ability to isolate and identify symptoms associated with OSA among women. The following reasons have been identified as barriers to diagnosis:

1. Daytime sleepiness can be incorrectly associated with depression, poor sleep quality from pregnancy factors, or other illnesses.
2. Women might be more reluctant to report snoring owing to a lack of awareness from their bed partner or an opinion of it being a masculine symptom.[44]

Table 2
Sleep apnea presenting symptoms

Higher Prevalence in Women	Equal Prevalence by Gender
Nonrestorative sleep, fatigue	Snoring
Morning headache	Daytime sleepiness
Insomnia	
Mood changes, irritability (features of depression)	
Sleep fragmentation; frequent awakenings	

3. Men might have more "classic" symptoms and increased severity of AHI, which can allow them to move quickly in pathways to treatment.
4. Women come to clinical interviews alone more frequently than men, possibly leading to underreporting of sleep sounds.[39]
5. Bed partners of female patients do not complain of snoring or observed apneic episodes.[45]

TREATMENT OF OBSTRUCTIVE SLEEP APNEA

Continuous positive airway pressure (CPAP) was first reported in 1981 and provides pneumatic splinting of the upper airway. It remains the most efficacious and, therefore, the first line of therapy for the majority of patients with OSA.[46,47] CPAP has proven to improve symptoms, normalize the risk of traffic and workplace accidents, and decrease the elevated sympathetic activity and risk for cardiovascular morbidities, especially arterial hypertension.[48,49]

Alternative therapies, including oral appliances, surgery, and positional therapies, have emerged, but have historically been reserved for patients who fail positive airway pressure therapy. CPAP more consistently diminishes AHI than oral appliance therapy (OAT); however, their results are comparable in symptom improvement and cardiovascular health outcomes.[50] In addition, compliance rates can be higher with OAT.[51] With an increased awareness of the variability in disease characteristics and population demographics, there is a growing sense that treatment options need to be more specified to the personal preferences and unique characteristics of the patient.[52] When used in combination with other therapies such as CPAP, surgery, weight loss, and positional aids additional reductions in AHI can be achieved. There are no reports in the literature of gender-specific treatment preferences for OSA.

PREDICTING THE SUCCESS OF ORAL APPLIANCE THERAPY

OAT varies tremendously in its ability to decrease the AHI across multiple studies. This variance can be attributed to definitions of success, degree of severity of OSA, types of appliances used, and methodology. However, an improved understanding would include recognition that the pathogenesis of OSA is not simply due to poor upper airway anatomy, but is also influenced by nonanatomic traits such as (1) airway collapsibility owing to poor pharyngeal muscle activity, (2) an oversensitive ventilator control system, and (3) a low respiratory arousal threshold.[53] Studies have shown the direct effect of OAT to enlarge the upper airway size,[54,55] which, although it is likely a key determinant of efficacy of OAT, might not be the only factor involved. It has been suggested that those with reduced upper airway collapsibility would gain the greatest benefit from OAT.[53] Women are believed to have a less collapsible airway,[56] and could therefore be better candidates for OAT, but further research in this area is needed.

The measures of success of OAT can be divided into a decrease in the AHI, improvement of oxygen desaturation events, and decrease in symptoms. Many studies have shown the benefits of the OAT versus placebo to decrease the AHI.[30,57,58] The success rates have been reported between 14% and 78%. The wide variance can be partially attributed to the percentage of milder forms of OSA in their subgroups, because greater efficacy of treatment has been reported in milder cases of OSA.[59–61] This finding would align well with female predispositions for milder forms of OSA. Success rates with more severe forms of OSA vary widely and range from 14% to 61%. Success of these forms are difficult to compare because the measures of success were not standardized.[62]

Efficacy with oral appliance therapy

To date, there is limited research in the area of gender-specific response to OAT. Marklund and colleagues[63] reported more success with OAT for women than men as measured by reduction in AHI to less than 10 (71% vs 51%). Based on the literature, it may be assumed that women had lower pretreatment AHI than men. It would have been interesting to see the net improvement in AHI by gender. A larger sample size of women in the study would also improve the validity of the outcomes.

BMI has not been consistently shown to be a good predictor of OAT success. A recent 10-year follow-up study found no effect of BMI on treatment success,[64] although others have found high BMI (>30) to negatively influence success of OAT.[63,65] There are no data on high BMI by gender and the relationship with efficacy of OAT to date.

The greatest predictor of OAT success in men was the presence of supine dependent sleep apnea with an odds ratio of 6.0 ($P<.001$), and mild levels of OSA.[63] In contrast, women who presented with non–supine-dependent OSA had an odds ratio of 6.1 of treatment success with OAT, and had greater success in milder forms of the condition.

Oral Appliance Effect on Sleep Apnea Symptoms

Although a dentist's focus lies primarily in decreasing the AHI and improving oxygen saturation with either an oral appliance or combination therapy, the myriad of symptoms associated with SDB can negatively influence quality of life and must also be addressed. The ability of OAT appliances to decrease these symptoms has not been measured as thoroughly as the objective measurement of change in AHI. However, it is these debilitating symptoms that often lead a patient to seek treatment and can ultimately influence their perceived benefit of therapy.

If the presenting symptom for SDB is daytime sleepiness, it has been shown that OAT or CPAP do not effectively reduce this symptom. Although women present with more sleepiness as a symptom before treatment, OAT or CPAP treatment do not have a strong effect on this symptom.[66–68] Perhaps this weak influence can be due to the presence of other causes of sleepiness, or the method of measurement of sleepiness.

Oral appliances have been found to decrease headaches as compared with placebo as well as to improve insomnia compared with baseline levels.[57] Although there has been case report evidence of the benefits of treatment of OSA in reduction of sleep bruxism,[66] this finding requires further study to show stronger effect relationships. The efficacy of oral appliances to reduce headaches and bruxism have not been studied relative to gender differences.

We should continue to seek a better understanding of the effectiveness OAT has on reduction of these symptoms, as well as examine differences in treatment effect on these symptoms based on gender. This research will help to provide insight on the impact our treatment will have on quality of life. This understanding is relevant not only to the practitioner, but also to the patient before initiation of therapy, and will aid in establishing realistic goals relative to outcomes.

Tolerance of Oral Appliance Therapy

The degree of tolerance of OAT studied by Marklund and colleagues[63] was not predictable based on the severity of the disease, presence of supine-dependent sleep apnea, age, or gender. The main issue is that tolerability and compliance are difficult to assess accurately owing to loss of patients returning for reevaluations, as well as compliance measures for OAT being predominantly by self-report.[63] Gender influence on adherence to OAT has not been evaluated as yet in the literature. There are varying reports on women's adherence to CPAP with studies reporting no relationship between gender and compliance,[69–71] and others showing women having poorer compliance than men.[72,73]

The causes reported for discontinuation of OAT regardless of gender are:

- Discomfort including excess salivation and awkwardness
- Poor effect on snoring
- Symptoms from craniomandibular system, periodontal disease, or change in occlusion
- Unrealistic expectations

SUMMARY

It is evident that there are notable differences in the frequency and severity of sleep apnea by gender. Although the prevalence in women is lower than men in middle-aged and older populations, the consequences of the disease are similar if not worse. The age of onset of the disease in women is later and is more closely related to key events in their reproductive life span, especially pregnancy and menopause. The consequences of OSA can be significant to the mother and fetus during pregnancy. BMI increases the risk for OSA among women in the younger and older age groups. Based on the literature, women tend to present with milder forms of OSA. However, it is believed that the incidence of OSA may not be accurately reported in the literature. It is possible that women are being misdiagnosed, and therefore, those with more advanced forms of the disease are not being evaluated in sleep centers. Without an awareness of these differences in presentation of the disease state, women can remain unrecognized and undiagnosed. Female-specific screening questionnaires should be developed and used not only in medicine, but in dentistry to target their history, findings more accurately, and improve treatment of the condition.

The common goal of medicine and dentistry is to pursue identification and management of individuals according to their unique characteristics. The results of this effort are to improve overall quality of life and health of the population we serve. Identifying phenotypic variations in our SDB population, especially in the subgroups of women during pregnancy, perimenopause, and menopause, will allow for improvement in the management of their condition.[52] More research on gender differences is needed in dental sleep medicine with a focus on treatment outcomes including efficacy of OAT, side effects, and long-term compliance. In addition, efforts should be spent in increasing our understanding of gender differences in symptoms of sleep apnea. Use of this gained knowledge in evolving improved gender-specific screening tools will ultimately lead to more women obtaining appropriate care. The importance of dentists contributing to this change cannot be underscored and could potentially improve the quality and length of life for their female patients.

REFERENCES

1. Reichmuth KJ, Austin D, Skatrud JB, et al. Association of sleep apnea and type II diabetes: a population-based study. Am J Respir Crit Care Med 2005;172(12): 1590–5.
2. Redline S, Budhiraja R, Kapur V, et al. The scoring of respiratory events in sleep: reliability and validity. J Clin Sleep Med 2007;3(2):169–200.

3. Eastwood PR, Malhotra A, Palmer LJ, et al. Obstructive sleep apnoea: from pathogenesis to treatment: current controversies and future directions: think tank series: OSA. Respirology 2010;15(4):587–95.
4. Senaratna CV, Perret JL, Lodge CJ, et al. Prevalence of obstructive sleep apnea in the general population: a systematic review. Sleep Med Rev 2017;34:70–81.
5. Young T, Palta M, Dempsey J, et al. Burden of sleep apnea: rationale, design, and major findings of the Wisconsin Sleep Cohort study. WMJ 2009;108(5):246–9.
6. Young T. Analytic epidemiology studies of sleep disordered breathing–what explains the gender difference in sleep disordered breathing? Sleep 1993;16(8 Suppl):S1–2.
7. Ye L, Pien GW, Ratcliffe SJ, et al. Gender differences in the clinical manifestation of obstructive sleep apnea. Sleep Med 2009;10(10):1075–84.
8. Franklin KA, Lindberg E. Obstructive sleep apnea is a common disorder in the population-a review on the epidemiology of sleep apnea. J Thorac Dis 2015; 7(8):1311–22.
9. Heinzer R, Vat S, Marques-Vidal P, et al. Prevalence of sleep-disordered breathing in the general population: the HypnoLaus study. J Lancet Respir Med 2015; 3(4):310–8.
10. Pengo MF, Won CH, Bourjeily G. Sleep in women across the life span. Chest 2018;154(1):196–206.
11. Ciano C, King TS, Wright RR, et al. Longitudinal study of insomnia symptoms among women during perimenopause. J Obstet Gynecol Neonatal Nurs 2017; 46(6):804–13.
12. Cohen LS, Soares CN, Vitonis AF, et al. Risk for new onset of depression during the menopausal transition: the Harvard Study of moods and cycles. Arch Gen Psychiatry 2006;63(4):385–90.
13. Mirer AG, Young T, Palta M, et al. Sleep-disordered breathing and the menopausal transition among participants in the sleep in midlife women study. Menopause 2017;24(2):157–62.
14. Bixler EO, Vgontzas AN, Lin HM, et al. Association of hypertension and sleep-disordered breathing. Arch Intern Med 2000;160(15):2289–95.
15. Izci-Balserak B, Keenan BT, Corbitt C, et al. Changes in sleep characteristics and breathing parameters during sleep in early and late pregnancy. J Clin Sleep Med 2018;14(7):1161–8.
16. Pien GW, Pack AI, Jackson N, et al. Risk factors for sleep-disordered breathing in pregnancy. Thorax 2014;69(4):371–7.
17. Pamidi S, Pinto LM, Marc I, et al. Maternal sleep-disordered breathing and adverse pregnancy outcomes: a systematic review and meta-analysis. Am J Obstet Gynecol 2014;210(1):52.e1-14.
18. Bourjeily G, El Sabbagh R, Sawan P, et al. Epworth sleepiness scale scores and adverse pregnancy outcomes. Sleep Breath 2013;17(4):1179–86.
19. Appleton S, Gill T, Taylor A, et al. Influence of gender on associations of obstructive sleep apnea symptoms with chronic conditions and quality of life. Int J Environ Res Public Health 2018;15(5) [pii:E930].
20. Lindberg E, Benediktsdottir B, Franklin KA, et al. Women with symptoms of sleep-disordered breathing are less likely to be diagnosed and treated for sleep apnea than men. Sleep Med 2017;35:17–22.
21. Kapsimalis F, Kryger MH. Gender and obstructive sleep apnea syndrome, part 1: clinical features. Sleep 2002;25(4):412–9.

22. Basoglu OK, Tasbakan MK. Gender differences in clinical and polysomnographic features of obstructive sleep apnea: a clinical study of 2827 patients. Sleep Breath 2018;22(1):241–9.
23. Subramanian S, Jayaraman G, Majid H, et al. Influence of gender and anthropometric measures on severity of obstructive sleep apnea. Sleep Breath 2012;16(4): 1091–5.
24. Vagiakis E, Kapsimalis F, Lagogianni I, et al. Gender differences on polysomnographic findings in Greek subjects with obstructive sleep apnea syndrome. Sleep Med 2006;7(5):424–30.
25. Shepertycky MR, Banno K, Kryger MH. Differences between men and women in the clinical presentation of patients diagnosed with obstructive sleep apnea syndrome. Sleep 2005;28(3):309–14.
26. Basoglu OK, Vardar R, Tasbakan MS, et al. Obstructive sleep apnea syndrome and gastroesophageal reflux disease: the importance of obesity and gender. Sleep Breath 2015;19(2):585–92.
27. Hesselbacher S, Subramanian S, Rao S, et al. Self-reported sleep bruxism and nocturnal gastroesophageal reflux disease in patients with obstructive sleep apnea: relationship to gender and ethnicity. Open Respir Med J 2014;8:34–40.
28. Ohayon MM, Li KK, Guilleminault C. Risk factors for sleep bruxism in the general population. Chest 2001;119(1):53–61.
29. Lavigne GJ, Goulet JP, Zuconni M, et al. Sleep disorders and the dental patient: an overview. Oral Surg Oral Med Oral Pathol Oral Radiol Endod 1999;88(3): 257–72.
30. Durán-Cantolla J, Alkhraisat MH, Martínez-Null C, et al. Frequency of obstructive sleep apnea syndrome in dental patients with tooth wear. J Clin Sleep Med 2015; 11(4):445–50.
31. Kato T. Sleep bruxism and its relation to obstructive sleep apnea-hypopnea syndrome. Sleep Biol Rhythms 2004;2(1):1–15.
32. Khoury S, Carra MC, Huynh N, et al. Sleep bruxism-tooth grinding prevalence, characteristics and familial aggregation: a large cross-sectional survey and polysomnographic validation. Sleep 2016;39(11):2049–56.
33. Smith MT, Wickwire EM, Grace EG, et al. Sleep disorders and their association with laboratory pain sensitivity in temporomandibular joint disorder. Sleep 2009; 32(6):779–90.
34. Cunali PA, Almeida FR, Santos CD, et al. Prevalence of temporomandibular disorders in obstructive sleep apnea patients referred for oral appliance therapy. J Orofac Pain 2009;23(4):339–44.
35. Sanders AE, Essick GK, Fillingim R, et al. Sleep apnea symptoms and risk of temporomandibular disorder: OPPERA cohort. J Dent Res 2013;92(7suppl): S70–7.
36. Guilleminault C, Chowdhur S. Upper airway resistance syndrome is a distinct syndrome. Am J Respir Crit Care Med 2000;161(5):1412–3.
37. Mohsenin V. Gender differences in the expression of sleep-disordered breathing: role of upper airway dimensions. Chest 2002;120(5):1442–7.
38. O'Connor C, Thornley KS, Hanly PJ. Gender differences in the polysomnographic features of obstructive sleep apnea. Am J Respir Crit Care Med 2000;161(5): 1465–72.
39. Quintana-Gallego E, Carmona-Bernal C, Capote F, et al. Gender differences in obstructive sleep apnea syndrome: a clinical study of 166 patients. Respir Med 2004;98(10):984–9.

40. Molarius A, Tegelberg A, Ohrvik J. Socio-economic factors, lifestyle, and headache disorders - a population-based study in Sweden. Headache 2008;48(10):1426–37.
41. Young T, Hutton R, Finn L, et al. The gender bias in sleep apnea diagnosis. Are women missed because they have different symptoms? Arch Intern Med 1996;156(21):2445–51.
42. Ambrogetti A, Olson LG, Saunders NA. Differences in the symptoms of men and women with obstructive sleep apnoea. Aust N Z J Med 1991;21(6):863–6.
43. Guilleminault C, Stoohs R, Kim YD, et al. Upper airway sleep-disordered breathing in women. Ann Intern Med 1995;122(7):493–501.
44. Lin CM, Davidson TD, Ancoli-Israel S. Gender differences in obstructive sleep apnea and treatment implications. Sleep Med Rev 2008;12(6):481–96.
45. Young TL, Evans L, Finn L, et al. Estimation of the clinically diagnosed proportion of sleep apnea syndrome in middle-aged men and women. Sleep 1997;20(9):705–6.
46. Sullivan CE, Issa FG, Berthon-Jones M, et al. Reversal of obstructive sleep apnea by continuous positive pressure applied through the nares. Lancet 1981;1(8225):862–5.
47. Elshaug AG, Moss JR, Southcott AM, et al. Redefining success in airway surgery for obstructive sleep apnea: a meta analysis and synthesis of the evidence. Sleep 2007;30(4):461–7.
48. Chobanian AV. National High blood pressure education program committee: seventh report of the Joint National Committee on Prevention, Detection, Evaluation, and Treatment of High Blood Pressure. Hypertension 2003;42:1206–52.
49. Marin JM, Carrizo SJ, Vicente E, et al. Long-term cardiovascular outcomes in men with obstructive sleep apnoea-hypopnoea with or without treatment with continuous positive airway pressure: an observational study. Lancet 2005;365:1046–53.
50. Marklund M, Verbraecken J, Randerath W. Non-CPAP therapies in obstructive sleep apnoea: mandibular advancement device therapy. Eur Respir J 2012;39(5):1241–7.
51. Gagnadoux F, Fleury B, Vielle B, et al. Titrated mandibular advancement versus positive airway pressure for sleep apnoea. Eur Respir J 2009;34(4):914–20.
52. Budhiraja R, Thomas R, Kim M, et al. The role of big data in the management of sleep disordered breathing. Sleep Med Clin 2016;11(2):241–55.
53. Edwards BA, Andara C, Landry S, et al. Upper-airway collapsibility and loop gain predict the response to oral appliance therapy in patients with obstructive sleep apnea. Am J Respir Crit Care Med 2016;194(11):1413–22.
54. Chan AS, Sutherland K, Schwab RJ, et al. The effect of mandibular advancement on upper airway structure in obstructive sleep apnoea. Thorax 2010;65:726–32.
55. Battagel JM, Johal A, Kotecha BT. Sleep nasendoscopy as a predictor of treatment success in snorers using mandibular advancement splints. J Laryngol Otol 2005;119(2):106–12.
56. Mohsenin V. Effects of gender on upper airway collapsibility and severity of obstructive sleep apnea. Sleep Med 2003;4(6):523–9.
57. Marklund M, Carlberg B, Forsgren L, et al. Oral appliance therapy in patients with daytime sleepiness and snoring or mild to moderate sleep apnea: a randomized clinical trial. JAMA Intern Med 2015;175(8):1278–85.
58. Petri N, Svanholt P, Solow B, et al. Mandibular advancement appliance for obstructive sleep apnoea: results of a randomised placebo controlled trial using parallel group design. J Sleep Res 2008;17(2):221–9.

59. Menn SJ, Loube DI, Morgan TD, et al. The mandibular repositioning device: role in the treatment of obstructive sleep apnea. Sleep 1996;19(10):794–800.
60. Rose E, Staats R, Virchow C, et al. A comparative study of two mandibular advancement appliances for the treatment of obstructive sleep apnoea. Eur J Orthod 2002;24(2):191–8.
61. Kushida CA, Morgenthaler TI, Littner M, et al. Practice parameters for the treatment of snoring and obstructive sleep apnea with oral appliances: an update for 2005. Sleep 2006;29(2):240–3.
62. Haviv Y, Bachar G, Aframian DJ, et al. A 2-year mean follow-up of oral appliance therapy for severe obstructive sleep apnea: a cohort study. Oral Dis 2015;21(3):386–92.
63. Marklund M, Stenlund H, Franklin KA. Mandibular advancement devices in 630 men and women with obstructive sleep apnea and snoring. Chest 2004;125(4):1270–8.
64. Chen H, Lowe A. Updates in oral appliance therapy for snoring and obstructive sleep apnea. Sleep Breath 2013;17(2):473–86.
65. Tsuiki S, Ito E, Isono S, et al. Oropharyngeal crowding and obesity as predictors of oral appliance treatment response to moderate obstructive sleep apnea. Chest 2013;144(2):558–63.
66. Verbruggen AE, Dieltjens M, Wouters K, et al. Prevalence of residual excessive sleepiness during effective oral appliance therapy for sleep-disordered breathing. Sleep Med 2014;15(2):269–72.
67. Antic NA, Catcheside P, Buchan C, et al. The effect of CPAP in normalizing daytime sleepiness, quality of life, and neurocognitive function in patients with moderate to severe OSA. Sleep 2011;34(1):111–9.
68. Oksenberg A, Arons E. Sleep bruxism related to obstructive sleep apnea: the effect of continuous positive airway pressure. Sleep Med 2002;3(6):513–5.
69. Riachy M, Najem S, Iskandar M, et al. Factors predicting CPAP adherence in obstructive sleep apnea syndrome. Sleep Breath 2017;21(2):295–302.
70. Gagnadoux F, Vaillant M, Goupil F, et al. Influence of marital status and employment status on long-term adherence with continuous positive airway pressure in sleep apnea patients. PLoS One 2011;6(8):e22503.
71. Budhiraja R, Parthasarathy S, Drake C, et al. Early CPAP use identifies subsequent adherence to CPAP therapy. Sleep 2007;30(3):320–4.
72. Joo MJ, Herdegen JJ. Sleep apnea in an urban public hospital: assessment of severity and treatment adherence. J Clin Sleep Med 2007;3(3):285–8.
73. Pelletier-Fleury N, Rakotonanahary D, Fleury B. The age and other factors in the evaluation of compliance with nasal continuous positive airway pressure for obstructive sleep apnea syndrome. A Cox's proportional hazard analysis. Sleep Med 2001;2(3):225–32.

Consideration for Contemporary Implant Surgery

Dean Morton, BDS, MS[a,*], Kamolphob Phasuk, DDS, MS[a], Waldemar D. Polido, DDS, MS, PhD[b], Wei-Shao Lin, DDS[a]

KEYWORDS

- Computer-guided surgery • Virtual planning • CBCT • Intraoral scan • Facial scan • Virtual patient • Dental implant

KEY POINTS

- The use of three dimensional (3D) radiographic imaging, such as cone beam computed tomography (CBCT), allows for the collection of accurate pretreatment diagnostic dataset. However, creating airspace around regions of interest is essential to provide clear outlines of varying structures during CBCT imaging.
- A static virtual dental patient can be created from the CBCT imaging and optical scanning systems for intraoral (IOS) and extraoral (EOS) imaging to facilitate prosthodontically driven implant planning process.
- A radiographic template or a virtual diagnostic wax-up is essential for a prosthodontically driven treatment plan.
- Although the use of computer-guided surgery can provide clinical advantages, an objective assessment of proposed treatment difficulty should be undertaken (Straightforward/Advanced/Complex) to reduce surgical complications.

Dental implant-based treatment has developed from a revolutionary option into a widely accepted treatment modality in dentistry. Studies have demonstrated long-term survival rates for dental implants,[1–4] and success criteria have evolved to include the esthetic outcome of the implant-prosthetic complex.[5] A lifelike implant supported or retained prosthesis, accompanied by healthy peri-implant tissue, has become the gold standard for dental implant treatment. Appropriate patient assessment from a prosthodontic, surgical, and radiographic perspective is now considered to be a pre-requisite for the achievement of a satisfactory clinical outcome. Computer-assisted

Disclosure Statement: The authors have nothing to disclose.
[a] Department of Prosthodontics, Indiana University School of Dentistry, 1121 West Michigan Street, DS-S408, Indianapolis, IN 46202-5186, USA; [b] Department of Oral Surgery and Hospital Dentistry, Indiana University School of Dentistry, 1121 West Michigan Street, DS-S408, Indianapolis, IN 46202-5186, USA
* Corresponding author.
E-mail address: deamorto@iu.edu

Dent Clin N Am 63 (2019) 309–329
https://doi.org/10.1016/j.cden.2018.11.010 dental.theclinics.com

options allow clinicians to realize the virtual prosthodontically driven surgical plan, facilitating predictable implant placement. Various methods, including the use of computer-aided design and computer-aided manufacturing (CAD-CAM) for surgical template design and fabrication are becoming more common place.[6]

The purpose of this article is to review fundamental concepts important to the use of computer-assisted options relating to implant surgery and to prosthodontic treatment.

THREE-DIMENSIONAL RADIOGRAPHIC IMAGING

Thorough pretreatment evaluation of the implant recipient site, and its associated anatomic forms and limitations is required. Visualization of the proposed prosthesis or prostheses and their relationship to the recipient site should be routinely incorporated to improve clinical outcomes and minimize complications. Although two-dimensional (2D) intraoral (**Fig. 1**) and panoramic (**Fig. 2**) radiographic imaging remains an option that is used extensively in daily dental practice, access to and use of three-dimensional (3D) radiographic imaging has dramatically enhanced options for data collection. The use of cone beam computed tomography (CBCT) has allowed for the collection of a more consistent and accurate pretreatment diagnostic dataset, with acceptable levels of radiation exposure and cost to the patients (**Fig. 3**). Unlike traditional fan-beam (medical) computed tomography (CT), CBCT uses a cone or pyramid-shaped beam to scan an entire 3D volumetric dataset in a single rotation using reduced x-ray tube power.[7] The lower power characteristic reduces the radiation exposure and the cost to the patient, but also decreases the contrast resolution of the resulting 3D volumetric dataset. This limits the suitability for the data gathered using CBCT with regard to soft tissue imaging including, for example, facial soft tissue contours.[8] Existing metallic restorations can also result in artifacts (including scatter) and compromise the diagnostic value of 3D volume gathered from CBCT imaging.[9] The reducing initial investment and maintenance costs of CBCT units, and the high spatial resolution of hard tissue structures, have greatly increased the application of CBCT in dentistry.[10,11]

CREATING AIR SPACE DURING 3D RADIOGRAPHIC IMAGING

Hounsfield units (HU) are proportional to the degree of x-ray attenuation, are allocated to each pixel, and represent the density of the tissue. HUs provide a universal standard

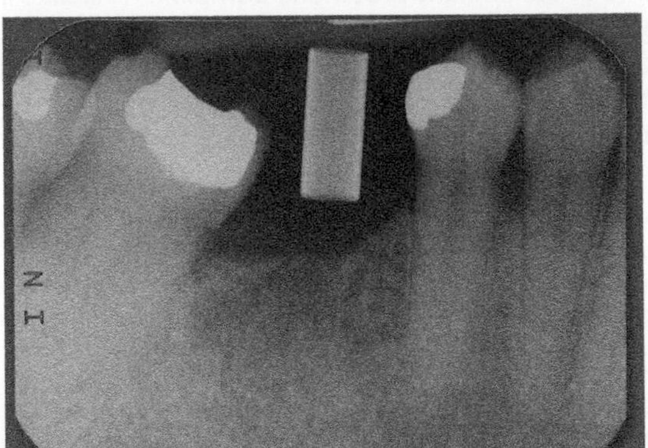

Fig. 1. Traditional 2D intraoral periapical radiograph with radiopaque marker to provide reference for the magnification.

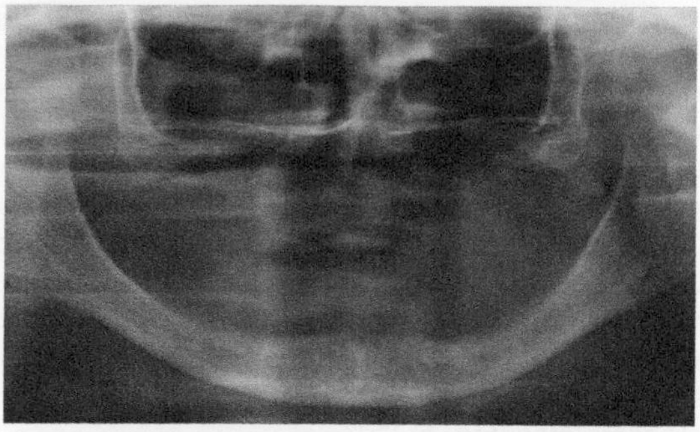

Fig. 2. Traditional 2D panoramic radiograph.

in medical CT imaging systems for scaling reconstructed attenuation coefficients. The degree of x-ray attenuation in CBCT imaging is presented as a gray scale (voxel value), and manufacturers do not have a standard system. However, different studies show a linear relationship between HU (CT imaging) and the gray scale (CBCT imaging), and it has been suggested that the gray scale can be used in determining the radiodensity changes.[12,13] The different radiodensity, for example, of cortical bone (1700 HU), denture acrylic resin (70 HU), tissue (50 HU), pure water (0 HU), and air (−1000 HU) affords clinicians a method by which a discernible comparison among different structures can be made. The larger the difference between HUs, the easier for clinicians to discern different structures using CBCT imaging. Obtaining a digital volume without proper air space separation in regions of interest can limit interpretation of information relating to hard tissues (such as bone and teeth). Airspace is required to provide a clear visualization of additional structures with similar radiodensity, such as soft tissues and denture acrylic resin, lips, cheeks and gingiva, and occlusal surfaces between opposing arches.[14,15]

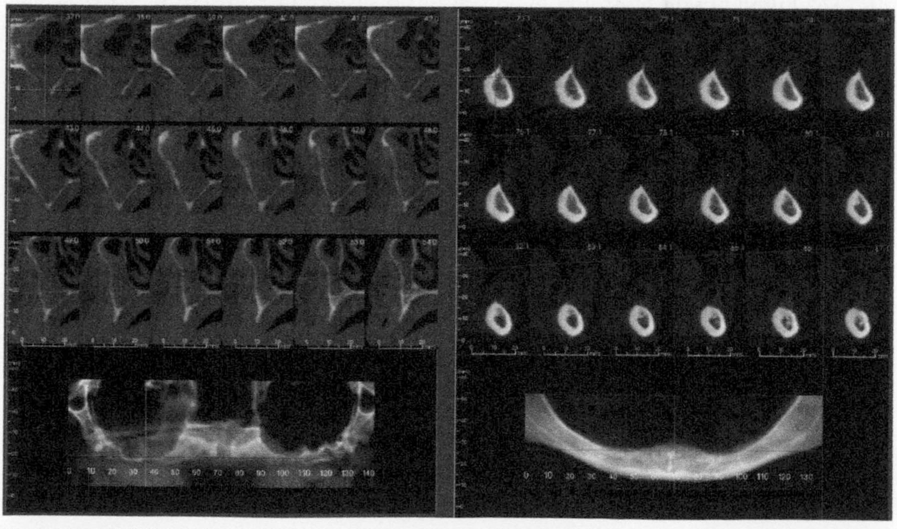

Fig. 3. 3D CBCT imaging provides more accurate diagnostic dataset to evaluate the surgical site.

Cotton rolls and soft tissue retractors are useful and simple tools that can be used to create air space around regions of interest to provide clear outlines of varying structures. For instance, cotton rolls can be placed between occlusal surfaces of opposing arches to create separation, and it can allow for clearer visualization of surface detail. Soft tissue retractors and cotton rolls can also be used to isolate the patient's cheeks and lips from adjacent alveolar ridges and gingiva, and facilitate improved distinction among various soft tissue structures (**Fig. 4**). When using removable dental prostheses as scanning aids during CBCT imaging, cotton rolls are needed to separate cheeks, lips, and tongue from the acrylic resin of the removable dental prostheses. This can greatly improve the clinician's ability to visualize the outline of proposed prostheses (the planned prostheses) without the need to duplicate existing prostheses into distinct radiographic templates (**Fig. 5**).[14,15]

CREATING A VIRTUAL DENTAL PATIENT FOR COMPUTER-GUIDED SURGERY PLANNING

A virtual dental patient can be created in computer-aided design and computer-aided manufacturing (CAD-CAM) and/or virtual implant planning software, thus replicating relevant anatomic structures and functional positions. These include the maxillofacial soft tissues (including muscles of facial expression and facial contour), maxillofacial hard tissues (such as skull and dentition), and intraoral soft tissues (such as edentulous ridge and periodontal or peri-implant soft tissue). Including the aforementioned CBCT imaging, different technologies can be used to collect 3D volumetric data to compose a desirable virtual patient for diagnostic purposes.[16] Current data acquisition technologies include CBCT imaging and optical scanning systems for intraoral (IOS) and extraoral (EOS) imaging. CBCT imaging generates data in the DICOM (Digital Imaging and Communications in Medicine) file format, a general standard format for handling, storing, printing, and transmitting information in medicine (ISO 12052:2017). IOS imaging uses proprietary file formats, or exports the 3D scan in Surface Tessellation Language file format, which consists only of the surface geometries of 3D objects without any color or texture information. EOS imaging can store the scan data in a proprietary format or as OBJ files (developed by Wavefront Technologies for its Advanced Visualizer animation package), an open geometry definition file format capable of storing 3D texture and color information.[16]

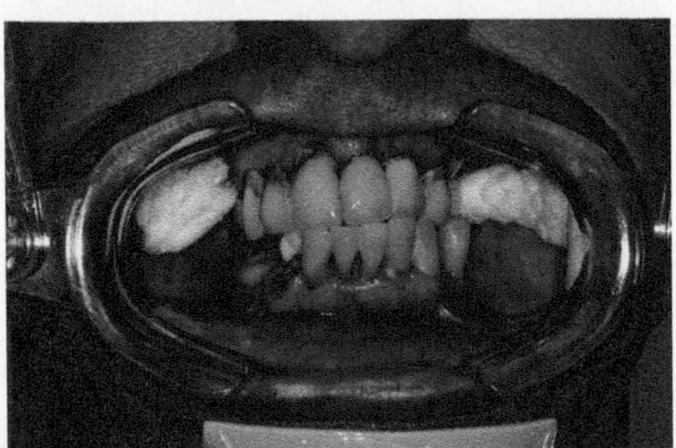

Fig. 4. Plastic retractor and cotton rolls can be used as effective tools to create air space around the region of interest during CBCT imaging.

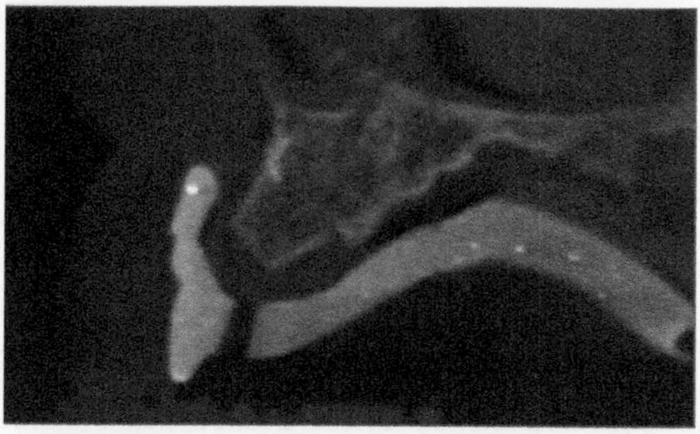

Fig. 5. Radiopaque material can be used to duplicate diagnostic waxing or existing prostheses into radiographic template. The outline of the radiographic template can serve as a reference for the intraoral soft tissue outline in the patient.

The triad of maxillofacial hard tissue, extraoral facial soft tissue, and the intraoral dentition and surrounding soft tissue is key to creating a virtual patient under static conditions. The high-resolution and scatter-free 3D volumetric dataset from IOS and EOS imaging (surface scan) can be used to supplement the diagnostic information from CBCT imaging to create a virtual dental patient for implant planning (**Fig. 6**). Currently, no readily available system allows for the visualization and duplication of functional movements of maxillofacial structures facilitating a complete 4D (dynamic)

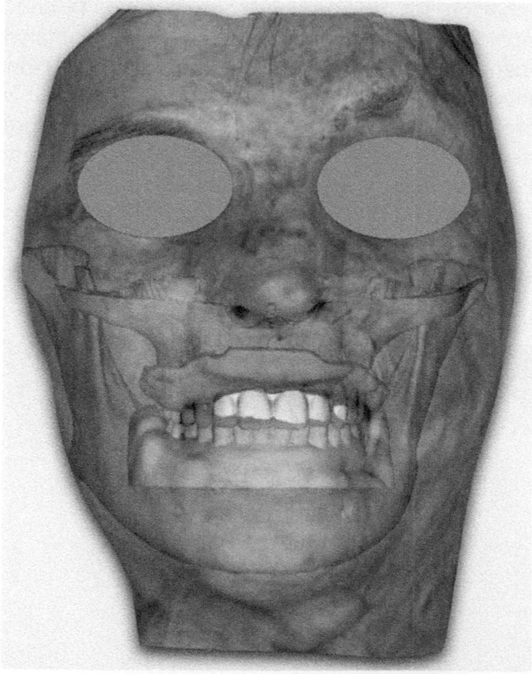

Fig. 6. The triad of maxillofacial hard tissue (CBCT), extraoral facial soft tissue (EOS), and the intraoral dentition and surrounding soft tissue (IOS) can be used to create a virtual patient under static conditions.

virtual dental patient, although this is under investigation. It is of future research interest to improve current technology and develop protocols to do so.[17,18]

IMPORTANCE OF DIAGNOSTIC WAX-UP FOR IMPLANT PLANNING

A prosthodontically driven treatment plan is needed to improve the possibility of a favorable treatment result.[19] The location and position of dental implants should follow the plan for the desired definitive restoration. Comprehensive oral examination, complete periodontal charting, and appropriate radiographic examination are vital for diagnosis and treatment planning. Conventionally, along with a good quality clinical photographs, appropriate diagnostic casts are obtained and articulated. The diagnostic wax-up and tooth arrangement of the desired definitive restoration or prosthesis are traditionally procedures completed in the laboratory (**Figs. 7** and **8**), and should follow sound prosthodontic principles. In many situations, appropriate soft tissue contours and prosthesis extensions are included in the diagnostic wax-up to reflect the desired outcome. The pink component of diagnostic wax-up represents the deficiency of hard and soft tissue (**Figs. 9** and **10**). This information is necessary for the designing of implant and tooth supported prostheses, and assessment of any potential tissue augmentation.[20]

THE USE OF RADIOGRAPHIC TEMPLATES

Traditionally, the diagnostic wax-up or satisfactory existing prosthesis can be duplicated and used to fabricate a radiographic template. Radiographic templates contain radiopaque materials (barium sulfate) and/or fiducial markers such as gutta percha or titanium rods, and transfer the proposed prosthesis design and contour, as well as proposed implant position, for radiographic capture (**Figs. 11** and **12**).[21] The patient wears the radiographic template during imaging (CBCT or otherwise), and the proposed prosthesis can then be visualized on a radiograph or planning software for the purpose of treatment planning. Cross-sectional radiographic images of edentulous areas incorporating radiographic markers also help to determine the need for augmentation procedures during or before dental implant placement (**Fig. 13**). The implant prosthesis and location of the access for screw retention can also be determined by using the information made available through effective use of radiographic templates.[22] A drawback of radiographic templates is the need for additional clinical and laboratory steps and associated costs needed for fabrication. The clinician is

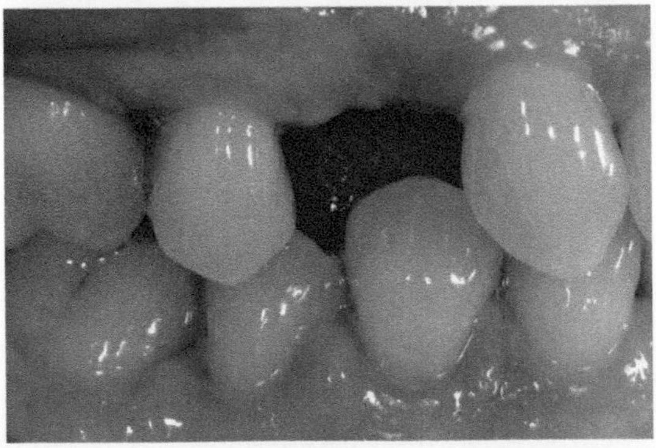

Fig. 7. In a partially edentulous patient receiving dental implant treatment, an analog or digital diagnostic waxing should be completed during the treatment-planning process.

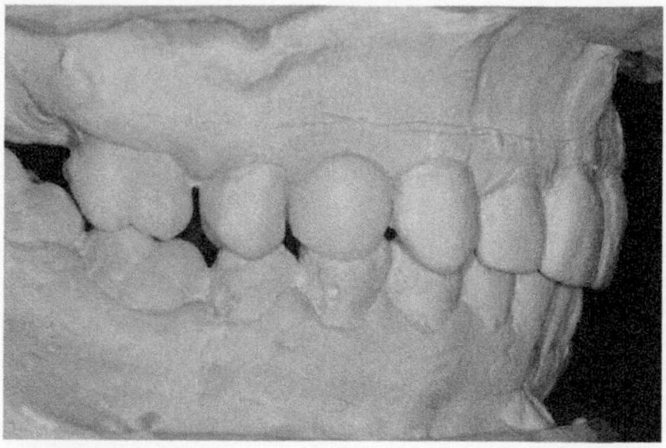

Fig. 8. An analog diagnostic waxing was completed for the maxillary first premolar to prepare for the dental implant treatment.

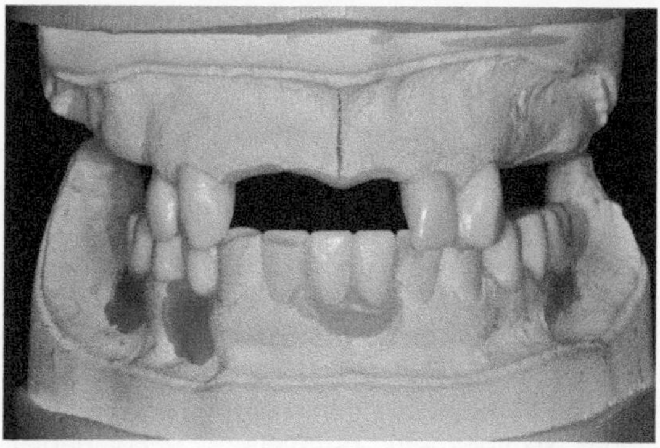

Fig. 9. The diagnostic waxing should accurately reflect the design and contours of desired definitive prostheses. When the soft or hard tissue defects are noted, the diagnostic waxing should illustrate the defects with a tissue-colored component.

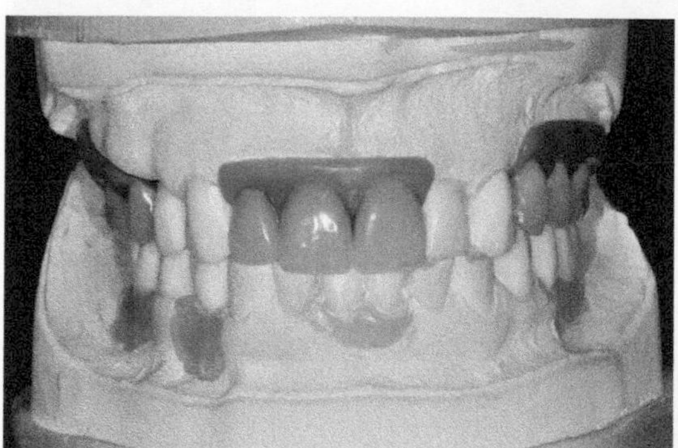

Fig. 10. When the definitive removable dental prostheses are desired, a flange should be added to the diagnostic tooth arrangement for the trial insertion to confirm the required lip support.

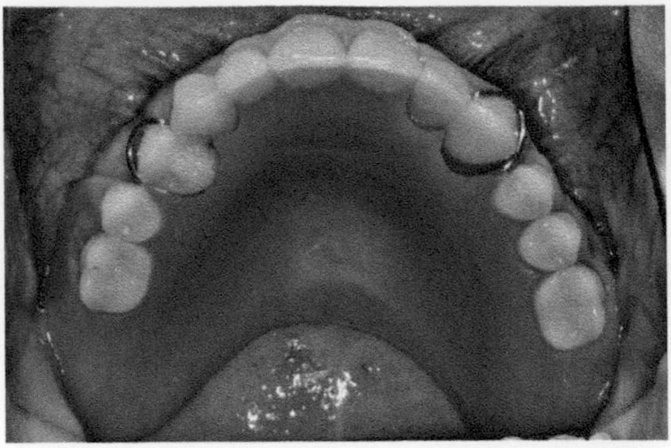

Fig. 11. Satisfactory existing prosthesis can be duplicated with radiopaque material as a radiographic template.

required to obtain duplicate diagnostic casts for the fabrication process and a second clinical appointment is often needed to confirm the fit of the radiographic template before imaging.

THE USE OF A VIRTUAL DIAGNOSTIC WAX-UP

Contemporary virtual implant planning software allows the 3D volumetric dataset obtained from IOS and/or EOS imaging (surface scans) to be superimposed over 3D rendering of DICOM files. When a radiographic template is used, the radiopaque fiducial markers can be recognized by the computer algorithm, and marker-based registration can superimpose all the datasets to facilitate planning for the computer-guided surgery. Newly improved surface-based registration methods provide the clinician with an opportunity to forgo the radiographic template and use available intraoral surface markers, including the surfaces of remaining teeth, to accomplish digital superimposition of various 3D volumetric datasets.[6,14,15] For partially dentate arches in particular, the IOS and EOS datasets can be merged with DICOM datasets, and provide clinicians with clearer scatter-free surface detail (**Figs. 14–17**). Once the surface-based registration is completed, a virtual diagnostic wax-up can be added

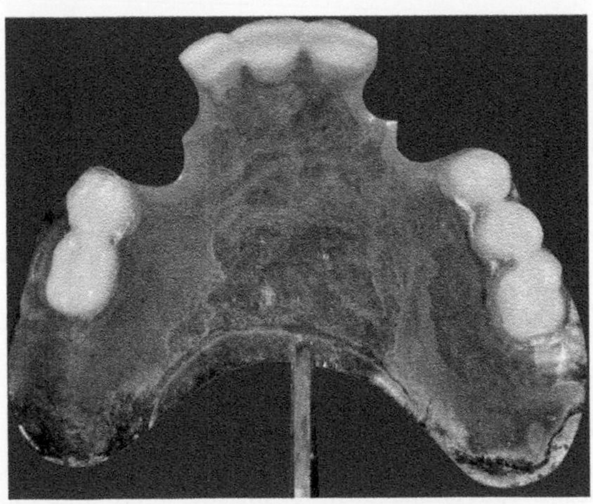

Fig. 12. The acrylic teeth are duplicated with barium sulfate.

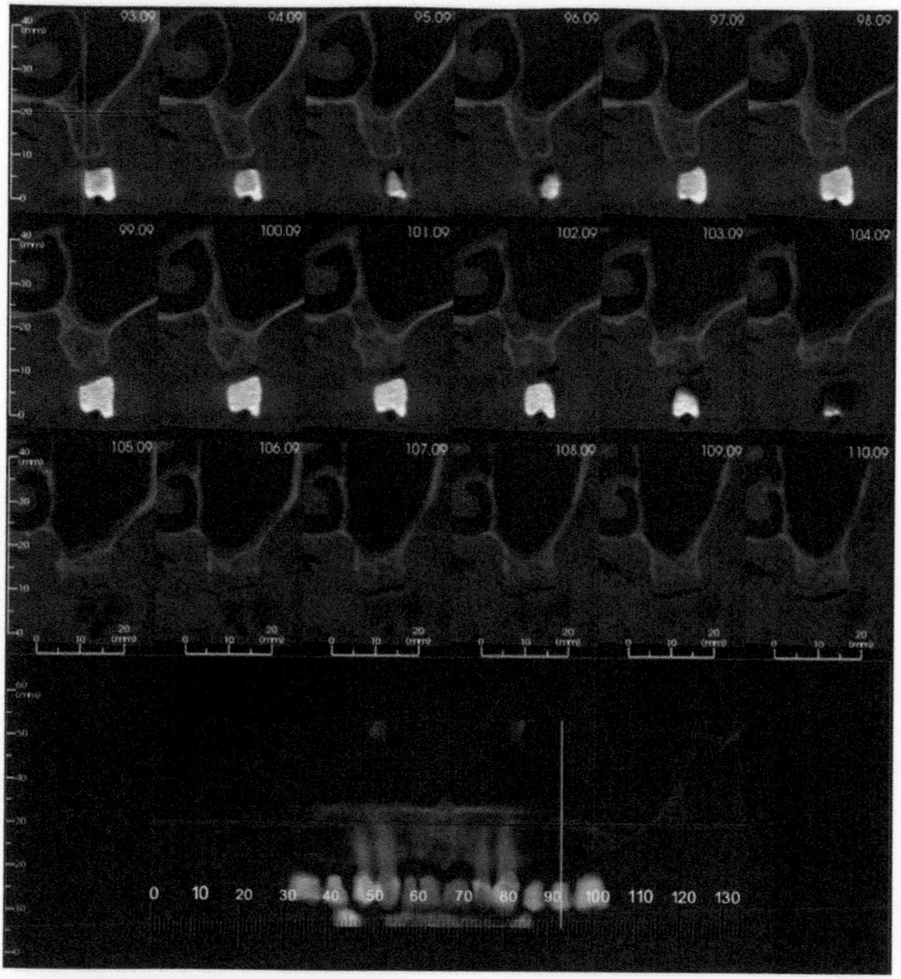

Fig. 13. The duplicate barium sulfate teeth are radiopaque and transfer the proposed prosthesis position onto the CBCT imaging.

to the dataset to formulate a prosthodontically driven computer-guided surgical plan (**Figs. 18** and **19**). The layers of DICOM 3D rendering, surface scan, and virtual wax-up can each be toggled on and off in the implant planning software, providing for a clear assessment of the dental implant site.[23,24]

DYNAMIC VERSUS STATIC COMPUTER-GUIDED SURGERY

Dynamic and static approaches are 2 options for computer-guided surgery. The dynamic approach (navigation systems) allows the tracking of surgical instruments and their relative positions to the patient in real time, and has the ability to update the virtual surgical instrument position within the patient's preoperative 3D CBCT imaging during surgery.[25,26] Navigation systems are based on optical tracking technology. The surgical drill coupled with tracking elements is tracked by an optical camera and the osteotomy/implant placement can be guided in the real time following the predefined surgical plan in the preoperative 3D CBCT volume. Dynamic computer-guided

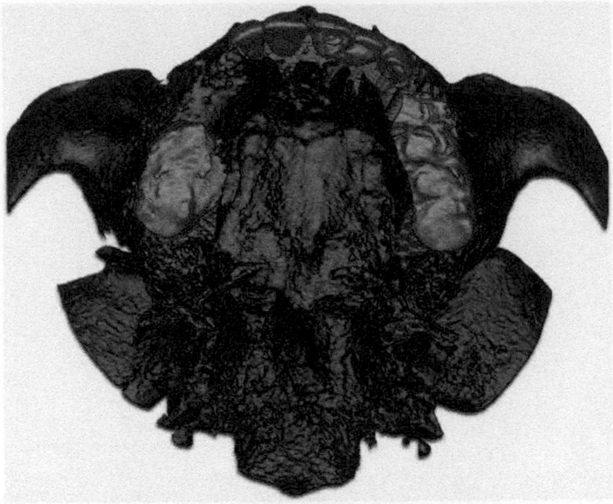

Fig. 14. The remaining dentition will often present scatter or artifacts in the DICOM dataset.

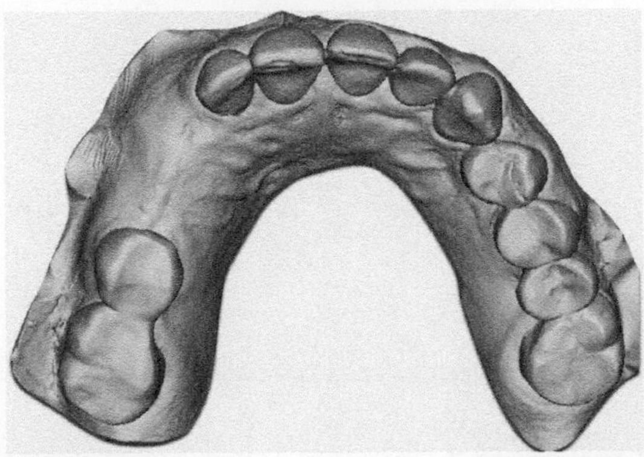

Fig. 15. Intraoral scan can provide scatter-free surface detail of remaining dentition.

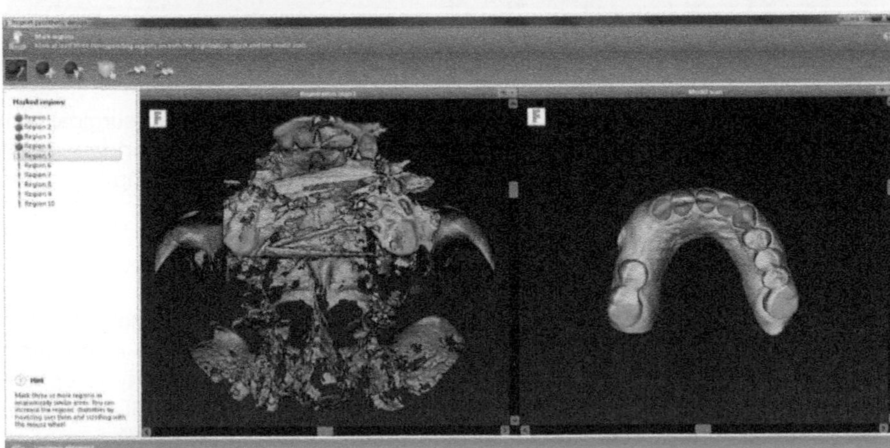

Fig. 16. Surface-based registration method can be used to register IOS and DICOM dataset by using common anatomic landmarks.

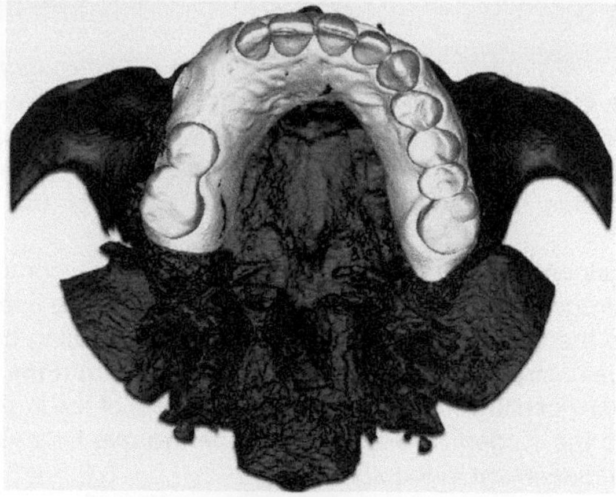

Fig. 17. Merged dataset containing maxillofacial hard tissue from CBCT imaging and the intraoral dentition and surrounding soft tissue from IOS.

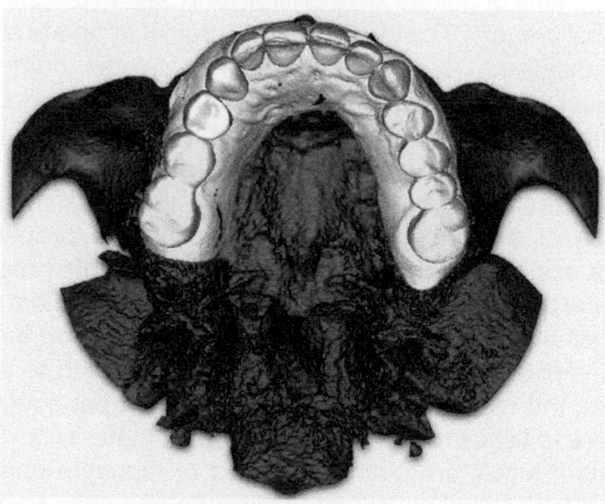

Fig. 18. The virtual diagnostic waxing can be added to the merged dataset to formulate a prosthodontically driven computer-guided surgical plan.

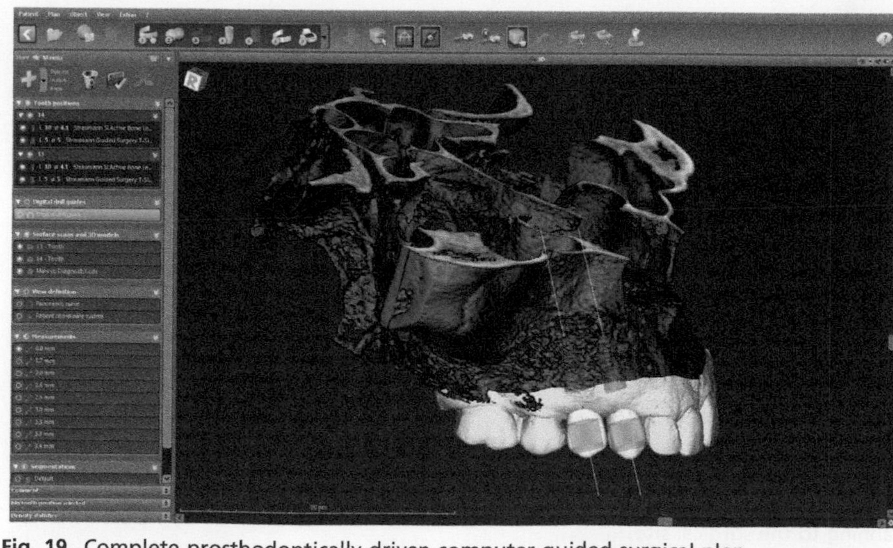

Fig. 19. Complete prosthodontically driven computer-guided surgical plan.

surgery has the advantage of changing the implant size, system, and location during the surgery (allowing inter-operative changes). When the patient has limited mouth opening, the dynamic navigation allows for implant placement by relying on the navigation screen to guide the osteotomy without the need for the clinician's direct visualization.[26]

Because of the uncomplicated nature and lower cost, static computer-guided surgery is used more frequently than dynamic. The static approach uses a surgical template that transfers the virtual surgical planning to the site, using coordinated metal sleeves and surgical instruments to guide implant placement (**Figs. 20** and **21**). The static approach does not allow for inter-operative changes of the implant size, system, and location during the surgery. It does not provide the real time visualization of the osteotomy/implant placement in the software.

IMPLANT SURGICAL TEMPLATE

Implant surgical templates or guides are a critical tool used to transfer the prosthodontic plan to the surgical arena.[27] The ideal implant surgical template should be descriptive rather than indicative. Descriptive surgical templates communicate implant placement to precisely defined depths and positions as defined by the diagnostic wax-up, while indicative surgical templates communicate to the surgeon areas whereby a dental implant should not be placed (**Fig. 22**).[22,28] One of the important components of the descriptive surgical template is the transfer of the prospective mucosal emergence of desired definitive restoration. The proper position of the desired cervical mucosal margin guides the surgeon to facilitate proper implant placement and any surgical augmentations (**Figs. 23** and **24**). The implant surgical template needs to be rigid, well-fitting, and stable in the patient's mouth during implant surgery. Various designs of implant surgical templates have been used to aid dental implant placement; however, the template should allow for the proper cooling of the surgical drills without interfere to tissue reflection.[29] Clear splint material (1–1.5 mm thickness) or clear acrylic resin (PMMA) are commonly used to fabricate conventional implant surgical templates due to the simplicity of fabrication and ease to modify.

CAD/CAM SURGICAL TEMPLATE

Computer technology has been introduced to implant dentistry in recent years and has become a vital tool for modern dental implant treatment. CAD/CAM technology can be facilitated in all phases of care including planning and execution. The IOS

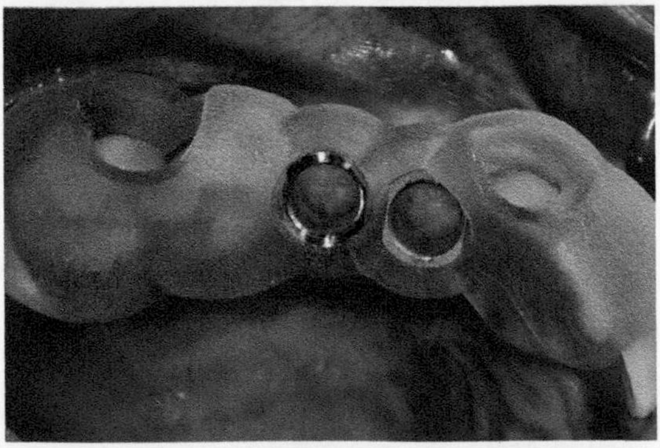

Fig. 20. The static computer-guided surgery uses a surgical template to transfer the virtual planning to the surgical site.

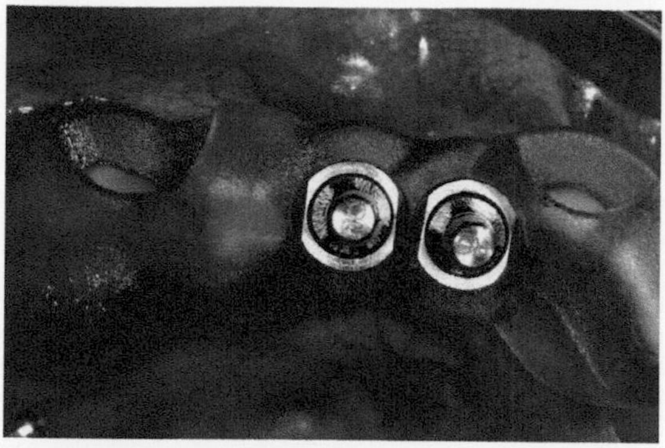

Fig. 21. Coordinated metal sleeves and surgical instruments are used to guide the implant placement.

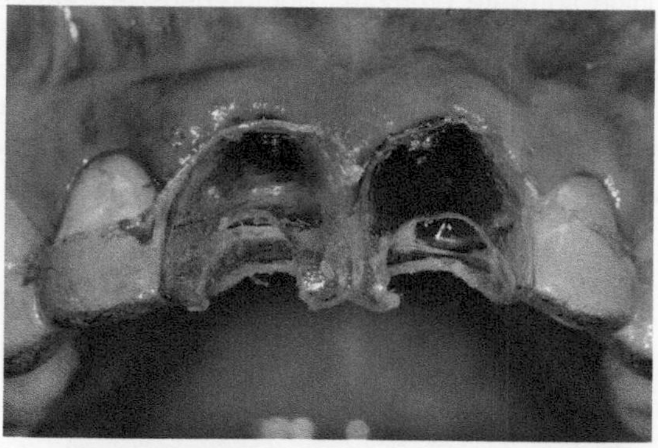

Fig. 22. Indicative surgical template only provides the general bordered area guiding the implant placement.

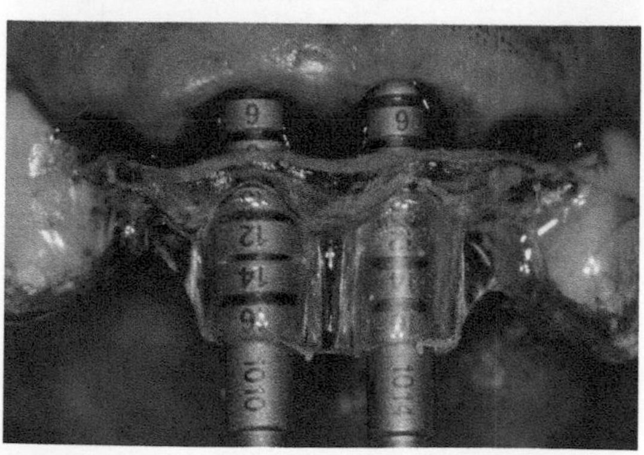

Fig. 23. Descriptive surgical template provides implant placement to precisely defined and positions as defined by the diagnostic wax-up.

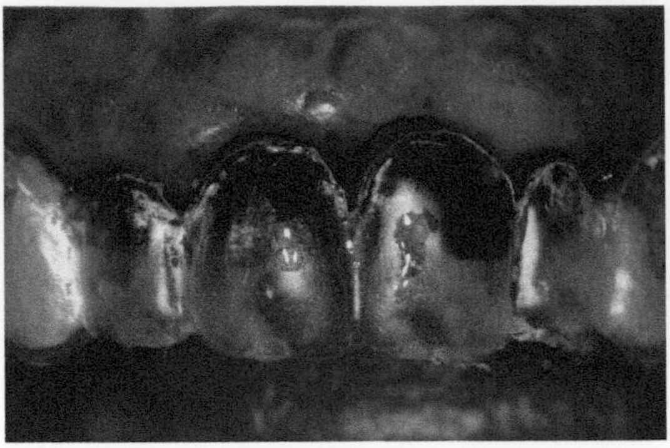

Fig. 24. A second surgical template can be used to provide the position of the desired cervical mucosal margin from diagnostic wax-up guiding proper depth of implant placement.

and CBCT are initially used in the diagnostic phase. Using the information garnered from IOS and CBCT, software can be used to undertake the diagnostic wax-up digitally. Implant planning software promotes comprehensive treatment planning and communication between the prosthodontic and surgical aspect of treatment. Guided surgical options for implant placement and site modification, using CAD templates manufactured via 3D printing or milling technologies, can enhance the accuracy and minimize intervention time (**Figs. 25–33**).[30,31] However, care should be exercised

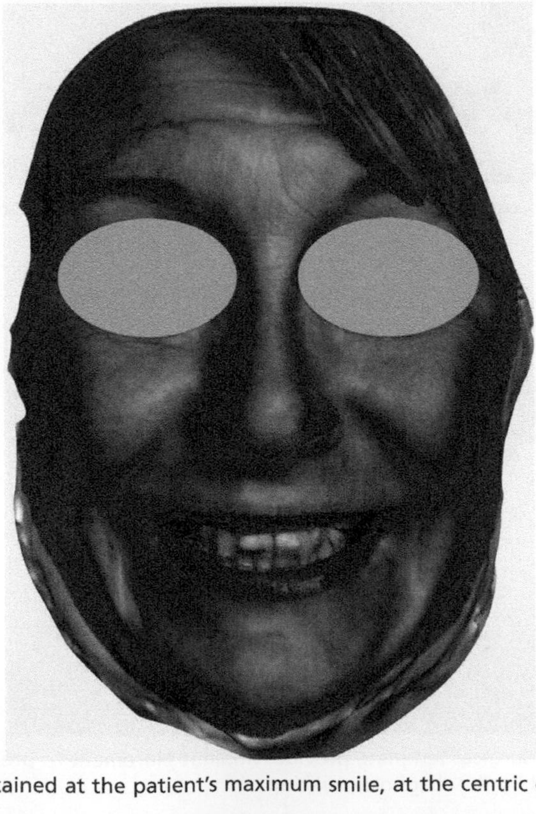

Fig. 25. EOS is obtained at the patient's maximum smile, at the centric occlusion position.

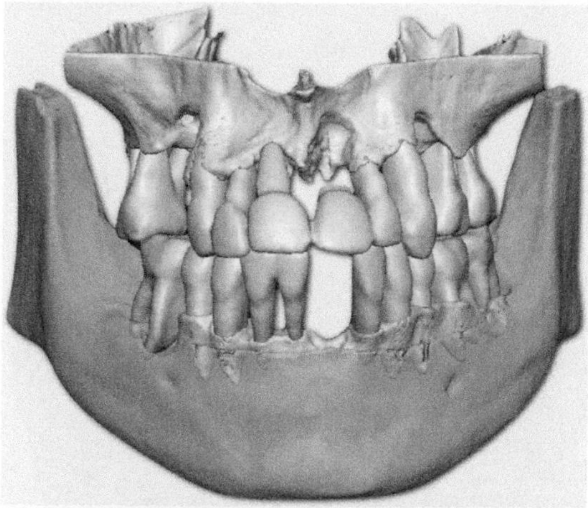

Fig. 26. CBCT imaging is obtained at the centric occlusion position.

when using guided surgery technology. Although the average error for guided surgery is low, maximum errors can be relatively high. In addition, it has been reported that, for guided surgery, the form of support (tooth, implant, and/or tissue) can influence accuracy.[32,33]

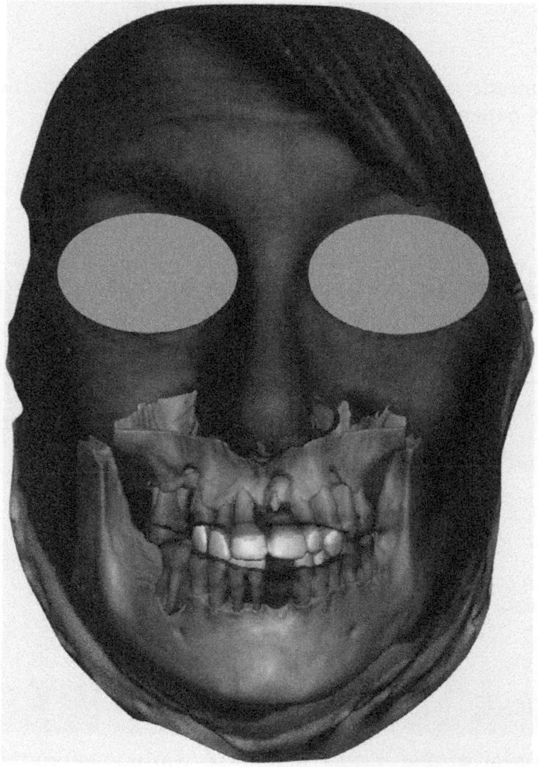

Fig. 27. EOS and CBCT dataset are merged using existing dentition as common landmarks.

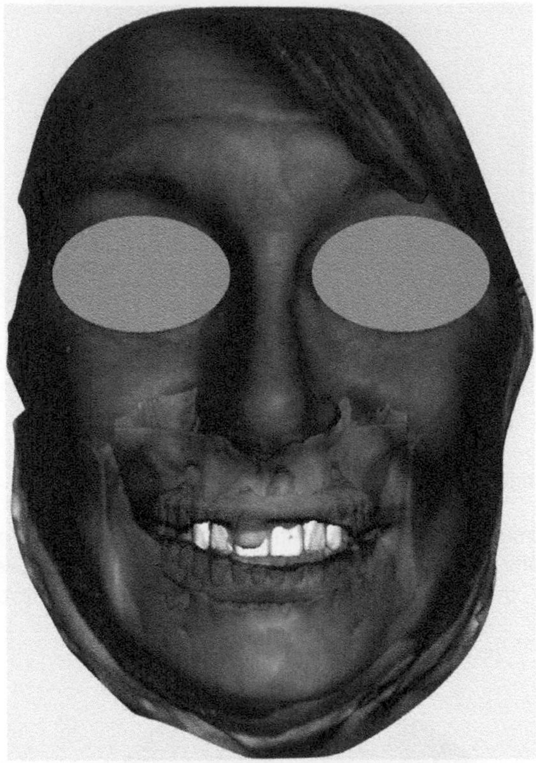

Fig. 28. Virtual diagnostic wax-up is completed and used as a diagnostic and communication tool among the patient, clinician, and dental technician.

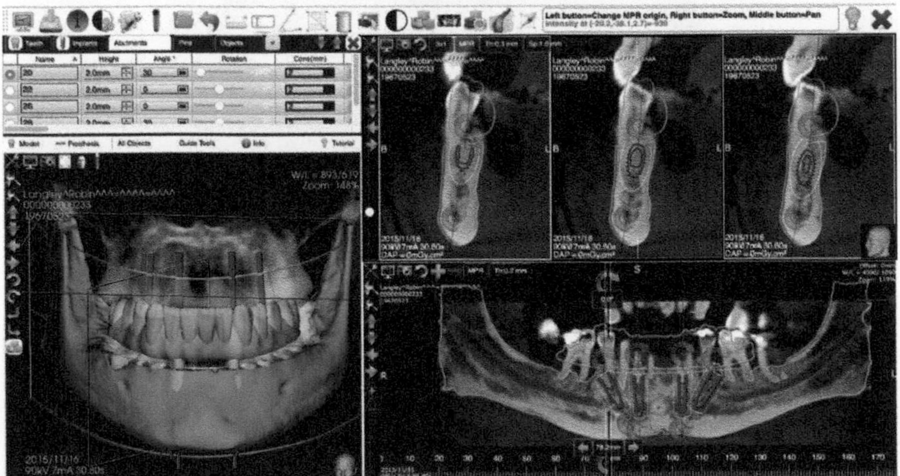

Fig. 29. After approval of the virtual diagnostic wax-up, a prosthodontically driven computer-guided surgical plan can be formulated.

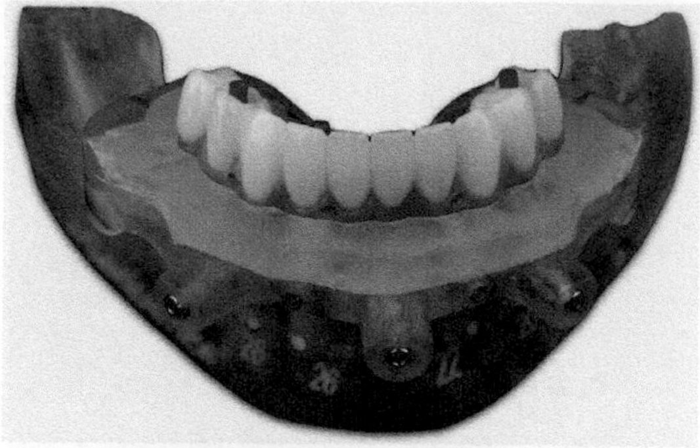

Fig. 30. CAD-CAM surgical template and interim prosthesis can be fabricated before the surgery for the immediate implant placement and provisionalization.

SURGICAL CONSIDERATIONS FOR COMPUTER-GUIDED SURGERY

The use of computer-guided surgery does not mean that all surgical details and preparation used in a conventional implant surgery should be neglected. The medical condition of the patient should be carefully evaluated, especially with regard to medications that the patient is taking, and possible negative interactions with the planned procedure. The level of complexity of the procedure should be carefully assessed from the perspective of surgical principles to reduce or completely avoid surgical complications. It is recommend that an objective assessment of proposed treatment difficulty be undertaken (Straightforward/Advanced/Complex) to help determine the relationship between clinician skill, education, and level of complexity.[34]

As for any surgery, including implant-related procedures, each office must prepare to perform the procedure following the current standards of care. Surgical setup and staff preparation is important, as is the use and maintenance of a sterile environment (including patient drapes and gloves) (**Fig. 34**).

An understanding of and a striving for aseptic technique is critical. Adequate lighting, suction, instrumentation, and surgically trained assistance is mandatory.[35] Infection control in the dental office should be followed at all times.[36] As stated by Bidra,[37] with the increase in the number of dentists with varying experience levels performing implant surgeries throughout the world, a surgical safety checklist may help standardize the perioperative workflow for implant and related surgeries in an outpatient (dental office) setting.

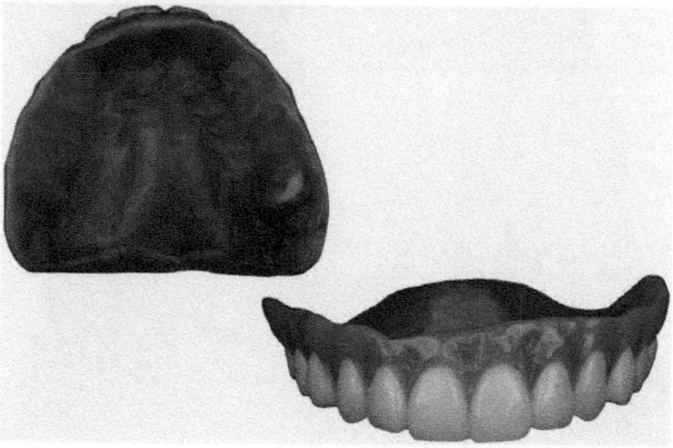

Fig. 31. CAD-CAM interim removable dental prosthesis.

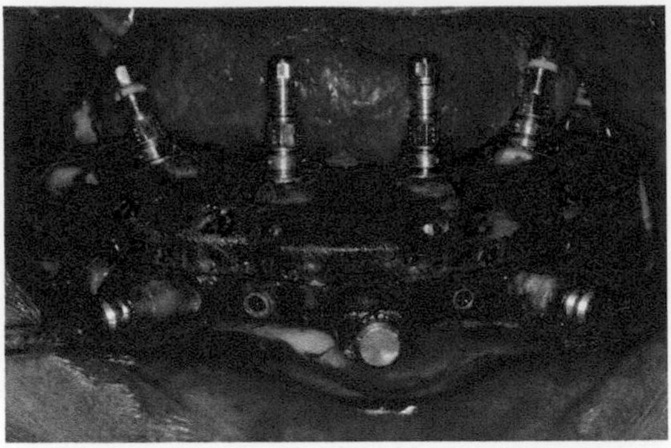

Fig. 32. Implants are placed under the guidance of surgical template.

Specific procedure-related aspects should also be taken into consideration. The soft tissue phenotype should be carefully evaluated to decide between a flap or a flapless surgery. Positioning and fixation of the guide with positional screws or stabilized in adjacent teeth should be also checked, once this is a vital step for the success of the implant positioning. Mouth opening and access, specially to the posterior areas of the maxilla and mandible should be checked also before the surgery is scheduled. Guided surgery templates can occupy a lot of space in the mouth, reducing visibility and access to the alveolar bone area, especially in the posterior region (see **Fig. 32**).

Selecting the appropriate treatment pathway is important to achieving predictable results when working with digital planning and computer-guided surgery. Lanis and colleagues[38] suggested consideration of 3 different pathways based on the presence or absence of patient reference information. Single or short span partially edentulous areas, with neighboring teeth, will be the more straightforward, for example, because the adjacent teeth are reference points to assist in the planning (analog or digital) and treatment execution. The absence of occlusal references for use during a virtual wax-

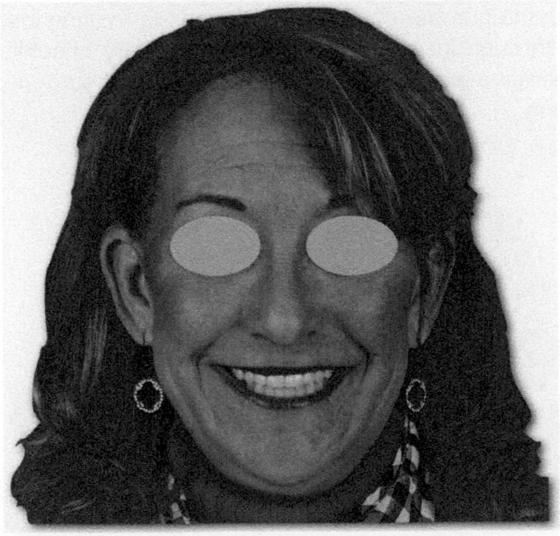

Fig. 33. The interim prostheses in situ.

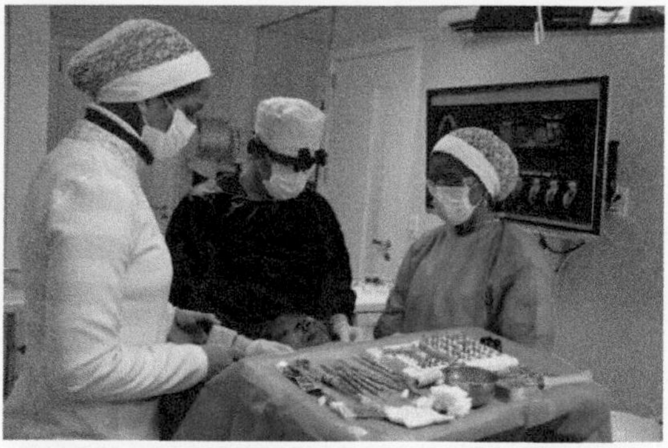

Fig. 34. Sterile setup for implant surgery.

up will add complexity. Patients presenting with no occlusal surface to reference bring an additional degree of difficulty.

SUMMARY

It is clear that implant placement surgery can range in difficulty from straightforward to complex. There are many contemporary aids available to clinicians that enhance the planning options available as well as improving intervention predictability. Even so, basic principles of surgical technique and management of the patient remain fundamental. The information discussed in this article assumes adequate training, experience, and skill on behalf of the clinician. It should be emphasized that use of technology in no way exempts clinicians from the responsibility to learn and gather adequate abilities before treating patients.

REFERENCES

1. Romeo E, Lops D, Margutti E, et al. Long-term survival and success of oral implants in the treatment of full and partial arches: a 7-year prospective study with the ITI dental implant system. Int J Oral Maxillofac Implants 2004;19(2):247–59.
2. Lai HC, Si MS, Zhuang LF, et al. Long-term outcomes of short dental implants supporting single crowns in posterior region: a clinical retrospective study of 5-10 years. Clin Oral Implants Res 2013;24(2):230–7.
3. Buser D, Mericske-Stern R, Bernard JP, et al. Long-term evaluation of non-submerged ITI implants. Part 1: 8-year life table analysis of a prospective multi-center study with 2359 implants. Clin Oral Implants Res 1997;8(3):161–72.
4. Simonis P, Dufour T, Tenenbaum H. Long-term implant survival and success: a 10-16-year follow-up of non-submerged dental implants. Clin Oral Implants Res 2010;21(7):772–7.
5. Papaspyridakos P, Chen CJ, Singh M, et al. Success criteria in implant dentistry: a systematic review. J Dent Res 2012;91(3):242–8.
6. Mora MA, Chenin DL, Arce RM. Software tools and surgical guides in dental-implant-guided surgery. Dent Clin North Am 2014;58(3):597–626.
7. Scarfe WC, Farman AG. What is cone-beam CT and how does it work? Dent Clin North Am 2008;52(4):707–30, v.
8. Kau CH. Creation of the virtual patient for the study of facial morphology. Facial Plast Surg Clin North Am 2011;19(4):615–22, viii.

9. Abramovitch K, Rice DD. Basic principles of cone beam computed tomography. Dent Clin North Am 2014;58(3):463–84.
10. Vandenberghe B, Jacobs R, Bosmans H. Modern dental imaging: a review of the current technology and clinical applications in dental practice. Eur Radiol 2010; 20(11):2637–55.
11. Jacobs R, Quirynen M. Dental cone beam computed tomography: justification for use in planning oral implant placement. Periodontol 2000 2014;66(1):203–13.
12. Razi T, Niknami M, Alavi Ghazani F. Relationship between Hounsfield unit in CT scan and gray scale in CBCT. J Dent Res Dent Clin Dent Prospects 2014;8(2): 107–10.
13. Mah P, Reeves TE, McDavid WD. Deriving Hounsfield units using grey levels in cone beam computed tomography. Dentomaxillofac Radiol 2010;39(6):323–35.
14. Scherer MD. Presurgical implant-site assessment and restoratively driven digital planning. Dent Clin North Am 2014;58(3):561–95.
15. Ganz SD. Three-dimensional imaging and guided surgery for dental implants. Dent Clin North Am 2015;59(2):265–90.
16. Joda T, Wolfart S, Reich S, et al. Virtual dental patient: how long until it's here? Curr Oral Health Rep 2018;5(2):116–20.
17. Kuric KM, Harris BT, Morton D, et al. Integrating hinge axis approximation and the virtual facial simulation of prosthetic outcomes for treatment with CAD-CAM immediate dentures: a clinical report of a patient with microstomia. J Prosthet Dent 2018;119(6):879–86.
18. Lin WS, Harris BT, Phasuk K, et al. Integrating a facial scan, virtual smile design, and 3D virtual patient for treatment with CAD-CAM ceramic veneers: a clinical report. J Prosthet Dent 2018;119(2):200–5.
19. Buser D, Martin W, Belser UC. Optimizing esthetics for implant restorations in the anterior maxilla: anatomic and surgical considerations. Int J Oral Maxillofac Implants 2004;19(Suppl):43–61.
20. Pollini A, Goldberg J, Mitrani R, et al. The lip-tooth-ridge classification: a guidepost for edentulous maxillary arches. diagnosis, risk assessment, and implant treatment indications. Int J Periodontics Restorative Dent 2017;37(6):835–41.
21. Pesun IJ, Gardner FM. Fabrication of a guide for radiographic evaluation and surgical placement of implants. J Prosthet Dent 1995;73(6):548–52.
22. Zitzmann NU, Margolin MD, Filippi A, et al. Patient assessment and diagnosis in implant treatment. Aust Dent J 2008;53(Suppl 1):S3–10.
23. Harris BT, Chen L, Lin WS. Digital imaging and prosthetic-driven implant planning: efficient, accurate, and reliable treatment. Compend Contin Educ Dent 2017;38(7):492–4.
24. Harris BT, Scarfe WC, Llop DR, et al. Using dental GPS to navigate implant placement. Compend Contin Educ Dent 2016;37(8):520–5.
25. Vercruyssen M, Fortin T, Widmann G, et al. Different techniques of static/dynamic guided implant surgery: modalities and indications. Periodontol 2000 2014;66(1): 214–27.
26. Block MS, Emery RW. Static or dynamic navigation for implant placement-choosing the method of guidance. J Oral Maxillofac Surg 2016;74(2):269–77.
27. The glossary of prosthodontic terms: ninth edition. J Prosthet Dent 2017;117(5s): e1–105.
28. D'Haese J, Van De Velde T, Komiyama A, et al. Accuracy and complications using computer-designed stereolithographic surgical guides for oral rehabilitation by means of dental implants: a review of the literature. Clin Implant Dent Relat Res 2012;14(3):321–35.

29. Arunyanak SP, Harris BT, Grant GT, et al. Digital approach to planning computer-guided surgery and immediate provisionalization in a partially edentulous patient. J Prosthet Dent 2016;116(1):8–14.
30. Tahmaseb A, Wismeijer D, Coucke W, et al. Computer technology applications in surgical implant dentistry: a systematic review. Int J Oral Maxillofac Implants 2014;29(Suppl):25–42.
31. Tahmaseb A, De Clerck R, Aartman I, et al. Digital protocol for reference-based guided surgery and immediate loading: a prospective clinical study. Int J Oral Maxillofac Implants 2012;27(5):1258–70.
32. Pozzi A, Polizzi G, Moy PK. Guided surgery with tooth-supported templates for single missing teeth: a critical review. Eur J Oral Implantol 2016;9(Suppl 1): S135–53.
33. Park C, Raigrodski AJ, Rosen J, et al. Accuracy of implant placement using precision surgical guides with varying occlusogingival heights: an in vitro study. J Prosthet Dent 2009;101(6):372–81.
34. Dawson A, Chen S, Buser D, et al. The SAC classification in implant dentistry. Berlin: Quintessence Publishing Co. Ltd; 2010.
35. Polido WD. Surgical setup for office-based Implant surgery. Basel (Switzerland): ITI Online Academy; 2016.
36. Sebastiani FR, Dym H, Kirpalani T. Infection control in the dental office. Dent Clin North Am 2017;61(2):435–57.
37. Bidra AS. Surgical safety checklist for dental implant and related surgeries. J Prosthet Dent 2017;118(3):442–4.
38. Lanis A, Llorens P, Alvarez Del Canto O. Selecting the appropriate digital planning pathway for computer-guided implant surgery. Int J Comput Dent 2017; 20(1):75–85.

Digital Workflows in the Management of the Esthetically Discriminating Patient

David L. Guichet, DDS

KEYWORDS

• Intraoral capture • Implant scan-bodies • Digital dentistry • CAD/CAM provisional • Hybrid abutments • Dental esthetics • CAD/CAM restorations

KEY POINTS

- Digital CAD/CAM workflows are used in the preview, prototype and definitive esthetic prosthodontic rehabilitation.
- New workflows allow for local CAD/CAM production of restorations for teeth and implants.
- Intra-oral capture can be used as an entry point into the digital workflow.
- CAD/CAM compatable materials in use are improving in esthetic and functional capabilities.

INTRODUCTION

The advent of digital pathways for the restoration of teeth and implants has matured in recent years.[1,2] Digital design software is now an important tool that can assist in the dental rehabilitation of the esthetically discerning patient.[3,4] When combined with direct digital capture of a patient's pretreatment and prepared teeth, digital design software is used to simulate the patient's eventual esthetic outcome. In addition, once approved by the patient and the dentist, the laboratory technician has the ability to convert these designs into durable precision restorations for use as prototypes of the patient's eventual definitive restorative designs. Testing these restorations in function allows the patient and the dental team to confirm or to modify the designs before manufacture of the definitive restorations.[5] The ability to efficiently design and manufacture esthetic and well-adapted restorations is now easier due to the advances in computer-assisted design and computer-assisted manufacturing (CAD/CAM) technology in the clinical and laboratory settings.

Disclosure: The author has nothing to disclose.
Private Practice, Providence Prosthodontics Dental Group, 1310 West Stewart Drive #202, Orange, CA 92868, USA
E-mail address: drdavid@guichetdental.com

Dent Clin N Am 63 (2019) 331–344
https://doi.org/10.1016/j.cden.2018.11.011
dental.theclinics.com
0011-8532/19/

Intraoral scanning has been suggested as providing improved efficiency and accuracy for clinicians and laboratory technicians.[6–8] Digital workflows for the design and manufacture of restorations have proved to be accurate and efficient in laboratories.[8,9] Simultaneously, new restorative materials used in digital manufacturing are proving to be safe and effective.[10–13] Esthetic performance is improving as manufacturers continue to adapt nontraditional materials such as translucent zirconia to the digital workflow. Technicians have become increasingly proficient with new colorants and new digital restorative designs and material manufacturing strategies.[14–16] This article is written to illustrate the clinical and laboratory digital workflows and material advances that have taken place that can be effectively used for the efficient dental management of the esthetically focused rehabilitation patient.

Many investigators have validated the accuracy of intraoral scanning for the restoration of individual teeth and quadrants.[17] Achieving cross-arch accuracy still presents a challenge when using intraoral scanning.[18–21] The full-arch scan is an assembly of multiple smaller individual images. The reconstruction of the images to create a full-arch surface scan relies on built-in software to stitch images together. Theoretically, this may present distortions and may result in a misfit in the full-arch splinted or long-span restoration. Investigators are working to understand and validate the trueness and accuracy of the full-arch scanned intraoral impression.[22,23]

However, when direct intraoral scanning is used in the individual tooth nonsplinted full-arch rehabilitation, the process yields highly accurate individual restorations with only minimal risk of discrepancy from cross-arch distortions.[24] Individual tooth size is smaller than the field of view of the scanner image size. Therefore, the actual dimension of the tooth is not extrapolated from stitching. Cross-arch imaging can only be achieved by stitching multiple smaller images, and therefore cross-arch distortions can and do exist. Multiple accurately fitting individual restorations made from intraoral scans are registered for the laboratory and remounted with physical interocclusal registrations on an appropriate physical articulator and adjusted before delivery. In addition, the restorations are commonly adapted intraorally at the time of try-in for remounting in the laboratory and adjusted again before final delivery.

The patient presented in this article was treated using a complete digital process for the diagnosis, design, and manufacture of the complete maxillary arch restorations on teeth and implants along with multiple opposing mandibular restorations. The mandibular restorations included all mandibular molars and several incisor teeth. Digital intraoral scans yielded 3-dimensional (3D) digital diagnostic casts. Consultation with the patient was performed regarding her needs and a treatment plan was developed to achieve the esthetic and functional goals the patient requested. Conservative full crown preparations were performed on all treated teeth and conservative inlay preparations were used for the mandibular second molars. Optical capture was used for all final impressions and interocclusal registrations including the optical capture of implant scan-body positions for 2 molar implants. Multiple single-tooth restorations including provisional restorations and implant abutments were digitally designed. The contour of the restorations was designed in collaboration with the patient and laboratory with the dentist and patient present in front of the design station. Minor esthetic adjustments were facilitated through this process. All abutments and restorations were produced in-house using a digital design station and a 5-axis milling system, including an additional prototype set of milled provisional restorations (Zirkonzahn). The definitive restorative designs were made from the same initial files as the prototype files. The design chosen for the crowns used minimally veneered zirconia, and a monolithic lithium disilicate (Emax, Ivoclar, Liechtenstein) material was chosen for the bonded ceramic inlays.

WHY USE A DIGITAL PROCESS?

The use of a complete digital workflow in the treatment of this patient resulted in increased efficiency, accuracy, and overall effectiveness not previously realized by this investigator when compared with conventional means. In addition, an enhanced overall experience for the patient was noted as compared with past patients receiving traditional treatment methods. Digital design and manufacture of restorations from an optical impression allows for both laboratory and clinical effectiveness that might not otherwise be possible. Once the data are received by the laboratory, no impressions have to be poured. Implant analogs do not have to be adapted to a physical impression and no soft tissue casts have to be created around the implant impression posts. No casts have to be separated. No dies have to be trimmed or ditched. All of these steps are performed digitally in a fraction of the time, including the addition of die spacer and undercut block out. Digital waxing from tooth libraries occurs rapidly because global changes can be made to adapt the tooth forms to the patient's tooth preparations in the virtual environment. Using a virtual articulator, adjustments can be made to the vertical dimension if needed and eccentric movements can be accomplished via the virtual articulation including the adaption of the digital restorative designs to prescribed average motion pathways.

Esthetics in tooth form, proportion, smile design, color, and texture can all be achieved via a digital tooth library and 3D modeling software. High-strength esthetic materials can be milled to make prototype provisional restorations. The milled provisional restorations have similar marginal accuracy as a final restoration and can serve to validate the impression accuracy, esthetics, and the interocclusal relationship on try-in. If the provisional is accepted by the patient or requires only minor modifications, then the delivery of the final restorations becomes a routine process because the final design files can be derived from the exact same files that created the provisional prototype. This can be done in collaboration with the patient. The definitive restoration files can be modified easily if desired and usually requires some modifications before final export for manufacturing. Moving from provisional acceptance to final restoration can be completed with confidence because the final restorations are not started from scratch, but rather they are improved versions of the same files. The manufacturing of the final crowns is performed digitally and robotically. Ceramists are able to input the most artistic effects in the finished result via a 0.8 mm facial cutback for conventional customized feldspathic porcelain layering. Ceramists now focus more on the artistry rather than managing the traditional porcelain buildup and compensations for feldspathic porcelain firing shrinkage and distortion.

DIAGNOSIS, PLANNING, TREATMENT CONFIRMATION, AND CLINICAL WORKFLOWS

The patient presented 7 years before treatment with a severely worn dentition. In addition, there were many broken down and carious involved teeth and restorations (**Figs. 1–5**). A treatment plan was developed to address these concerns and also to address the etiological factors causing the destructive process. She was also interested in lightening her teeth and improving her overall smile while maintaining a natural color and appearance in order to match her untreated teeth. It was determined that in order to control the color and shape of the teeth a maxillary arch reconstruction would be indicated. The mandibular arch would receive multiple crowns as needed to control the occlusion and manage the excessive spacing. For many of the mandibular teeth,

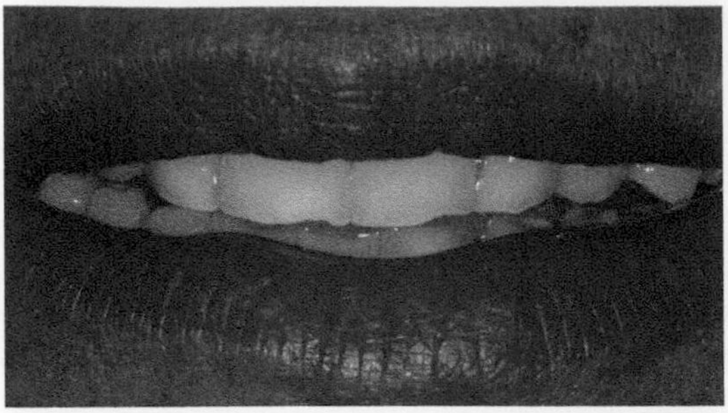

Fig. 1. Relaxed smile of the patient's pretreatment condition revealing worn dentition.

bleaching and direct composite restorations were indicated. The patient delayed the overall plan and had the maxillary right first and second molars extracted and wide-diameter implants placed. After waiting several years, the patient returned and requested to initiate the rehabilitative plan.

Updated intraoral and extraoral photographs were made. Esthetic consultation was performed and treatment time and expectations were discussed and agreed on. Preliminary composite restorations and in-house bleaching with light activated carbamide peroxide was performed.

The patient was then appointed for tooth preparation and was treated with the assistance of an MD anesthesiologist using intravenous sedation. The 3Shape Trios Color scanner (3Shape Inc., Copenhagen, Denmark) was used for impressioning. The scanner software prescription was filled out including the implant locations, type of abutment designs and restorative material, and the design and shade desired for each restoration. Direct intraoral 3D optical scans of the unprepared teeth were made and stored. Local anesthetics were administered in the maxillary arch. Tooth preparations were performed using a minimally invasive thinly reduced crown preparation design described by Guess.[25] Tissue displacement was accomplished using retraction cord, and local hemorrhage control was achieved using 3M ESPE Astringent Retraction Paste. Implant scan-bodies (Biodenta) were positioned on the implants in the maxillary right first and second molar positions. Final maxillary tooth preparation scans were completed and confirmed as well as scans of the implant scan-bodies (**Fig. 6**). The scan data were copied, stored, and secured from automatic deletion. The patient received direct chairside provisional

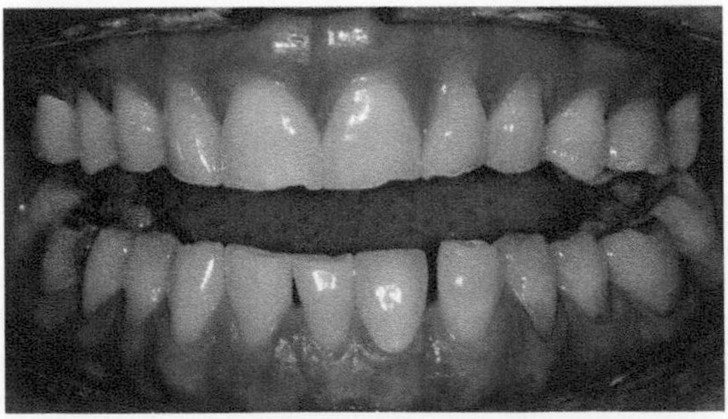

Fig. 2. Retracted open-mouth view of the pretreatment condition revealing worn, carious, and fractured dentition with mandibular anterior spacing.

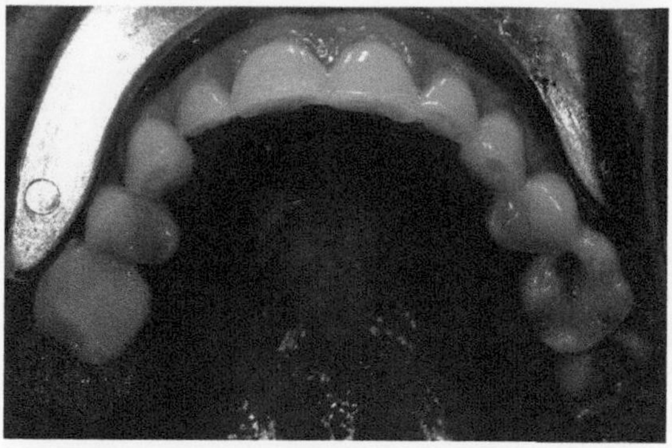

Fig. 3. Maxillary arch image of the pretreatment condition.

restorations created from a bisacryl material (Integrity Shade A1, Dentsply) using an irreversible hydrocolloid impression made before tooth preparation. The trimmed and polished provisional restorations were cemented with Temp Bond temporary cement (Kerr Dental).

One week later the patient was treated using a similar protocol for the lower arch. On completing the tooth preparations and tissue retraction, direct intraoral optical scan impressions were made of the mandibular crown preparations of teeth numbers 19, 20, 22, 23, 24, and 30. Mesio-occlusal inlay preparations were performed on teeth numbers 18 and 31. Interocclusal registrations were then made in centric relation using digital optical scanning, with the patient wearing an anterior silicone jig in the centric relation position at the desired vertical dimension of occlusion. In addition, intraocclusal registrations were also made by traditional physical means. A silicone anterior jig was made at the same vertical dimension of occlusion as the patient's pretreatment condition and confirmed using of the patient's molar implant restoration (Exabite II NDS VPS Bite Registration Creme, GC America Inc., IL, USA). The jig was trimmed to allow visual access to the buccal aspects of the tooth preparations in order to facilitate direct optical scanning of the teeth at the desired treatment position to register the interocclusal relationship. Once optical interocclusal scanning was completed a physical interocclusal registration was made by adding additional silicone material to the anterior silicone jig using a trimmed aluminum tray (Panadent Bite Tray: Panadent Corporation, Colton, California, USA). The centric-relation registration was confirmed clinically and transferred to the laboratory. All digital data

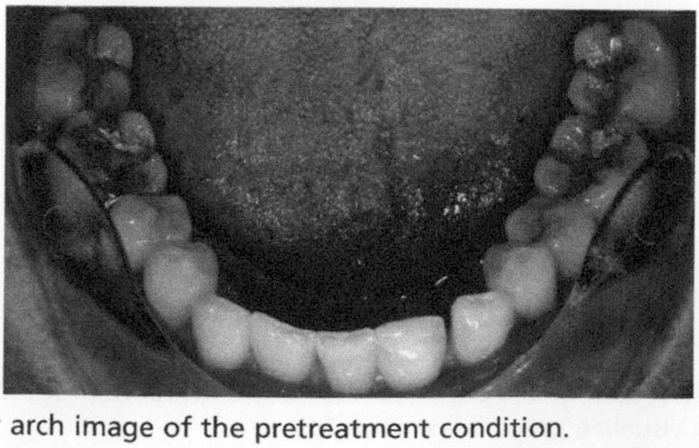

Fig. 4. Mandibular arch image of the pretreatment condition.

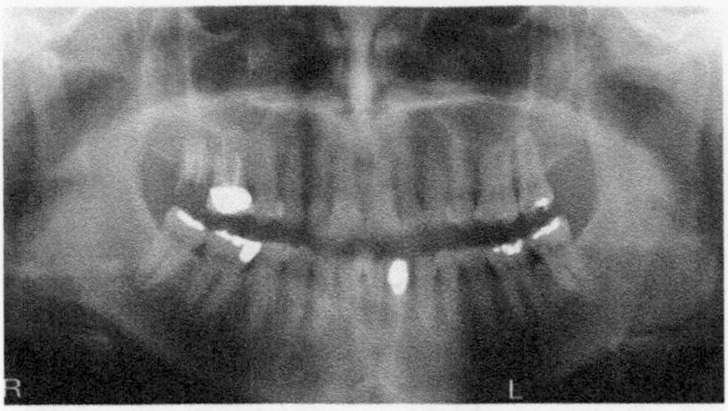

Fig. 5. Pretreatment panoramic radiograph reveals worn, carious, and fractured teeth.

were stored and transmitted via the Internet to the digital dental laboratory for processing. Cloud access to the data also was accessible via a secure Web Portal and an integrated iOS app (see **Fig. 6**; **Figs. 7** and **8**).

INTRAORAL SCANNING VALIDATION

Cross tooth validation of digital intraoral scanning has been well established for crown restorations by various investigators.[7,26] Quadrant scans or half-mouth scan accuracy has also been evaluated and shown to be accurate. Full-arch intraoral scanning accuracy has been shown to be less accurate than vinyl polysiloxane for the full-arch scan, but equal in accuracy to polyether and more accurate than alginate. Cross-arch accuracy remains to be evaluated for splinted versus nonsplinted restorations. German Gallucci studied the use of intraoral scanning in the mandibular full-arch splinted restoration.[27] The patient treated in this article received multiple single-tooth nonsplinted restorations, for which there is well-established cross tooth trueness and accuracy validations. Also, the cross-arch trueness and accuracy of the intraoral optical impressioning system used in this instance were proved to be as accurate as polyether impression material as previously mentioned. Polyether historically served as a trusted standard for multiple single-tooth restorations for years.

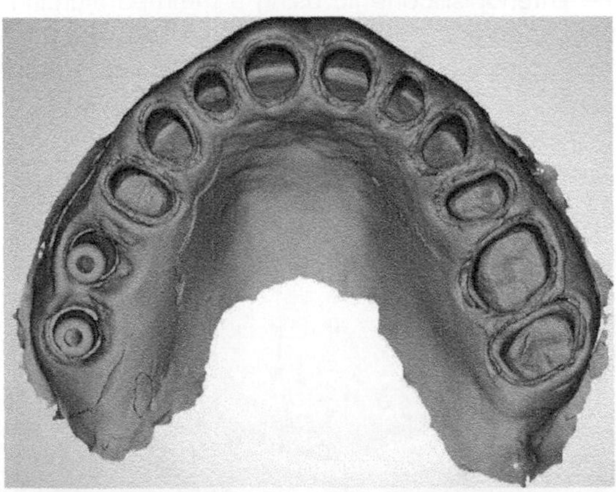

Fig. 6. Intraoral optical scan of the patient's maxillary arch tooth preparations and implant scan-bodies used to visualize preparation margins.

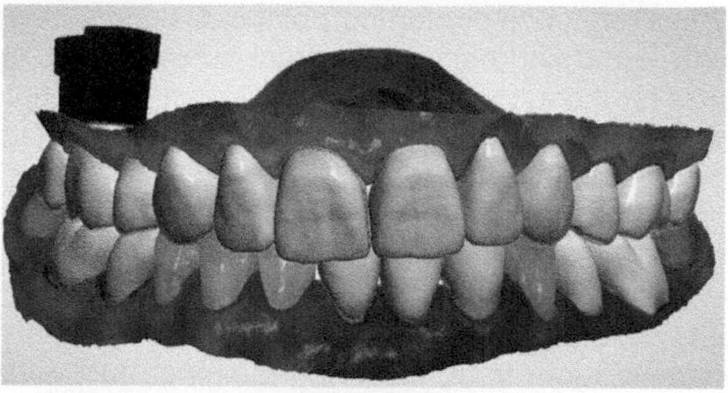

Fig. 7. Facial view of the design files used to produce full-contour CAD/CAM PMMA provisional restorations. PMMA, polymethyl methacrylate.

DENTAL LABORATORY INTERACTION AND DIGITAL WORKFLOWS

The laboratory received and accepted the patient's pretreatment and treatment scans. The technician team also confirmed the accuracy of the scan visually using onscreen magnification of the marginal details and interocclusal relationship. The 3Shape Dental System software (3Shape, Copenhagen), which is bundled with the laboratory scanner system, was used to open the case, process the optical scans, and develop the restorative designs. The software prescription form was filled out. Tooth preparations were identified and "Anatomy Cutback Crown" designs using minimally veneered zirconia material designated. Two-piece hybrid zirconia abutments were selected using titanium bases.[28] A split-file design strategy was chosen to indicate that the hybrid zirconia abutments and the corresponding implant crowns would be separated digitally creating 2 stereolithograph (STL) files per implant restoration.[29,30] One STL would be for the abutment and the other would be for the corresponding crown to be seated over the abutment. Inlays were used for the lower second molar restorations and Emax CAD lithium disilicate material was selected.

MERGED DIAGNOSTIC AND FINAL SCANS USED AS DESIGN REFERENCE

Diagnostic scans of the patient's pretreatment condition were previously made before the tooth preparations were initiated. These scans were visualized in the digital design

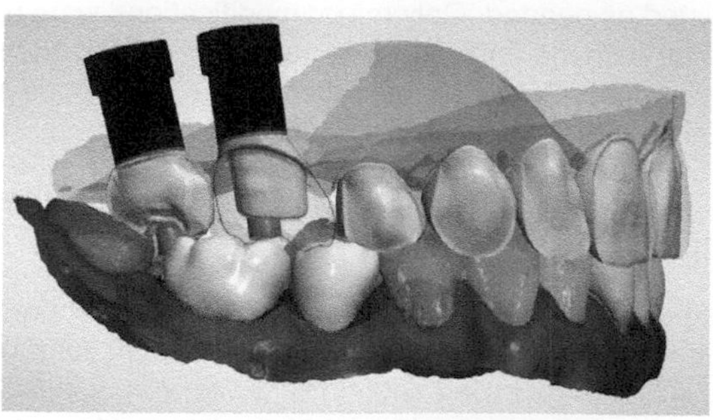

Fig. 8. Lateral view of the final digital restorative designs. Transparency reveals CAD/CAM abutments and Ti-bases on the preparation scan combined with the implant analogies. A split-file abutment/restoration workflow was used with anatomy cutback. All teeth and implant restorations are modified to include 0.6 mm facial digital cutback. All interproximal and occlusal contacts are included in the design file.

software and used as a reference or starting point in making subsequent corrections to the patient's tooth forms and occlusal contact scheme. This step facilitates the digital design process for the future idealized provisional restorations and final restorations. A transparency toggle allows one to visually bring in the diagnostic (prepreparation) scans into the digital design environment.

Next, the digital cast and die preparation was performed. All tooth preparation margins were identified and digital die spacing was completed, including the identification of the individual path of insertion and the elimination of preparation defects and/or undercuts. Virtual teeth from the software library were selected according to the patient's facial form and anatomic tooth form, including reference to the patient's untreated teeth of the opposing arch. The initial virtual teeth were positioned over the tooth preparations and implants and manipulated to optimize occlusal and esthetic relationships with reference to the patient's pretreatment condition. Before adapting the digital tooth forms from the tooth library, changes can be made to the arch form globally and/or regionally. Once the positions were approved, the tooth forms were adapted to the preparations. Final adjustments in interproximal contact form and occlusal contact positions were completed (see **Fig. 7**).

COMPUTER-AIDED DESIGN/COMPUTER-AIDED MANUFACTURING PROVISIONAL RESTORATION DESIGN AND MANUFACTURE

The patient's approval of the esthetics during the provisional phase is crucial. In order to esthetically and functionally test the virtual tooth designs, a full-contour splinted prototype restoration design file, STL, was exported for milling. Now that the CAD design of the provisional was complete, the next step would involve the CAM process. The CAM milling process includes multiple distinct steps. The software steps include material registration, restoration nesting, and tool-path calculation. A shade A1/B1 95 mm polymethyl methacrylate (PMMA) resin disc was selected and registered in the software (Zirkonzahn, Gais, Italy). Nesting of the design file (STL) in the registered material was accomplished and horizontal supports were added. The associated computer numerical control tool path calculations were performed with the final bur diameter designated at 0.3 mm ultrahigh resolution. The PMMA disc was placed in the mill with the correct burs loaded in the bur holder and the program was run using the M1 Wet Heavy 5-axis mill (Zirkohnzahn, Gais, Italy). Following several hours of milling, the provisional restorations were inspected, removed from the disc, finished, and polished. The patient was appointed and the milled provisional restorations were delivered and adjusted as needed. Only minor modifications were made to the provisional restorations for esthetic form and occlusal function and the mandibular treatment position was verified. These modifications were performed together with the patient at the design station. Patient acceptance was confirmed.

COMPUTER-AIDED DESIGN/COMPUTER-AIDED MANUFACTURING DEFINITIVE RESTORATION DESIGN

A final esthetic shape and shade consultation was then accomplished together with the patient and ceramist and digital dental technical team. All modifications to the provisional restoration were recorded and similar edits were subsequently made digitally by reopening the original provisional crown design files. These same crown design files were further modified to become the final restoration STL design files through a very efficient process of making minor edits. The final restorations were no longer splinted as they were in the provisional restoration. The full-contour anatomy was digitally reduced to incorporate 0.7 mm facial "anatomy cutback" to make room for veneering ceramic. The designs were finalized and individual restoration STL files were exported together with the abutment design STL files (see **Fig. 8**). The final material selected for the crowns was Prettau Anterior zirconia from Zirkonzahn. The abutments were made of the most opaque version of zirconia from the same manufacturer in order to block out the influence of the metallic color from the titanium abutment base. The appropriate zirconia discs were selected and registered in the software. The STL files were nested and supporting bars were added. The milling strategy for zirconia includes tool path calculations at a 25% magnification. This compensates for the 20% shrinkage that occurs during sintering. In addition, the master cast and die STL files were exported for printing, including the recess spaces for the implant analogs. Printed master casts were relieved, implant analogs were added, and the casts were mounted using an arbitrary face-bow and centric relation occlusal registration using an adjustable Denar D5A articulator set to anatomic averages.

Following the milling stage, the 25% magnified green state "anatomy cutback" crowns were removed from the disc, finished, and then infused with aqueous color liquids shade B1. The liquids were allowed to dry and the appropriate sintering cycle was completed for the crowns and abutments, respectively. The final sintering temperature for Prettau anterior was 1500°C and the sintering cycle lasted 4 hours per the manufacturers recommendations. The crown margins were finished and adapted to the dies and the printed casts. Occlusal adjustments were made on the physical articulator. Feldspathic porcelain was then layered to the facial aspect of the crowns (Shade 1M1) and fired at 930°C. Occlusion was again adjusted and the crowns were prepared for try-in and delivery (**Figs. 9** and **10**).

The patient was appointed, the provisional restorations were removed, and the teeth were cleaned of residual cement. The abutments were delivered and torqued to manufacturer's recommendations of 35Ncm (**Fig. 11**). All restorations were tried in and checked for marginal accuracy, contact tightness, and occlusal contact accuracy before final cementation.

The digital workflow in this rehabilitation created very accurate outcomes. No internal adjustments were required. The interproximal contact tightness was confirmed with 10 um Mylar strip as described by Campagni.[31,32] No interproximal adjustments

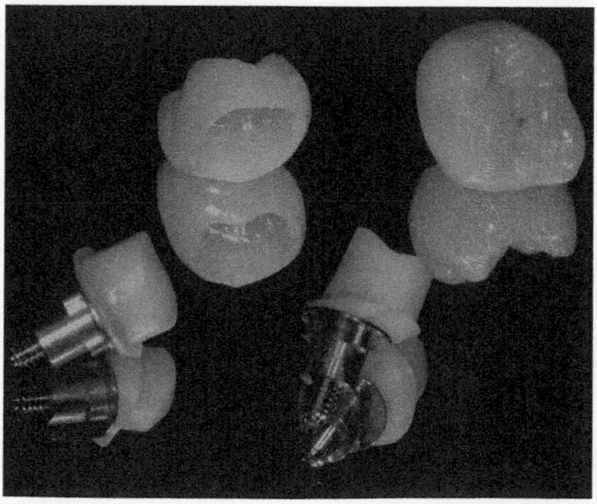

Fig. 9. Final hybrid implant abutments with simultaneously designed split-file/minimally veneered zirconia restorations ready for delivery.

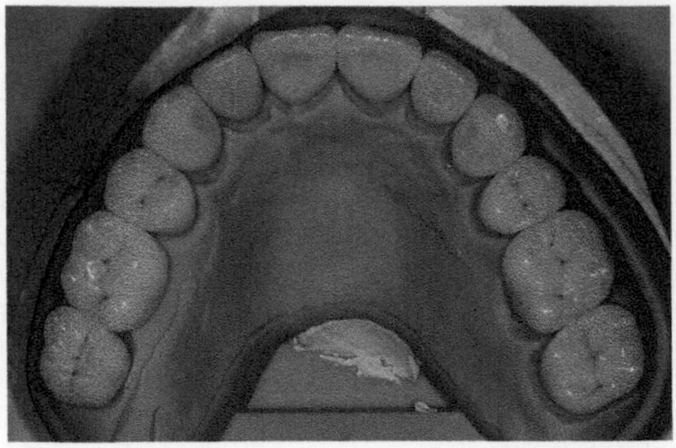

Fig. 10. Hybrid abutments and restorations seated on a digitally printed master cast. The cast design incorporating space for implant analogs and gingival cutout to receive the abutments and restorations.

were required and all contacts held Mylar without tearing. Only minor occlusal adjustments were performed.

During the try-in phase the cement was chosen based on the desired shade and the resistance and retention form of the tooth preparations. The patient expressed a preference for a light shade. A self-adhesive resin reinforced glass ionomer luting cement shade white opaque was chosen for the complete crown restorations (RelyX Unicem Aplicap, 3M ESPE). The restorations were prepared for delivery using Ivoclean (Ivocllar, Schaan, Liechtenstein) according to manufacturer's recommendations. The lithium disilicate restorations were delivered with an adhesive resin cement (Multilink, Ivoclar, Schaan, Liechtenstein).

Following delivery, the patient had all remaining cement removed and was reappointed for 1 week and 1 month after treatment visits (**Figs. 12–15**). The patient was reexamined to confirm a stable nonchanging treatment position without evidence of muscular dysfunction. A new full-mouth set of radiographs and photographs were made and slight occlusal refinements were made as needed. Evaluation of the soft tissue response to the restorations was made and all restorations were evaluated for the possibility of cement retention. The patient also received dental hygiene prophylaxis and was encouraged to maintain her home care and bleaching regimen

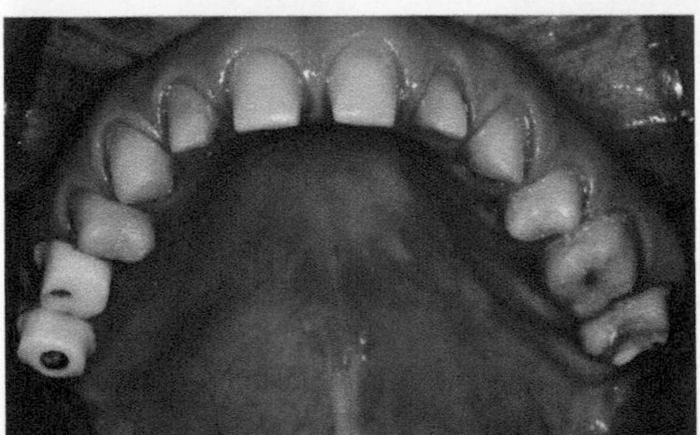

Fig. 11. Maxillary arch tooth preparations with custom CAD/CAM abutments; torqued to manufacturer's recommendations of 35Ncm.

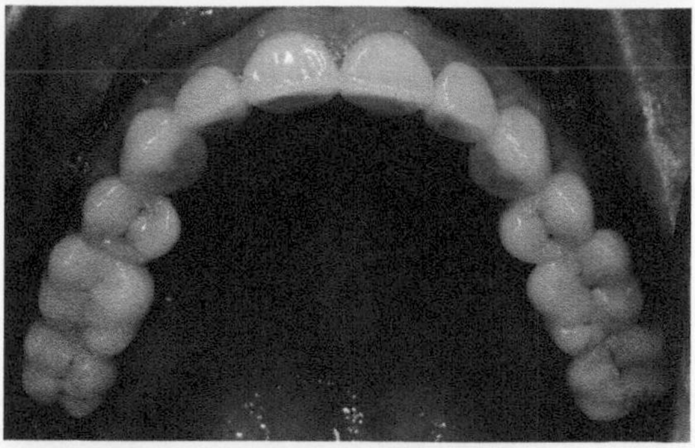

Fig. 12. Maxillary arch with definitive minimally veneered zirconia restorations in place.

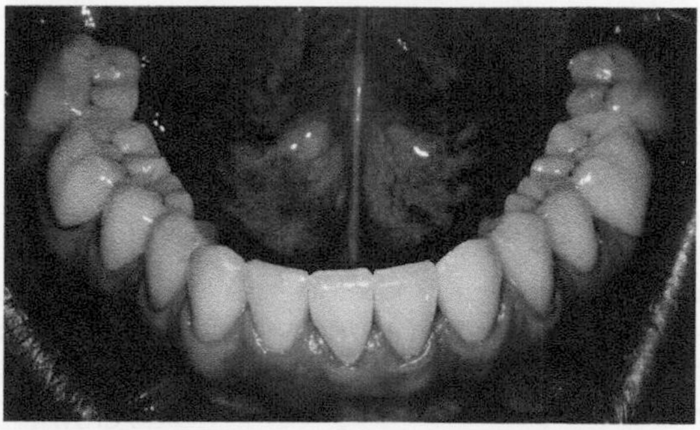

Fig. 13. Mandibular arch following the delivery or several minimally veneered zirconia restorations, second molar lithium disilicate inlays, and numerous conservative composite resin restorations.

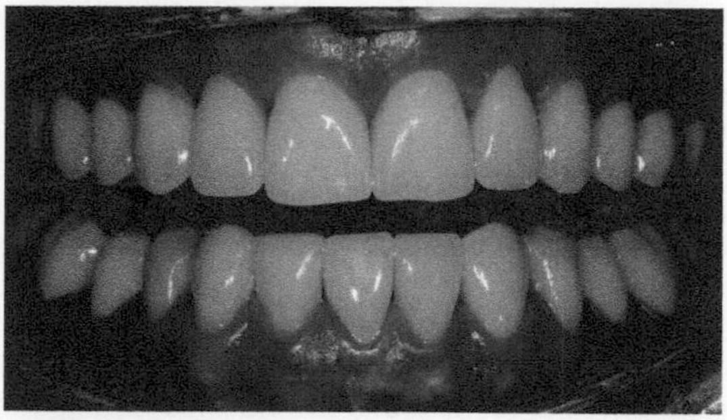

Fig. 14. Facial view of the restorations.

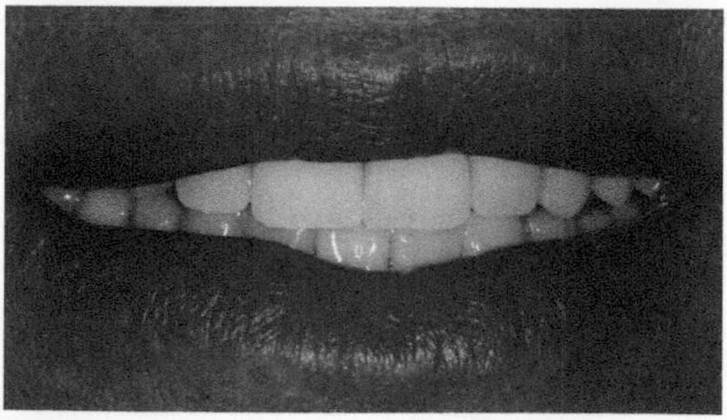

Fig. 15. Facial view of the patient revealing a relaxed semismiling tooth display.

for best results. Patient acceptance of the final treatment result was confirmed. Finally an occlusal splint was created and delivered to the patient. Oral hygiene instructions were confirmed and an appropriate recall schedule was established. The patient has been followed without incident for 30 months at the time of writing this article.

SUMMARY

This patient treatment presentation is a clinical testament to the accuracy of this complete digital uninterrupted CAD/CAM approach to the management of the esthetically discriminating complete-mouth rehabilitation patient. The treatment presented in this article used a complete digital workflow. All steps from diagnosis to delivery involved a linear uninterrupted digital process. These steps included the optical capture of the pretreatment condition, teeth preparations, the implant positions, model design and creation, provisional restoration design and creation, digital articulation, implant abutment design and abutment milling, and final restorative design and crown manufacture. At no time was the patient rescanned or were components in the laboratory rescanned and reentered into the digital design system.

Because all steps in the data capture, digital design, and computer-aided manufacturing process were completed digitally and linked, it was critical that all the steps in the process were validated and proved to be acceptable and without presenting risk to the patient. In this instance, the investigator used protocols that were either well established and/or could be verified before delivering any device or material product to the patient. In short, there was minimal treatment time required to produce the restorations, confirm the esthetics, and deliver the treatment result. As compared with traditional approaches, there was a notable improvement in the accuracy of fit as evidenced by the accurate marginal adaptation and contact tightness without the need for internal or external adjustment. The advent of computer-enabled 3D imaging, computer-aided design, and computer-aided manufacturing (CAD/CAM) in industry has led to a change in the way that dental restorations are planned, created, and delivered. Simultaneously, advances in materials were required to take advantage of these digital design and manufacturing changes. Adapting these technologies to dentistry has not been intuitive. Software has been developed requiring dentists and dental technicians to work with unfamiliar tools in an unfamiliar and sometimes unforgiving work environment. Ideally, clinical and laboratory workflows in the digital world would mirror those used in the physical workplace.

This analogy to past techniques is not required however. The familiar steps used traditionally in making physical restorations are not necessarily the best process in the digital environment. In order to make the best use of the digital design and manufacturing processes, one may need to adapt oneself to the new procedures. Learning and understanding the strengths and limitations of the new processes allows one to take full advantage of the new process and use it to its optimal utility and effectiveness.

REFERENCES

1. Duret F, Preston JD. CAD/CAM imaging in dentistry. Curr Opin Dent 1991;1(2):150–4.
2. Guichet D. Digitally enhanced dentistry: the power of digital design. J Calif Dent Assoc 2015;43(3):135–41.
3. Coachman C, Paravina RD. Digitally enhanced esthetic dentistry - from treatment planning to quality control. J Esthet Restor Dent 2016;28(Suppl 1):S3–4.

4. Silva BP, Mahn E, Stanley K, et al. The facial flow concept: an organic orofacial analysis-the vertical component. J Prosthet Dent 2018. https://doi.org/10.1016/j.prosdent.2018.03.023.
5. Moscovitch MS, Saba S. The use of provisional restorations in implant dentistry: a clinical report. Int J Oral Maxillofac Implants 1996;11(3):395–9.
6. Lee SJ, Gallucci GO. Digital vs. conventional implant impressions: efficiency outcomes. Clin Oral Implants Res 2013;24(1):111–5.
7. Ahlholm P, Sipilä K, Vallittu P, et al. Digital versus conventional impressions in fixed prosthodontics: a review. J Prosthodont 2018;27(1):35–41.
8. Koch GK, Gallucci GO, Lee SJ. Accuracy in the digital workflow: from data acquisition to the digitally milled cast. J Prosthet Dent 2016;115(6):749–54.
9. Sailer I, Mühlemann S, Fehmer V, et al. Randomized controlled clinical trial of digital and conventional workflows for the fabrication of zirconia-ceramic fixed partial dentures. Part I: time efficiency of complete-arch digital scans versus conventional impressions. J Prosthet Dent 2018. https://doi.org/10.1016/j.prosdent.2018.04.021.
10. Keren H, Caro S. The best material. Dent Labor; 2009.
11. Sailer I, Fehér A, Filser F, et al. Five-year clinical results of zirconia frameworks for posterior fixed partial dentures. Int J Prosthodont 2007;20:383–8.
12. Neves FD, Prado CJ, Prudente MS, et al. Micro-computed tomography evaluation of marginal fit of lithium disilicate crowns fabricated by using CAD/CAM systems or the heat-pressing technique. J Prosthet Dent 2014;112(5):1134–40.
13. Moscovitch M. Consecutive case series of monolithic and minimally veneered zirconia restorations on teeth and implants: up to 68 months. Int J Periodontics Restorative Dent 2015;35(3):315–23.
14. Batson ER, Cooper LF, Duqum I, et al. Clinical outcomes of three different crown systems with CAD/CAM technology. J Prosthet Dent 2014;112(4):770–7.
15. Tan JP, Sederstrom D, Polansky JR, et al. The use of slow heating and slow cooling regimens to strengthen porcelain fused to zirconia. J Prosthet Dent 2012;107:163–9.
16. Blatz M, Bergler M, Ozer F, et al. Bond strength of different veneering ceramics to zirconia and their susceptibility to thermocycling. Am J Dent 2010;23(4):213–6.
17. Ender A, Zimmermann M, Attin T, et al. In vivo precision of conventional and digital methods for obtaining quadrant dental impressions. Clin Oral Investig 2016;20(7):1495–504.
18. Ender A1, Attin T2, Mehl A. In vivo precision of conventional and digital methods of obtaining complete-arch dental impressions. J Prosthet Dent 2016;115(3):313–20.
19. Hack GD, Patzelt S. Evaluation of the accuracy of six intraoral scanning devices: An in-vitro investigation. ADA Prof Prod Rev 2015;10(4):1–5. Available at: https://www.beldental.cz/upload/useruploads/files/ke_stazeni/evaluation_of_the_accuracy_of_six_intraoral_scanning_devices.pdf.
20. Mangano FG, Veronesi G, Hauschild U, et al. Trueness and precision of four intraoral scanners in oral implantology: a comparative in vitro study. PLoS One 2016;11(9):e0163107.
21. Park H-N, Lim Y-J, Yi W-J, et al. A comparison of the accuracy of intraoral scanners using an intraoral environment simulator. J Adv Prosthodont 2018;10(1):58–64.
22. Treesh JC, Liacouras PC, Taft RM, et al. Complete arch accuracy of intraoral scanners. J Prosthet Dent 2018;120(3):382–8.
23. Kim RJ, Park JM, Shim JS. Accuracy of 9 intraoral scanners for complete-arch image acquisition: a qualitative and quantitative evaluation. J Prosthet Dent 2018. https://doi.org/10.1016/j.prosdent.2018.01.035.

24. Tsirogiannis P, Reissmann DR, Heydecke G. Evaluation of the marginal fit of single-unit, complete-coverage ceramic restorations fabricated after digital and conventional impressions: a systematic review and meta-analysis. J Prosthet Dent 2016;116(3):328–35.
25. Guess PC, Selz CF, Voulgarakis A, et al. Prospective clinical study of press-ceramic overlap and full veneer restorations: 7-year results. Int J Prosthodont 2014;27(4):355–8.
26. Chochlidakis KM, Papaspyridakos P, Geminiani A, et al. Digital versus conventional impressions for fixed prosthodontics: a systematic review and meta-analysis. J Prosthet Dent 2016;116(2):184–90.e12.
27. Papaspyridakos P, Gallucci GO, Chen CJ, et al. Digital versus conventional implant impressions for edentulous patients: accuracy outcomes. Clin Oral Implants Res 2016;27(4):465–72.
28. Zeller S, Guichet D. Accuracy of three digital workflows for implant abutment and crown fabrication using a digital measuring technique. J Prosthet Dent 2018. https://doi.org/10.1016/j.prosdent.2018.04.026.
29. Kapos T, Evan C. CAD/CAM technology for implant abutments, crowns and superstructures. Int J Oral Maxillofac Implants 2014;29(suppl):117–36.
30. Parpaiola A, Norton MR, Ceccianato D, et al. Virtual abutment design: a concept for delivery of CAD/CAM customized abutments — report of a retrospective cohort. Int J Periodontics Restorative Dent 2013;33(1):51–8.
31. Campagni WV. The final touch in the delivery of a fixed prosthesis. CDA J 1984; 12:21–9.
32. Guichet D, Yoshinobu D, Caputo A. Effect of splinting and interproximal contact tightness on load transfer by implant restorations. J Prosthet Dent 2002;87: 528–35.

Printed and bound by CPI Group (UK) Ltd, Croydon, CR0 4YY
03/10/2024
01040480-0017